KT-406-340

Nursing Models for Practice

Education Centre Library
Southend Hospital, Prittlewell Chase
Westcliff-on-Sea, Essex SS0 0RY
Tel: 01702 385090
or ext 5090

WITHDRAWN
FROM STOCK

Tl

Al
FA

Exe
Ade
Adju

Ba

Form

Ma

Profe

Carto

208552

EDINBU

BUTTERWORTH-HEINEMANN

An imprint of Elsevier Limited

© Reed Educational and Professional Publishing Ltd 1986
© Elsevier Limited 2003
© 2005, Elsevier Limited. All rights reserved.

The right of Alan Pearson, Barbara Vaughan and Mary FitzGerald to be identified
as authors of this work has been asserted by them in accordance with the
Copyright, Designs and Patents Act 1988

No part of this publication may be reproduced, stored in a retrieval system, or
transmitted in any form or by any means, electronic, mechanical, photocopying,
recording or otherwise, without either the prior permission of the publishers or a
licence permitting restricted copying in the United Kingdom issued by the
Copyright Licensing Agency, 90 Tottenham Court Road, London W1T 4LP.
Permissions may be sought directly from Elsevier's Health Sciences Rights
Department in Philadelphia, USA; phone: (+1) 215 238 7869, fax: (+1) 215 238 2239,
e-mail: healthpermissions@elsevier.com. You may also complete your request
on-line via the Elsevier homepage (http://www.elsevier.com), by selecting
'Customer Support' and then 'Obtaining Permissions'.

First edition 1986
Second edition 1996
Third edition 2005

ISBN 0 7506 5442 2

British Library Cataloguing in Publication Data
A catalogue record for this book is available from the British Library

Library of Congress Cataloging in Publication Data
A catalog record for this book is available from the Library of Congress

Note
Knowledge and best practice in this field are constantly changing. As new
research and experience broaden our knowledge, changes in practice, treatment
and drug therapy may become necessary or appropriate. Readers are advised to
check the most current information provided (i) on procedures featured or (ii) by
the manufacturer of each product to be administered, to verify the recommended
dose or formula, the method and duration of administration, and contraindications.
It is the responsibility of the practitioner, relying on their own experience and
knowledge of the patient, to make diagnoses, to determine dosages and the best
treatment for each individual patient, and to take all appropriate safety
precautions. To the fullest extent of the law, neither the publisher nor the
authors assume any liability for any injury and/or damage.

The Publisher

The publisher has made every effort to obtain permission to reproduce all
borrowed material.

ELSEVIER   your source for books,
journals and multimedia
in the health sciences

www.elsevierhealth.com

The
publisher's
policy is to use
**paper manufactured
from sustainable forests**

For B
Senior
Projec
Projec
Desig
Illustr

Printed in China

Contents

Preface

Nursing Models for Practice was initially developed in the mid-1980s to be used by practising nurses. The second edition was substantially expanded in content in response to a growing number of schools of nursing prescribing it as required reading for undergraduate and pre-registration students, but the style was deliberately designed to appeal to a wider audience. The book continues to be popular in UK and Australian undergraduate nursing schools, and many of the lecturers using it have suggested a number of additional pedagogical features designed to assist students to develop their own study programme. In response to this feedback the text has been extensively updated and rewritten and two new chapters (Nursing as Theory Laden Practice and Developing an Evidence Base for Nursing Practice) have been added. These additional chapters give a brief social history of modern nursing, consider the theoretical bases of contemporary practice, overview the evidence based practice movement and compare evidence with theory. The style has been modified to meet the needs of students; and each chapter now includes learning objectives, learning exercises and study questions.

As the delivery of health services continues to grow and develop, and the role of nurses and nursing increases in complexity, the theorising of nursing as a practice and knowledge enterprise of the 1970s and 1980s has been replaced with a blurring of roles between health professionals and a focus on the multidisciplinary nature of knowledge and practice. To some extent, this offers nursing an opportunity to take its rightful, equal place with other health professions in developing and applying knowledge that improves the health and well-being of individuals and communities. Multidisciplinary teamwork is based on equal participation of all members of the team; and thus, each member of the team brings a particular perspective. Medical practitioners, psychologists and social workers (and all other members of the health team) bring a perspective that is informed by their views of the world, the nature of health and illness, the role of their own profession within the multidisciplinary team, and the knowledge or science of their own profession. Nursing and nurses have been plagued with the tendency for the community – and nurses themselves – to think that their role is to acquire and apply the science of others and thus that their contribution to health caring relates only to doing. Such a proposition does not, of course, reflect the reality of the complexities of modern health care. Nurses (and doctors, physiotherapists, etc.) do apply the knowledge and science of many disciplines; but, in doing so, they modify it in action; and there is a complex theoretical base to intelligent, sensitive nursing that gives nurses a distinctive knowledge perspective that is of much use to other members of the multidisciplinary team.

Thinking about nursing and organising these thoughts to communicate with others is the stuff of theorising. Nursing models represent this theorising of nursing practice and are of fundamental importance in learning how to practice and in organising and delivering nursing care. This book sets out to describe the role of models, theories, knowledge and science in professional nursing in a simple, practical way. We hope that it becomes a useful foundation for students and practitioners of nursing.

Alan Pearson, Melbourne, Australia
Barbara Vaughan, Oxford, UK
Mary FitzGerald, Gosford, Australia
2005

Acknowledgements

Our thanks must go to the very large number of people who have made use of this text since publication of the first edition, many of whom have offered us valuable feedback, which has guided the production of this edition. Without their help we would have been less able to judge what additions and alterations were needed and what has stood the test of time and should still be included. It is only through our continued contact with such people that we have been able to gain insight into the needs of nurses who are exploring the use of models in practice, and we thank them for their support.

Thanks must also be offered to the authors of the original books, whose ideas we have summarised and to the following, who have given permission to reproduce figures in this text:
- The Open University
- Little, Brown and Co.
- John Wiley & Sons
- Churchill Livingstone
- Sage Publications
- Discovery International Publishers
- W.B. Saunders
- Colorado Associated University Press

Chapter 1

Nursing as Theory Laden Practice

LEARNING OBJECTIVES

On completion of this chapter, the reader will be able to:

1. Define theory
2. Discuss the role of theory in nursing
3. Describe the relevance of nursing theory for practice
4. Discuss the historical influences on contemporary approaches to nursing theory

INTRODUCTION

Developing models which attempt to describe the practice of nursing has occupied the energies and minds of some of nursing's leaders for over 30 years. Many of the models developed over this period are referred to in the nursing press, on courses for nurses and in places where nurses work. But what are models, what purpose do they serve (if any) and what value do they have in the practice of nursing? Do we really need to spend time and energy on thinking about such things when there are so many people to be nursed, so little time and so many obstacles to be overcome in actually getting the work done? And since there are a wealth of other things to learn before we can nurse effectively, is it not better to develop skills and gain knowledge first, leaving this theorising about what nursing is and what nurses do until there is time for it?

We believe that thinking about nursing and trying to construct a picture to represent these thoughts is a crucial beginning, not only in learning how to nurse, but also in actually nursing. This book is simply a collection of thoughts about the subject, which takes a practical approach in order to share them with others. In the following chapters the role of models in practice and the effects they may have on nursing care are discussed. We give a basic explanation of what a model actually is. Then these ideas are briefly linked to the process of nursing and approaches to work organisation to show how models are inextricably part of the real nursing of people.

NURSES, NURSING AND THEORY

For many nurses and students of nursing, nursing theory and the development of nursing models often seem to have little relevance to the complexities of the contemporary health system. In this chapter we explore the nature of nursing theory and its relationship with modern nursing.

Nursing is essentially a practice; it is primarily concerned with the frontline delivery of health care to individuals and communities. Because of this practical imperative of nursing, its theoretical base is frequently, at worst, denied or, at best, forgotten. At its simplest level 'nursing theory' used to mean those things about nursing work which were taught in the classroom, and this meaning is still commonly held by many in nursing today. Some nursing lecturers (and students!) still talk about 'theory hours', referring to classroom time, and 'clinical hours', which implies that anything occurring in a practical situation is ostensibly atheoretical (that is, 'without theory'). Nursing theory however, like any other theory, is not simply that which is not practical. All planned human practices are grounded on some kind of theoretical premise, and theory itself is most often essentially practical in intent. In this book we hope to dispel the notion that nursing theory is boring – or impractical – or irrelevant to nursing practice or the delivery of nursing services.

There is a widespread misconception that, as nursing is practical, theoretical discussion is pretentious and irrelevant. 'Good' nursing theory is nothing more or less than the result of serious thought about the nature and processes of nursing. The Macquarie Dictionary (1982) suggests that theory is:

a logical group of statements used as principles to explain something

Theory is therefore seen as a formulation of ideas; a conceptualisation of the real with the purpose of understanding it; but it takes many forms. This is best described by Tripp (1987), who says:

The whole idea of theory is a very confused one. Different people use it in different ways to mean quite different things. The idea of theory is further confused as it is frequently opposed to the equally diffuse idea of practice.

The term theory is used indiscriminately and linked to quite disparate intellectual activities and knowledge. On examination of the literature, you are quite likely to find terms such as:

- grand theory
- critical theory
- personal theory
- local theory
- normative theory
- practical theory
- espoused theory

All of the above have differing approaches, which appear to have commonality solely in the fact that they claim to be 'theoretical'. One way of making sense of this plethora of terms is to group them according to the purpose they serve. For example:

- epistemological theories
- grand theories
- local theories
- metatheories

The first group, the 'epistemological theories', are essentially procedural in the sense that they suggest ways of perceiving and investigating the world. Although these theories may have originated within a discipline, their perspectives inform all branches of human understanding. Amongst these we can include the critical theorists (such as Habermas), the structural theorists (such as Levi-Strauss), the phenomenological theorists (such as Schutz) and the relativity theorists (such as Einstein). This is by no means an exhaustive list and I am sure you could name many more.

The second group, the 'grand theories', are substantive in that they are concerned with explicating particular features of the world. They are normally located within particular disciplines in a way that epistemological theories are not. The purpose of this group is to account for major trends and phenomena in such general terms that individual instances are lost in the production of broad patterns. Amongst the grand theories are to be found the major theories of the natural sciences (such as the steady state theory of the universe), psychological theories (such as labelling theory) and sociological theories (such as reproduction). Again, this list can be added to. Just think about the major disciplines and some of the theories that have emerged from them.

'Local theories' is the name attributed to the third group. These are also substantive but apply to particular situations or individuals, and are locked into narrow confines of space and time. Local theories serve specifically to explain events for particular individuals and particular situations. As such, these theories often involve perceptions of particular assumptions and biases. So, local theory does not have to be 'correct' in any locality other than its own. What is important, however, is that it works in the particular circumstance in which it is used.

A fourth and somewhat different grouping is that of the 'metatheories'. In short, a metatheory is a theory about theory, in much the same way as metacommunication is communication about communication. The work in this area is essentially philosophical, and although it has been an issue since the time of the Ancient Greeks, it is only relatively recently that it has been seen to be of consequence either to issues of knowledge or of action.

Many nurses interested in theorising suggest that if you take a broad view of the role of theory, the development of nursing theory will advance both nursing and an understanding of nursing by the rest of the community.

The current devaluing of nursing theory seems to stem from a preoccupation with grand theory, or the extant theoretical literature on conceptual models for practice. Furthermore, the role conceptual models of nursing have played in clarifying practice has been oversimplified and marginalised, and the fact that nursing practitioners draw on rich theoretical traditions is dismissed. This may be largely due to the dominant view that personal, local and action theory does not exist, but this is not the only basis for rejection of an intellectual component to nursing practice. Nursing academics contend that the opposition to a theoretical development of nursing stems from:

- misunderstandings of what constitutes theory;
- power relations between nurses, other health professionals and other disciplines;
- professional and academic arrogance;
- the gendered conception of nursing and nursing work;
- the reverence of nurses for the knowledge bases and theories of other disciplines and professions;
- the unexplained anti-intellectual bias of nurses themselves.

From our perspective, nursing is a complex professional activity that is expressed in practical service, but draws on sophisticated, integrated theoretical understanding. Nursing theory is not rhetoric; such a label serves to devalue nursing and is most frequently used as a device to control and subjugate nursing in line with dominant discourses about science, health and gender relations. Consider the complexity of language used in nursing specialties and compare that to the so-called 'jargon' of nursing theory. The former is far more loaded with specialist terms known only to those who work within the specialty concerned. Yet this language is sanctioned while the language surrounding nursing theory is scorned. This dismissal of serious thought through the pejorative use of the term 'jargon' relegates nursing thinkers to a realm of insignificance. Cody and Mitchell (2002) and Roy and Fawcett (2002) suggest that, although nursing has its own sophisticated theoretical base, nursing theory has not developed as well as it could and this is, in part, because of nursing's historical development.

A HISTORICAL PERSPECTIVE ON NURSING KNOWLEDGE

It is useful, in considering nursing theory, to trace nursing's historical development and juxtapose this with knowledge development and the way nurses may have approached theory and theorising over time. To do so is difficult because much of the written history on nursing is shrouded in the political position of the writers of nursing history. If you have an interest in this, there are a number of contemporary works on how written nursing history may have distorted our understanding of the emergence of current assumptions about the nature of nursing work, the role of the nurse and the genderisation of the profession.

Throughout the ages, human beings have experienced ill health and have strived to maintain or regain health. It follows, then, that the act of nursing has probably always occurred. Mothers and fathers have always nurtured their young, and men and women have helped each other to be healthy. As various civilisations emerged, sometimes thousands of years ago, helping the sick, fighting disease and sickness, and searching for ways to prevent ill health and cure illness all became specialised in different ways.

The development of the two, now powerful, professions of medicine and nursing arose out of this search. In Western countries, modern medicine and nursing were only formally established in the nineteenth century and while medicine made great strides in mapping out the domain of medical knowledge, nursing, until recent times, tended to focus on practical activity, the values of service to others and selflessness, and the personal characteristics of nurses, such as kindness and gentleness.

In the past 100 years nursing knowledge has been shaped by those approaches which were dominant in wider society. Thus, the rise in scientific thought tended to encourage the generation of nursing knowledge through scientific methods. Current interest in new age philosophy in Western countries, and the belief in traditional philosophies and religions in Eastern countries (for example, Buddhism, Islam, etc.), appear to be influencing knowledge development at the moment.

THE EMERGENCE OF NURSING AS A FIELD OF KNOWLEDGE

Modern nursing has, until recently, focused on *doing* nursing – that is, on the practical skills nurses use in their day-to-day practice, such as lifting patients, dressing wounds, giving medications and managing intravenous infusions. However, nurses throughout the ages have developed and drawn on a wide range of knowledge to underpin these activities. In the past 80 years, nurses in many countries have sought to clarify the nature of nursing a person and to 'map out' what constitutes nursing theory.

Theory is something that arises out of *theorising*. Theorising is something that we all engage in for most of the time. It is an attempt to bring the experience of thinking to speech. So, whenever a nurse *thinks* about a patient, a nursing action or about nursing people and then explains these thoughts to another, she or he will interpret these thoughts, make judgements, draw conclusions and express a theoretical understanding of the phenomena in question.

In the professional and academic worlds, different groups of people have worked together and developed quite specific ways of thinking about the world: i.e. of theorising. These groups have developed certain rules to be applied to theorising so that the whole group can follow a similar path or apply an agreed-upon *discipline* to think about, explore and examine phenomena that lead to the development of theory.

These groups of people – such as sociologists, physicists, psychologists, historians – are now referred to as *disciplines* because they all apply a certain discipline or set of rules in defining their interests and in thinking about, theorising and researching this interest. Nurses, too, have developed a distinctive approach to viewing the world. They use a professional language which non-nurses are unfamiliar with; they think about the people they care for in a way that is different from other health workers; and they use knowledge from a wide variety of sources in ways that differ from those of other professional practitioners. Nursing also has a specific interest focus – how people experience health and illness and how to support people as they experience these phenomena.

Until recently, however, nursing has not been seen, by nurses or society as a whole, as a discipline. The thoughts and practices of nurses have largely been seen as the practical application of knowledge derived from other disciplines. Knowledge and knowing are complex concepts and nursing knowledge is related to, but different from, other kinds of knowledge. Contemporary nursing is rapidly developing its own disciplinary approaches to nursing knowledge and theory, focusing largely on the knowledge that is embedded in nursing action.

Tracing nursing's historical development in terms of its theoretical basis cannot be separated from the development of the broader human sciences. Thus, in the Middle Ages and the Renaissance, nursing knowledge was aligned to the teachings of the Church and was usually linked to a religious life. Nursing was not gendered and nurses were amongst the most educated and literate in society. The period of The Enlightenment led to massive changes in Western thought and to the general demise of 'non-scientific' knowledge. The effects of this era on nursing's own theoretical base and its development are still visible.

Nightingale occupies a particular and special place in the historical discourse of nursing (Pearson and Taylor, 1996; Pearson et al., 1997). When she is treated critically, she is still a figure of importance precisely because she represents the shift in nursing practices around the late nineteenth century. Nightingale is an icon, a symbol invoked when discussion turns – as it inevitably does – to the training of nurses in hospitals. But when she is used by historians as a symbol of the transition from untrained nurses to more efficient nursing practices, the implication is that she caused the change to occur. Certainly some of Nightingale's work had an impact in the colonies. Yet there is evidence that change was occurring prior to this in some hospitals, and certainly that the ideal of efficient nursing was prominent before it became widespread. The historical space of nursing pre-Nightingale is filled only by stereotypes of the 'dissolute nurse', and no investigation of nursing practices, good or bad, is conducted.

Keneley (1988) agrees that the nineteenth century romanticisation of nursing through the image of Nightingale, 'an angelic heroine with cool hands on a fevered brow', explains the respectability and popularity of nursing despite poor conditions in hospitals. She concludes that a gruelling and arduous job was perceived as so ladylike – the right occupation for a woman – by the community that nurses found it difficult to improve their conditions, and hospitals took advantage of this positive image.

The changing concept of 'woman' in the nineteenth century, and the eventual dominance of the image of woman as the 'angel at the hearth', has been well documented. New nurses became part of this descriptive metaphor of femininity (Trembath and Hellier, 1987). Nursing then came to have a 'middle-class' image but attracted women from working-class backgrounds.

In their text Gender at Work, Game and Pringle (1983) marry sociological theories with historical perspectives when discussing nursing. Their perspective is also politically engaged; the model of 'conflict and resistance' leads them to conclude that the main problem for women health care workers is that female nurses are still seen as 'handmaidens' and their struggle is still over divisions of work/labour and the hospital hierarchy, together with the space of the ward.

What can we conclude, then, from this race through history?

- Early nursing knowledge in the northern hemisphere was related largely to the humanities and was grounded in the Christian value of service to others.
- The modernisation of nursing in the late nineteenth century mirrored changes in medicine, and nursing knowledge was linked to that of the good housekeeper and the obedient helper.
- Nursing knowledge for most of this century was drawn from medicine and the domestic sciences.
- The struggle for recognition by nurses coupled with the gendered nature of nursing work generated a rejection of positivism, rationalism and empiricism in the 1970s and the vigorous, creative pursuit of new paradigm thought.

Nursing has a rich history; this history has given rise to the widespread allegiance to a wealth of 'theories' about the human condition, health and illness, and the practice of nursing. Critically examining our own ideas and openly discussing them with each other may reveal fascinating insights into our own theoretic and intellectual traditions as an occupation and a discipline.

CONCLUSION

How we come to know nursing, and how nursing knowledge is structured, are inextricably linked with our past. The study of knowledge and knowing (technically referred to as *epistemology*) raises and answers questions about '… the origin, the nature, the methods, and the limitations in knowledge development and outlines the various criteria by which knowledge is accepted' (Meleis, 1985, p. 55). Nursing has been interested in these kinds of issues for at least the past 40 years.

In pursuing this interest, nurses are intensely concerned with knowledge in as much as it relates to practice. Given that nursing is a practical discipline and that practice is in itself complex and sophisticated, nurses who are interested in the pursuit of nursing knowledge have a complicated task ahead of them!

Pearson (1992) argues that the only 'respectable sort of theorising' has, until recently, been that which is driven by the natural and physical sciences, and this has led to a gap between theory and practice. In this scenario, practice is seen as inferior to theory, and both are seen as quite separate. Nurses in the universities and colleges, and nursing researchers, have become the 'thinkers' and the practitioners the 'doers'. He suggests that this gap between theory and practice only exists if we adopt a view of knowledge which deliberately separates the two. Theory and practice, in the practical world of nursing, are not, and could never be, separate. Both inform and interact with each other. Pearson cites Carr and Kemmis (1987) as follows:

> A practice … is not some kind of thoughtless behaviour which exists separately from theory and to which theory can be applied. Furthermore, all

practices, like all observations, have theory embedded in them and this is just as true for the practice of theoretical pursuits as it is for practical pursuits.

(Pearson, 1992, p. 220)

He goes on to say that 'nurses could no more nurse without reflecting upon (and, hence theorising about) what they were doing than theorists could produce theory without engaging in the sort of practices distinctive of their activity'. The position that we take on nursing knowledge in this book is based on the previous discussion.

- Nursing knowledge is a distinct field of knowledge which is characteristically developed by nurses in practice.
- Nursing is not the application of knowledge from other disciplines. Whilst nurses use the knowledge of other disciplines, they transform this knowledge in practice so that it becomes substantively different in form.
- Nursing theory comes from nursing practice and takes different forms: personal theory, local theory, grand theory, epistemological theory.
- Nursing theory is constructed by nurses – it is not to be found elsewhere.

Based on this, we are of the view that nursing is theory laden. Nurses continually deal with theory: they value the theory generated and described by those from other disciplines; they consider the theory generated and described by other nurses; and they theorise about nursing themselves, and describe personal and local theory to each other.

This chapter has explored the nature of theory and considered how nursing thought has been shaped historically by looking beyond the confines of romantic, uncritical histories.

Learning exercises

Consider your own nursing career and think about the following questions. You may like to jot down your answers so you can refer back to them at a later date.

1. How has nursing theory been presented to you? Has interest in what is nursing theory and its development altered over time (i.e. changed as you have taken different pathways through your career)?
2. Write down what you know about nursing's history. Concentrate, if you can, on the following eras:
   Nursing until 1750
   Nursing 1751–1850
   Nursing 1851–1950
   Nursing from 1950 until now
3. Note your answers to the following questions on a piece of paper:
   What are the three eras of nursing described in this chapter?
   What does this chapter tell you about the development of nursing knowledge?

continued

Learning exercises *(cont.)*.

4. How do you see the development of nursing practice and nursing theory progressing between now and the year 2010?
5. Think about the following question: What forces currently shape nursing thought and nursing practice?

Study questions

1. What is theory?
2. List three examples of a theory, in any sphere of activity, that has influenced action.
3. Describe two theories generated in the field of psychology that are applicable to nursing practice.
4. Describe two theories generated in the field of microbiology.
5. Describe two theories generated in the field of nursing that are applicable to nursing practice.
6. Discuss the influence of one nursing theorist on your understanding of nursing.

Chapter 2

Developing an Evidence Base for Practice

LEARNING OBJECTIVES

On completion of this chapter, the reader will be able to:

1. Define evidence based practice
2. Discuss the advantages of evidence based practice for nursing
3. Describe the systematic review process
4. Critically appraise evidence
5. Relate evidence based practice to nursing models

EVIDENCE BASED PRACTICE

Basing practice on the best available evidence has become a highly valued aspiration for nurses, doctors and other health professionals in the past decade. This chapter focuses on contemporary approaches to evidence based practice (EBP) as evidence is always generated from a specific theoretical perspective. Our intention is to briefly describe the essential features of evidence based practice and to demonstrate the need to take a position on 'what counts as evidence'.

There is, of course, nothing new in the general idea that the care or interventions delivered to patients or clients should be in line with the most up-to-date results of research, and nursing leaders have been exhorting nursing to engage in 'research based practice' for at least 50 years. There is considerable evidence, however, that nurses do not apply research findings in their practice. Pearson *et al.* (1997, p. 4) have cited quite a number of examples of this. As to why this is so, Lathlean (1989) suggests the following:

- a nurse may be unaware of the research findings;
- a nurse may not understand the findings;

- a nurse may not believe the findings;
- a nurse may not know how to apply them; and finally
- a nurse may not be permitted to apply the findings.

The evidence based practice movement is able to afford considerable assistance to nurses to improve research utilisation in practice. It recognises that it is unrealistic to expect busy health professionals to have the time to stay abreast of all the latest research. Hence, one of its key strategies is the development of condensed information that summarises the results of a systematic review of evidence on a topic that includes the meta-analysis or meta-synthesis of research results. This involves a trained researcher or a team of researchers gathering all the available research papers on a given question and systematically reviewing them for reliability and validity; that is, assessing their quality. Systematic reviews can provide the raw material for establishing clinical guidelines and assist in identifying gaps in existing research, often discovering that there has been no research (or none of sufficient quality) on a given question.

We believe that evidence based practice has much to offer nursing and there is a rapidly expanding literature on evidence based practice in nursing; Cullum *et al.* (1997) see much potential in the evidence based approach for nursing. Much work has originated in the United Kingdom, but there is a growing awareness in the United States too. In Australia, there has been considerable development of the infrastructure underpinning evidence based health care generally, and nursing in particular.

Most health professions are increasingly embracing the concept of evidence based practice, and many use evidence based guidelines to inform practice. In the UK, Australia, Canada and the USA, considerable resources have been invested in high-quality, high-cost research and development programmes to develop evidence based clinical guidelines. At an international level, the Cochrane Collaboration has linked R&D sites across the world to review and analyse randomised clinical trials from an international perspective, and to generate reports to inform practitioners, influence practice and be a resource in the development of consensus guidelines.

The practical application of rigorously reviewed evidence is now promoted through the development and dissemination of practice guidelines in most developed health care systems. Clinical practice guidelines consist of statements to assist practitioner and patient decisions about appropriate health care for specific clinical circumstances, and are systematically developed on the basis of consensus within expert groups.

Evidence based practice is now almost institutionalised in most industrialised countries, and many of these countries have established centres for evidence based health care, evidence based medicine and evidence based nursing. (For example, there are Cochrane Centres in all of these countries and centres for evidence based nursing in the United Kingdom and North America; the Joanna Briggs Institute, based in Australia, has collaborating centres throughout Australia and in China, New Zealand, Thailand, the UK and Spain.)

WHAT IS EVIDENCE BASED PRACTICE?

Simply defined, evidence based practice is the combination of individual clinical or professional expertise with the best available external evidence to produce practice that is most likely to lead to a positive outcome for a client or patient. Although medicine and nursing are the health care occupations most advanced in the evidence based practice movement, the ideas and arguments are common to all professionals who work in health care. Sackett *et al.* (1996) contend that evidence based medicine had its philosophical origins in the mid-nineteenth century in Paris. They define it as being 'the conscientious, explicit and judicious use of current best evidence in making decisions about the care of individual patients' (p. 71).

These concepts are not without controversy, however. The most controversial issue relates to the current focus on evidence of effectiveness. The dominant approach to the systematic review of evidence favours the meta-analysis of the results of randomised controlled trials (RCTs); indeed, the RCT is conceptualised as the 'gold standard' in evidence of effectiveness, with other quantitative methods ranked as lower in quality in terms of evidence, and the results of interpretive and critical research not regarded as high-quality evidence. Critics of the prevailing privilege of the RCT and quantitative research cite the arguments inherent in critiques of traditional science and the emergence of new paradigms for knowledge. Whilst the RCT is probably the 'best' approach to generating evidence of effectiveness, nurses, medical practitioners and other health professionals are concerned with more than cause and effect questions, and this is reflected in the wide range of research approaches utilised in the health field to generate knowledge for practice.

Although its proponents would argue that evidence based practice is not limited to the utilisation of the results of traditional research, there has been considerable emphasis on RCTs and meta-analyses, especially in medicine and by the Cochrane Collaboration. This has drawn criticism from those professions who regard qualitative research methods as equally valid forms of research and, thus, generators of legitimate evidence for practice. The result is that qualitative research is rendered invisible in systematic reviews. These are a key tool in the evidence based practice movement. The question here becomes one of what is acceptable research in terms of generating knowledge that amounts to evidence for the purpose of informing practice. There are currently different views on the subject, and these generally align with the various positions that characterise the long-standing debate between qualitative and quantitative researchers. This is clearly not an easily resolved argument, but it is vitally important in terms of ascertaining the value of research-generated 'evidence' to health care practices.

Of equal importance is the view that it is much more important that practice be well grounded in theory than in research. Many health professionals argue that, although it is important to be aware of and mindful of the results of research, the 'evidence' this offers has a tendency to become obsolete, and this is especially so in the case of technical evidence.

Pearson (1999) argues for a pluralistic approach when considering 'what counts as evidence' for health care practices, and Evans and Pearson (2001) suggest that the inclusion of both (or either) qualitative

Table 2.1   QARI levels of applicability of evidence

Feasibility	Appropriateness	Meaningfulness	Effectiveness
Immediately practicable	Acceptable and justifiable, within ethical guidelines	Provides a rationale for practice development	Effectiveness established to a degree that merits application
Practicable with limited local training or modest additional resources	Acceptable after minor revision	Provides a rationale for local regional or national reform	Effectiveness established to a degree that suggests application
Practicable with extensive additional training or resources	Acceptable after major revision	Provides a rationale for practice relevant research	Effectiveness established to a degree that warrants consideration of applying the findings
Practicable with significant national reforms	Acceptable after development of new ethical guidelines	Provides a rationale for advocating change	Effectiveness established to a limited degree
Impracticable	Ethically unacceptable	Evidence unlikely to make sense to practitioners	Effectiveness not established

Source: From NH&MRC (1995), *Guidelines for the Development and Implementation of Clinical Practice Guidelines*, 1st edn. Canberra: Australian Government Publishing Service.

II: Evidence obtained from at least one properly designed randomised controlled trial.

III-1:   Evidence obtained from well-designed controlled trials without randomisation.

III-2:   Evidence obtained from well-designed cohort or case–control analytic studies, preferably from more than one centre or research group.

III-3:   Evidence obtained from multiple time series with or without the intervention. Dramatic results in uncontrolled experiments (such as the results of the introduction of penicillin treatment in the 1940s) could also be regarded as this type of evidence.

IV: Opinions of respected authorities, based on clinical experience, descriptive studies, or reports of expert committees.

This hierarchy of evidence was designed to assess the validity of recommendations for clinical guidelines and focuses on the results of quantitative research to determine the effectiveness of treatment. A broader frame is frequently used to assess levels of evidence related to Therapy/Prevention, Aetiology/Harm, Prognosis, Diagnosis and Economic analyses. Although their hierarchy of evidence takes a broader view of evidence, it, like the NHMRC, renders all evidence that is not quantifiable as invalid for use in practice. Pearson (2004), in reporting on the group-oriented development of a system to examine evidence generated through qualitative methods, argues for an approach that differs from the conventional approach of linking the trustworthiness of evidence to specified research design. For qualitative evidence, he sets out three levels of credibility:

● unequivocal
● credible
● not supported

Unequivocal relates to evidence beyond reasonable doubt, which may include findings that are matter of fact, directly reported/observed and not open to challenge.

Credible relates to interpretations that are plausible in light of data and the theoretical framework, and can be logically inferred from the data. Because the findings are interpretive, they can be challenged.

Not supported is when neither of the previous two apply, and when most notably findings are not supported by the data.

There is little point in accumulating evidence to answer a question if we cannot then use that answer to benefit our patients. Remember, evidence based practice involves the integration of best available evidence with your own clinical expertise. When it comes to deciding whether or not to incorporate into practice a particular activity or intervention, some or all of the following considerations will be relevant.

- Is it available?
- Is it affordable?
- Is it applicable in the setting?
- Would the patient/client be a willing participant in the implementation of the intervention?
- Were the patients in the study or studies that provided the evidence sufficiently similar to your own to justify the implementation of this particular intervention?
- What will be the potential benefits for the patient?
- What will be the potential harms for the patient?
- Does this intervention allow for an individual patient's values and preferences?

So, as well as needing to define levels of evidence for practice, there is also a need to establish levels of applicability. Pearson (2003) reports a hierarchy of applicability of evidence (Table 2.1).

APPRAISING THE EVIDENCE

All evidence needs to be subjected to rigorous appraisal. Given that EBP aims at the use of best evidence, it is important to note that the use of poor-quality evidence may lead to outcomes that are less than desirable for patients.

Critical appraisal of evidence is probably the most difficult component of EBP. Many checklists have been developed to appraise quantitative reports, and different checklists are currently used for the appraisal of a variety of quantitative research designs (for example, randomised controlled trials, cohort studies and descriptive studies). The major aim in critically appraising experimental or quantifiable data is to limit bias and thus establish the validity of a study. From a quantitative perspective, sources of bias include selection bias, performance bias and attrition bias, and validity is assessed by establishing the extent to which study design and conduct address potential bias.

This focus on limiting bias to establish validity is antithetical to the philosophical foundations of qualitative approaches to inquiry. Emden and Sandelowski (1999) suggest that validity, in quantitative terms, measures those things that it purports to render generalisable. In social inquiry, however, they argue that validity is perceived in a different way, as criteria of rigour for qualitative research.

There is much dissent in the literature on the appropriateness of establishing criteria to assess the validity of qualitative research. However, Pearson (2003) takes the view that a transparent approach to appraising qualitative research is central to its ongoing credibility, transferability and theoretical potential. Popay *et al.* (1998) are unequivocal in their assertion that the development of standards for assessing evidence from qualitative research is both possible and desirable.

Students and practitioners of nursing interested in critically appraising a research paper or a systematic review can utilise a training module on the worldwide web called the Rapid Appraisal Protocol Internet Database (RAPid). RAPid is a program developed for nurses, midwives and allied health professionals by the Joanna Briggs Institute and is based on the CATmaker program developed by the Centre for Evidence Based Medicine in Oxford, UK, by Douglas Badenenoch, David Sackett and Sharon Straus. Like CATmaker, RAPid is designed to organise, conduct and archive an evidence summary of a single study of an intervention or professional activity, or of a completed systematic review. Unlike CATmaker, RAPid can be used to summarise evidence from a wide range of sources, including the results of quantitative and qualitative studies, expert opinion published by respected bodies and reports that draw on consensus. RAPid is designed to assist individual practitioners and undergraduate and postgraduate students to acquire the skills of posing relevant questions about the feasibility, appropriateness, meaningfulness or effectiveness of an intervention or professional activity, and to pursue this question through applying the basic steps of the comprehensive systematic review process. (RAPid can be accessed via the Joanna Briggs Institute website, www.joannabriggs.edu.au)

RAP MAKER

RAP maker is the software component of RAPid; it is where the type of paper (systematic review or single study) is selected. Once the type of paper is chosen, RAPPERS are prompted to choose the type of study or review the selected paper represented, and are then expected to use the program to appraise the paper, critiquing the study type, its methods, findings and applicability. Each aspect of appraisal and data entry is conducted in real time in RAP maker, using tools and methods established by the Joanna Briggs Institute. RAP maker facilitates study type recognition, data extraction and construction of a final report, which is then submitted on-line to the RAPid library for independent critique, then uploading for worldwide access.

THE RAPid LIBRARY

The RAP library (an *internet database*) is a readily available resource, accessible 24 hours a day via the internet. The library promotes the transfer of knowledge, increases the pool of resources available to health care professionals and students, and is frequently updated with new RAP sheets. Each RAP sheet has a limited lifespan, and students can access sheets with a view to update, or create a new RAP to supplement existing resources. The benefits of the RAP library are that it is possible to readily identify areas of practice not currently covered by the library and to address gaps, conduct updates or contribute on a similar topic using a different study design. RAP sheets are only loaded in the library after undergoing external appraisal via the Institute. The RAP library is fully indexed and has advanced search features, including date, keywords, subject headings and sentence strings.

CONCLUSION

EBP and Nursing Models, Evidence and Theory

High-quality nursing requires both a grounding in the beliefs, values and knowledge that underpin nursing practice, and the use of the best available evidence in practice. There is thus no conflict between nursing theory and evidence based practice. There are, however, important issues for nursing surrounding the notion of what constitutes high-quality evidence. The classical, scientific medical model (largely not adhered to by most doctors these days) only regards the results of highly controlled trials that generate findings that are statistically significant as valid evidence. The theoretical bases of nursing are much more inclusive in what they regard as appropriate sources of evidence on which nursing decisions can be made.

Learning exercises

1. Think of an area of your practice, and the way you practice. Would you change your practice to accommodate the evidence?
2. What aspects of evidence based practice have the potential to harm nursing in a political sense?
3. Think of a person you nursed recently and try to recall some of the questions you asked yourself and passed over either because time did not allow you to seek the answer or because there was no ready access to the answer. What were the consequences of not having that information? Do you believe this had an impact on the care of the person involved? In each case, if you had been able to pursue the answer, would the information have been available?
4. Find a research report on a topic of your choice and appraise it using RAPid.

Study questions

1. Define evidence based practice.
2. Define 'evidence'.
3. List the steps in the systematic review process.

Chapter 3

Models for Practice

LEARNING OBJECTIVES

On completion of this chapter, the reader will be able to:

1. Define the term 'nursing model'
2. Discuss the role of models in practice professions
3. Identify the ways in which nursing models can influence practice

A MODEL – WHAT IS IT?

Although the term 'model' was comparatively controversial in nursing in the 1970s and 1980s, the use of models in other walks of life at that time was certainly not. The word 'model' was frequently used in every-day language and models were seen in areas of both work and play. Models are, of course, things which are not the real thing, but which match or represent reality as closely as possible. Those plastic models of aeroplanes given to little children are certainly not capable of flying to faraway places, but the people who construct the kits try hard to make them as similar to the real thing as possible. The elaborate models constructed by architects in an attempt to explain a new building are totally unreal in terms of size, but their purpose is to faithfully represent the reality of the building. Such models are three-dimensional representations of reality made out of raw materials such as mini-bricks, metal and plastic.

In contrast, models for practice, work or activity have as their raw materials ideas, beliefs, knowledge and other less tangible building bricks. They are abstract models but their essence is the same. Models for nursing were initially greeted with much scepticism by nurses in the

1970s, but by the end of the 1980s they figured prominently in nursing practice and nursing education. Due to the rapid developments in medical science, and nursing's increasing interest in research and science, models began to be put aside by the end of the twentieth century and, to some extent, became much less central in nursing practice. Tierney (1998) was prompted to question whether nursing models were extant or extinct, but concluded that models in themselves would always exist, though the degree of formality and credibility ascribed to them may, indeed, vary according to the dominant concerns of nurses at a given point in time.

The essence of models for practice will be explained in Chapter 4, but it is useful to start with a basic understanding of a practice model – a descriptive picture of practice which adequately represents the real thing. Constructing such pictures – composed of ideas and values and written down in a clear way – is at first sight quite a new exercise for nurses. But of course individuals have painted such pictures about what they think reality is since the human race began. Furthermore, all nurses have a picture in their heads about what nursing actually is and what nurses do, and they base this picture on their ideas and values. Yet making such views explicit, talking and writing about them, and sharing them with others, is not an activity which is commonly found among nurses.

Lawler (1991) argues that this is partly because we have not, to date, had an adequate language to describe nursing since much of what we deal with is in the 'private' domain of life. O'Brien and Pearson (1993) suggest that, as nursing is an 'oral' culture, nurses do not commit their thoughts to formal, written explanations of practice. Thus, while actual models have always existed in our minds, being asked to make them explicit, to share them with others or to consider other people's views is a new experience for many.

Figure 3.1   All nurses have a picture in their head of what nursing actually is.

THE ROLE OF MODELS IN PRACTICE

All thinking people possess views of the world, their work and the subject of their work – in the case of nursing, the patients or clients. In occupations that involve service to other people, these views give direction to the people who work in them, if they construct models from beliefs about the patient/client and from current knowledge related to those beliefs. In teaching, for example, various writers describe teaching models which give different views about people and how they learn (e.g. Sterling, 2001). Some emphasise the belief that learners need to be told clearly what the teacher requires them to know and do, and that if this happens learning will take place. Others emphasise the belief that learners themselves need to decide what they wish to know and be able to do; they consider that learning takes place if the teacher allows this to happen and provides the resources learners appear to need to achieve their own objectives. Yet others suggest that skills cannot be taught but coached through reflection on experience. There are, of course, many other components to teaching models, and many other beliefs about teaching. However, these three basic but different sets of beliefs, derived from different theories of learning, serve to give an example of the need for some agreement on a model in an institution which sets out to help people learn. If the model based on setting learners objectives, and then giving them the material that is needed to achieve the objectives, is agreed on, it will give direction to the way in which the institution is run. It will influence the use of the school building, the library resources, the teaching aids and the actual behaviour of the teacher. The first approach would require efficient copying facilities to print out objectives for learners, and a good supply of set texts recommended by the teachers. If the second model, based on more active student involvement, is followed, less of these facilities may be required but more private study areas and a wider selection of books would be essential. And in the third model, access to real work experience by both students and teachers would be a prerequisite.

In nursing, the care given to patients or clients is also influenced by the model held by the people who give the care. However, in very many settings, no generally agreed model is held. In a team of nurses, for example, one nurse may align nursing very closely with the work of doctors and aim for the efficient carrying out of medically prescribed care. In this instance less emphasis will be placed on non-medical acts such as organising social activities or transport for visitors who are unable to make their own way to hospital, or exploring feelings and providing information in order for patients to participate in decision making. Another nurse may emphasise just those things and see the more medically related tasks as being important but no more so than social or educative activities. Yet another nurse may value tidiness and order and concentrate on clean and tidy patients and ward areas. There may be one nurse who spends much time on watching and supporting an elderly patient while she dresses herself, while another will consistently dress the patient because she sees 'doing things' for people as being a part of nursing.

If you reflect on this for a moment, we suspect that it actually describes at least one area where you have worked as a nurse or seen nursing, even if you are fairly new to this work. Although all of the nurses described are fictitious and have no names, you can probably fit them to people you know. Of course, all nurses are individuals and the past that belongs to them, the way they were brought up by their parents, the place they came from and their social background as a whole influence how they behave and what they value. As Allen (1985) suggests, all our realities are influenced and limited by our socio-historical backgrounds, which cannot be ignored. Furthermore, all of these things go towards the model for nursing practice on which we base our real work of caring for people. But some of the differences between the nurses in this fictitious team could at least be recognised, and the impact of the varying perspectives on patient care acknowledged. The strengths of each nurse could be better channelled if the team were to consider different descriptions of what nursing is, and after discussion agree on generally basing practice on one, or an agreed combination of two or more, descriptions. Models of nursing practice are such descriptions. It is irrelevant which model or combination of models is agreed upon as long as agreement is reached.

Achieving agreement demands that the team as a whole consider each individual nurse's beliefs about patients and nursing work. It leads to a number of possible advantages. If a team of nurses agree to base their practice on a generally accepted model, it will:

1. Lead to consistency in the sort of care received by patients and thus to a continuity of care patterns and treatments;
2. Give rise to less conflict within the team of nurses as a whole;
3. Make sense of the nursing given by the team (other health care workers involved, such as doctors, physiotherapists and ancillary staff, will understand better the logic behind the care);
4. Give direction to nursing care within the area, since the goals of nursing work will be understood by the whole team;
5. Act as a major guide in decision and policy making because the components of the model chosen can act as a guide against which to check decisions;
6. Act as a guide for the criteria on which new team members are selected.

As an example, let us consider a team of nurses who all agree that the model constructed by Orem (1980, 1991) should provide a basis for practice in their work. Orem's model is described in Chapter 9. It focuses on the nurse striving to help the patient or client to care for him or herself. Thus, the nurse concentrates on helping patients to do things for themselves rather than doing everything for them, a principle known as self-care (Furlong, 1995). If patients are unable to be independent in this way, however, nurses will act for them or on their behalf. Orem's model is, of course, more complex, but this specific component serves for this example. If self-care is the aim of nursing, patients are seen as having the right to care for themselves whenever possible, should they so wish. Nurses who agree to apply this model will value knowledge and skills related to promoting or giving self-care. The relationship of such a view of nursing to the six possible advantages listed above can be demonstrated.

Orem – self care model

To begin with, it can be assumed that all nurses in the team would consistently try to step back and support patients in doing things themselves whenever possible. They would only 'do' care when the patients are unable to help themselves. This does not mean that they would abdicate responsibility for care, but form a different type of relationship with the patients or clients in which they can contribute to deciding who does what. Stretched to its logical conclusion, some patients may take their own medications, give their own tube feeds, take and record their own observations, or dress and undress themselves, even if it takes longer than when the nurse does it (Day, 1995). Similarly, provision of information to help patients gain knowledge of their condition and contribute to informed decisions about their treatment would be fundamental within this approach to practice. Acceptance of this by the whole team may then lessen the current situation in which, for example, patients know they will have to dress themselves when Nurse White is on duty, but will be dressed by the nurse when Nurse Green is on duty. If the self-care model is agreed upon, care will be similar all the time, with only minor variations that will always arise because of differences between individual nurses.

Less conflict may also occur because the nurse who steps back and allows patients to be independent will be less likely to be seen as lazy or slow. Other members of the health team will also begin to understand that nurses in this area all value independence as a patient's right. Because self-care is accepted as the overall goal of nursing, this will give direction to the way work is organised, to the assessment, planning, implementation and evaluation of care, and to the relationship between the nursing team and other workers. The self-care goal could be used usefully as a yardstick when decisions need to be made about issues such as choices of new equipment, alterations in drug-giving procedures or patterns of work organisation. For example, when making policy decisions on how drugs should be given, options can be discussed alongside the beliefs about self-care. If nurses always retain control of drugs and do not allow patients to take personal responsibility for their safe administration, does this enhance the promotion of self-care? If it does not, then questions must be asked about how the procedure can be satisfactorily modified to promote self-care.

In the event of having to choose new equipment, the choice may be between a new disposable bedpan system or two commodes. The team may again weigh up the merits of the choice on the basis of which would be more likely to assist patients to achieve self-care.

The final point mentioned was that a model for nursing practice can be used as a guide for selecting the criteria on which a new member of staff will be appointed. If a group of nurses working together are in a position to be quite clear about the values on which they base their practice, and the goals that they are trying to achieve, there is an opportunity for both the applicant and the interviewers to discover whether they share these values and goals. Hopefully this would lessen the likelihood of someone who would not fit in being appointed to a team who have well-established, albeit flexible, views of the service that they are offering.

It is possible to go on listing all kinds of different examples, but the reasons why a team needs to agree on a model are probably becoming evident. Selecting a nursing model demands that the team agree on the nature and purpose of the work they are carrying out, and on a view about the people to whom they offer that service, namely the patients or clients. These are essential prerequisites for effective nursing.

We could, of course, leave the system of giving care unchanged. Nurses could carry on giving care to those who need it, in the way it occurs to them personally. However, if there are six nurses looking after one patient, whether in a hospital or at home, the chances are that the care will be based on up to six different models. Furthermore, none of these models may be appropriate for that patient. There is even likelihood that confusion will arise, especially for the patients or clients. It will lead to care which is disjointed and to a patient having to adjust to six nurses rather than six nurses adjusting to one patient.

Actual agreement among those six nurses on a broad picture of what they consider to be the role of the nurse, the needs of the patient and what it is they are trying to achieve will in the end lead to successful care, a satisfied patient and a united team. Furthermore, within a system of primary nursing (Manthey, 1992), where a single qualified nurse takes continual responsibility for the care planning of a named patient, continuity of care giving in his or her absence becomes much easier to achieve if there is a widely shared understanding of nursing.

All of this may seem to be highly theoretical, and it cannot be denied that nursing is really very practical. But theory guides all practice, all

Figure 3.2 An agreed model stops confusion.

living, even if this is not overtly recognised. There is an old saying that there is nothing so practical as a good theory. The practical, observable movement of the car from one point to another only happened because someone worked on the theory which led to the development of the internal combustion engine, just as our everyday dependence on electricity, telephones or microwaves has arisen from basic theories.

In this book we hope to share our understanding of models in relationship to practical nursing. It is our belief that all nursing is already based on models for practice, but that at the moment nurses find it difficult to explain and share their ideas with others because they are hidden in their minds rather than explicit. The issues that need to be raised are therefore very broad, and may initially seem to be outside what is normally considered to be important to nurses. That is why we began by saying that this book is a little different. It is intended to be used both personally and professionally. On a personal level, the book aims to help individual nurses to clarify their thoughts about nursing work and how they relate to it. Within clinical teams or a class of students, its purpose is to promote creative thinking about developing real nursing with the help of models for practice.

Bear with us then, if the following chapters bring up words or ideas which have been, up until now, unfamiliar or which seem inappropriate, and if the rest of the book generates more questions than clear answers. That state is the beginning of the thinking and questioning attitude which nursing demands.

Learning exercises

1. Consider how nursing practice would generally be described by the general public and compare this 'lay model' with your experience of practice.
2. What, in your experience, are the dominant elements of nursing practice?
3. Think of a time, in your experience, when a group of nurses (or – if you have yet to work in the nursing team – a group of any people who are engaged in a common task or process) had difficulty in working together. To what degree could this have been due to conflicting models of practice held by different members of the team?

Study questions

1. Define a 'nursing model'.
2. Describe the role of models in nursing practice.
3. List the advantages of identifying an agreed model in a nursing team.

Chapter 4

The Basis of Models

LEARNING OBJECTIVES

On completion of this chapter, the reader will be able to:

1. Define the terms concept, theory and paradigm
2. Discuss the components of nursing models
3. Examine the relationship between a nursing model and the delivery of nursing care

THE ELEMENTS OF A MODEL

We have already talked about the building bricks that go towards making up a nursing model. A model house constructed by an architect is made up of the components of that house, and represents the shape of the rooms, the slope of the roof and the relationship of one part to another. It is not a real house, but it accurately represents reality, and the successful construction of a house is only assured if time is spent initially on the careful creation of a model. A nursing model is made up of the components or ideas that go towards making up nursing – what it is, the beliefs and values, and the theories and concepts on which it is built. While these words are often viewed with some caution by many people, they are in fact the building bricks of what each one of us believes nursing is. All of us already hold beliefs, have values, and understand the theories and concepts on which we base our practice. In order to be able to share our ideas with others, a brief explanation of each of these terms is necessary.

PHILOSOPHIES AND BELIEFS

Throughout the ages there have been people who have publicly stated their views about the world, about people, and about what is right and wrong. While a few have made these statements publicly, all of us do, in fact, hold such beliefs. It is these beliefs which guide the whole of our lives. Bertrand Russell wrote in 1961 that 'Ever since men became capable of free speculation, their actions in innumerable important respects have depended upon their theories as to the world and human life, as to what is good and what is evil.' From what Russell says it becomes fairly evident that what you believe about people, society and life will affect the way you behave. So philosophy can be interpreted as the pursuit of wisdom or knowledge about the things around us and what causes them. A philosophy is an explicit statement about what you believe and about what values you hold. These values and beliefs will, in turn, affect the way you behave.

Stevenson (1974) takes two well-known philosophical stances, that of Christianity and of Marxism, and makes a simple comparison to demonstrate this point. The Christian view of people is that they are made in the image of God, who created and controls the universe. The goal or purpose of human lives is to fulfil God's purpose, and their state is dependent on their relationship with God. On the other hand, Marx suggested that the universe is fundamentally material and that nothing exists beyond it.

Our moral ideas and values are determined by the society in which we live. If the Christian belief is followed, the way forward lies in God's ability to forgive and regenerate in His image. The Marxist view, however, holds that an individual cannot change without fundamental changes in society. Two people holding these opposing views will ultimately behave in quite different ways – one seeking to develop in the image of God and the other seeking to change society in order to influence the way individuals behave.

Take a concrete example with which we are all familiar. We have already said that there are different views about how we learn, and our

Figure 4.1 Beliefs and values influence your views of life.

experience of 'being taught' clearly confirms this. There is the teacher who will stand before a class and lecture, who will 'deposit' a body of information for us to absorb because he or she believes that as the holder of expert knowledge on a given subject, his or her role is to hand on this knowledge to others. This is something we have all experienced at some time in our educational careers. Alternatively, there are those teachers who believe that people learn more effectively if they discover things for themselves. Their approach may be through guiding seminars prepared by students, and through involvement and discussion with very active participation on the part of the whole group. The development of the notion of practice development and the use of reflection on action has gained popularity, with active encouragement to gain insight into our actions in the real world and hence deepen our understanding of practice. One explanation for these different styles of teaching is that the beliefs of the varying types of teachers are based on completely different theories of learning, namely expository learning, discovery learning and reflective learning, which are derived from different philosophies.

In the same way, we are all familiar with nurses who behave in different ways in the same situation. An example of this is nurses' feelings about the use of high-technology medicine for very elderly patients with the aim of preserving life at all costs. One group of nurses will consider that, whatever the circumstances, if such treatment is available it should be given. Another view may be that the use of such treatment depends upon the individual circumstances of each patient, and that patients have a right to choose whether or not to receive treatment which in itself may be traumatic, their decision being based on their own views about the quality of their lives. Similar debates rage around both active and passive euthanasia, and the right to die as well as the right to live (Shamash, 1995). The argument may be seen as being related to quantity versus quality, but in our current society is also influenced by market forces as demonstrated by the Oregan experience (Honigsbaum, 1992), where the views of the community were sought in deciding how health care should be rationed. These variations in views are fundamentally based on a belief system about nature and life itself but are, it can be suggested, inevitably also influenced by external factors which impact on health services delivery.

In talking about philosophies, it becomes evident that they are made up of the views or ideas about the subject being discussed. Relating this to nursing, there are two questions that have to be asked. First, what are the specific subjects that we need to consider and clarify in relationship to nursing? Second, what ideas or theories do we hold in relationship to these subjects?

Concepts

A concept of a particular subject is the way in which it is viewed. It is a classification system applied to a particular area. Yet not all of us would classify things in the same way. This becomes very obvious when you try to find your way through a colleague's filing system and end up saying in exasperation 'I'd never have put it there'. Yet to the person who established the filing system, it is the obvious place. Thus, as cells are units of the body, so concepts are units of the mind which help us to put thoughts and ideas into some sort of order to make sense of the world.

Nursing itself may be seen as a very large collection of concepts, that is those things which individuals consider are important to nursing, which nurses need to know about and to develop theories about. It may be worthwhile to stop here for a minute and consider what major concepts you think are related to nursing. Hopefully they will be very similar to the ones identified by the people with whom you work. Otherwise there may be terrible confusion in trying to find your way about the filing system of each other's thoughts.

The most commonly identified concepts which have been discussed in relationship to nursing are those concerned with beliefs about people, society, the environment, health and nursing itself. A philosophy of nursing usually makes statements about each of these subjects.

Theories

The next stage of the game is to try to work out how the concepts fit together in practice, and this is the stage at which theories have to be considered. Theories are proposals that give a reasonable explanation to an event. They are ideas about how or why something happens. Returning to the example of teaching that we gave earlier, there are different theories about how people learn – none of which is proved absolutely. Once proved beyond reasonable doubt, a theory is considered to be a law, although as our state of knowledge advances even some ideas that were viewed with certainty, such as the constancy of gravity, are being challenged. Hence individuals must make knowledgeable judgements about the theories they accept, and where possible to test their theories or support them by facts. However, it must always be remembered that with the passage of time and the advancement of knowledge, theories may change and develop. As Lather (1986) so aptly comments:

> The search is for theory which grows out of context embedded data, not in a way which rejects prior theory but in a way which prevents it from distorting the logic of evidence. Theory is too often used to protect us from the awesome complexity of the world.

An example of this is that previously there was a theory in nursing that rubbing skin vigorously prevented the formation of pressure sores. With the advancement of time, and with it the acquisition of new knowledge, it became known that this theory is inaccurate and that in fact rubbing is potentially harmful. So new theories, based on an understanding of the anatomy and physiology of skin and the circulation of blood, have been proposed and widely accepted. In the same way the old habit of dry dressing has been superseded by our understanding of the moist environment required for tissue regeneration. Similarly, with new knowledge about the nature of people and views of health, theories about what nursing is and how it may be practised have developed.

There are two ways in which theories can be developed. First, someone may come up with an idea and wonder whether it is related to practice. For instance, with the current interest in complementary therapies the question of whether or not they are of any value to nurses, and through them to patients, may be asked. This type of theory is known as a deductive theory. It takes ideas that are already established in other fields and considers ways in which they may be related to nursing practice. Theories from both the physical and behavioural sciences have been applied to nursing in this way, although they may be transformed through use in practice. For example, theories about bonding between parents and children have been applied in a deductive way and have altered the practice of nursing in both obstetric and paediatric services.

Alternatively, it may be observed through practice that patients in one situation seem to recover more quickly than patients in another, and a nurse may set out to discover if this is true. This is known as an inductive theory, that is a theory that arises out of practice. Inductive theory building does not depend on an already established theory, but involves generating new ideas through exploring practice, identifying concepts and relating them to establish theory anew. For example, close observation of people approaching death led to the identification by Kubler-Ross (1969) of stages through which people appear to progress at this time. Recognition of these phases or stages has assisted nurses in understanding and helping people to progress towards their own death or the death of another. Similarly, Benner's (1984) views on the development of expert practice arose initially out of observation of practice. Both deductive and inductive approaches to theory development are valid and necessary for the advancement of nursing practice.

While conceptual models attempt to describe nursing as it is, theory attempts to systematically describe and predict. Whilst we recognise that theory has multiple meanings and is complex in its development, in purely simple terms theory can be seen as that which arises out of theorising – that is systematically thinking through a set of related concepts and theories and identifying possibilities. As we discussed in Chapter 1, theory also takes various forms, such as personal theory, local theory, grand theory, epistemological theory, metatheory. As Tripp (1987) says:

> The whole idea of theory is a very confused one. Different people use it in different ways to mean quite different things. The idea of theory is further confused as it is frequently opposed to the equally diffuse idea of practice. These difficulties are reflected, for instance, in the way in which the term 'theory' is used in the names of so many quite disparate intellectual activities and knowledge.

The crux of the debate on the relationship between theory and practice in nursing is the strongly held view of some that theory bears no relationship to the reality of practice. The suggestion here is that no practice is 'atheoretical', but the theory used may not be made explicit or comply with textbook theory. This does not mean to say that it is wrong, but that it is different.

Why this view should be so prevalent in nursing leads us on to yet another interesting analysis of theory – that is paradigms, which guide us in our search for knowledge and therefore for theory.

Guiding paradigms

A paradigm is defined by Chin and Jacobs (1987) as:

> ... *a generally accepted world view or philosophy, a structure within which the theories of the discipline are organised.*

Botha (1989) suggests that these world views give rise to assumptions in disciplinary groups which influence practice, research and therefore theory quite profoundly. For example, some people believe that everything which matters can be measured, and if ideas cannot be tested through controlled experiments their influence in practice should be less strong. While the widespread move to increase so-called 'evidence based practice' based on such a view is to be applauded, there is a risk that less well-defined concepts such as hopelessness (Welch *et al.*, 1994), which do not lend themselves readily to measurement, will be ignored within health care. To explore this idea further, it is useful to consider the three dominant paradigms of today and consider what influences they each have on theory and its relationship with practice.

In doing so we draw largely on the work of Allen *et al.* (1986) and Heath (1998) in an attempt to explore the assumptions which underlie the prevailing paradigms and their relationship to theory, method and practice.

The positivist paradigm

Positivism, sometimes known as logical positivism, or the empirico-analytical paradigm, attempts to view the world objectively in order to manipulate and control it. Vaughan (1992) says of positivism:

> *Its basic premise is concerned with identifying cause and effect and in so doing, being able to identify generally applicable theories which can hold good in a multitude of circumstances.*

Consequently, theory is generated through the use of controlled observation and experimentation of that which can be measured, in an attempt to confirm explanations. Thus the theorist starts off with a theoretical idea which is then transformed into a hypothesis, to be tested using objective methods. If the hypothesis is confirmed, it is then assumed that this will occur in the same way in the future. Thus the event and its results become predictable. For example, someone following the positivist regime may instigate a new regime for preoperative bowel preparation (a theoretical idea) with a view that it would lead to a cleaner bowel on which to operate (the hypothesis). Half the patients undergoing surgery would be randomly selected to receive the new preparation, and the cleanliness of the bowels at surgery of each group would be assessed.

There is no doubt that areas of nursing knowledge for practice are amenable to such an approach, especially those which relate to physiological processes, and that closing the curtain on this view is inappropriate for nursing. For example, much has been learned about management of the perineum during labour using a controlled trial (Sleep, 1984). Similarly different methods of treating venous ulcers have been assessed from a positivist stance (Duby *et al.*, 1993), as also one aspect of the study exploring the efficacy of nurse-led in-patient services (Griffiths and Evans, 1995). It is equally inappropriate, however, to conclude that this is the only view, yet it still predominates in nursing and other areas of health care, overly influencing our conception of theory.

The positivist paradigm is concerned with quantitative theory which aims at control. It is seen as distinct from practice, and in order to maintain objectivity, ways of ensuring distance between theory and the subtle, non-quantifiable subjective components of practice are actively sought. Theory is developed and then tested in a controlled environment which, as Schon (1987) suggests, does not always reflect the 'swampy lowlands' of reality. However, if the theory is supported through meta-analysis (that is review of a number of studies assessing the same thing), then it becomes nearer to a law which is generalisable when the same events occur in the future. If one adopts a positivist stance, then theory and practice become separated, practice driven by theory but not generating theory.

There is no doubt that positivism is still the dominant paradigm in health care, but while this stance should never be underestimated it must be remembered that it is not the only world view available to nurses.

The interpretive paradigm The interpretive paradigm is grounded on different assumptions and methods. It assumes that the meaning of events and feelings to an individual person is valid data. Rather than using objective, quantifiable methods to gather information, this paradigm involves listening to people or watching what they do and using the human imagination and understanding of those participating in order to interpret their meanings. True knowledge is viewed as dependent upon whether or not the participants accept them, rather than on whether they will identify cause, predict outcome or allow control (Fay, 1975). Thus it is as much concerned with the 'experience' of illness, something which is of critical importance to nurses, as with the cause and treatment of disease.

In this paradigm, the theories are built upon the basis of the understandings which arise out of the people studied, rather than testing a predefined hypothesis. Theory is seen as '... a skeletal, deprived view of reality that is drawn from everyday practical activity and knowledge' (Allen *et al.*, 1986). For example, looking at preoperative preparation from a different stance there may be a concern about nutritional status. In order to help patients, detailed attention would be paid to the factors which people perceive have enhanced or inhibited their ability to eat a balanced diet in order to gain insight into how help may be offered. Theory is not generalisable, although knowledge of interpretative theory can and is used in order to understand and hence guide practice. Essentially theory is seen to be already embedded in practice, although not made explicit.

In this paradigm, practice and theory are inextricably linked and formal theory, i.e. that which is documented and accessible but derived from knowledge embedded in practice, is used to guide the novice but is transformed and refined by the expert (Benner, 1984).

The critical paradigm The critical paradigm goes beyond the narrowness of both positivist and interpretative paradigms. The critical paradigm seeks to generate theory from action or practice in order to help people change things they would like to change. Vaughan (1992) suggests that the critical paradigm:

> ... is primarily concerned with emancipation of self. They [Habermas, 1971; Giroux, 1983, etc.] argue that rather than directly adding to world knowledge, critical theory is concerned with the ability to act rationally, to make decisions in the light of available knowledge, to gain a greater understanding of self. It is primarily concerned with controlling the knowledge gained through technical and interpretative enquiry, using actions to realise personal, social and professional goals.

The critical paradigm unambiguously integrates theory and practice totally. Theorist-practitioners aim at raising their own and others' consciousness through collaboratively analysing and seeking understandings of the real circumstance, and searching out alternative ways of seeing the situation. This paradigm involves a 'transaction' between theory and practice, and therefore welds the two together. The focus is on 'theory in action' or action theory. This perspective on theory offers us as nurses the opportunity to translate the frequently voiced rhetoric about the interrelationship between nursing theory and nursing practice into the real world of practice. Thus armed with knowledge about preoperative eating habits and the efficacy of differing bowel preparations, local actions would be taken to explore practice options, for example to consider ways in which flexible access to a range of different types of foods could be achieved and whether a balance was found between the acceptability to those concerned of the bowel cleansing regime and its effectiveness.

The driving influence on what we view as legitimate theory is grounded in our philosophical (world view) and epistemological (view of knowledge) position at that time. In the positivist paradigm, theory is deductive and aims to predict and control. Methods are objective and quantitative. In the interpretative paradigm, theory is inductive and concerned with exposing implicit meaning. It aims at understanding. Interpretive methods are not objective but may be both quantitative and qualitative as long as the aim is to describe and understand, rather than to manipulate and control. The critical paradigm, like the interpretative, is inductive and aims at emancipation of knowledge and practice. It is concerned with the relationship between meaning and the social notions of autonomy and responsibility. Methods are not objective but may be either quantitative or qualitative.

Although many people will favour one or another of these three perspectives, it must be said that all three have much to offer and a wide-ranging respect for the differing views can only help us to enhance our understanding of people and practice. Returning to models for nursing and the way in which nurses practice, the very foundations of these models and approaches to practice lie in an individual's philosophy or beliefs about nursing. This in turn is based on how each individual classifies nursing and the subjects related to it, as well as the theories believed to be true, which are shaped by each individual's own life experiences and the dominant paradigms of the day. Over a period of time every nurse has developed such a model. Nursing has reached a stage in its development where it is possible to be explicit about these thoughts and to share them with others.

COMPONENTS OF MODELS

The notion that what nurses believe actually affects the way in which they behave has been emphasised throughout this chapter. The model of nursing on which practice is based contains the theories and concepts of that practice, and the theories and concepts reflect the philosophies, values and beliefs about both human nature and what it is that the nursing you offer is trying to achieve. There are a plethora of texts that examine and analyse models (cf. Stevens, 1984; Fawcett, 1989; Chinn and Kramer, 1999; Kim and Kollak, 1999; Watson, 1999; Fitzpatrick and Whall, 1996; Marriner-Tomey and Alligood, 2002) and an approach to evaluating models is discussed in Chapter 17. For a detailed examination of extant nursing models from a range of perspectives, these texts are worthy of pursuit. In this book, we take a practical approach to exploring the nature and roles of nursing models and, from our perspective, there are, as a starting point, three basic components of any practice model (see Fig. 4.2).

1. The beliefs and values on which the model is based, related to:
   (a) the person;
   (b) health; and
   (c) the environment.
2. The goals of practice or what the practitioner aims to achieve.
3. The knowledge and skills the practitioner needs to develop in order to gain these goals.

There are similarities in any model of an occupation like teaching or nursing, where the subject of concern is a person rather than an object. What is apparent in all cases is the need to explore each of these components not only from your own perspective but also when reviewing the work of others.

Beliefs and values

Any occupation concerned with the provision of a human service has to adopt a stance about the nature of people, how they behave and the environment in which they live. This stance will underpin any model of

Figure 4.2 Components for a model in practice.

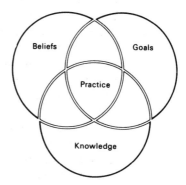

that occupation. For those working in health care the 'product' is health which, as anyone working in that field will know, can be viewed in many different ways. Hence clarity about views on health is also critical. And because people do not exist in isolation but as part of a community and of society itself, the issues of community and society must also be considered. Just as a carpenter must understand the nature of wood, his essential raw material – how pliable or durable it is and how it reacts with other materials – so any person who is dealing with a human service must have some understanding of how people, or the recipients of their service, function, not just as physical but also as social beings living within a community, and as psychological beings with feelings and relationships.

Compared to the complexity of human nature, wood is a relatively simple subject, and there are many confirmed facts or laws about the way in which it will behave. For example, it is indisputable that unseasoned wood will alter its shape in a fairly predictable way as it matures.

The huge range of individual differences among people makes it impossible for those who work with them to be anywhere near as certain about all aspects of human behaviour. There are no such things as 'truths' about human nature. However, there are many theories which give different explanations of it, and in any occupation or discipline which involves practice, particular theories are adopted as beliefs on which to base that practice. Different occupations focus on specific aspects of humanity according to the service they offer. For example, teaching models will always focus on beliefs about how people learn. In sociology, the emphasis is on how people relate to each other and in psychology, on how they behave. Western health care has traditionally emphasised the biological aspect of human beings based primarily on the positivist paradigm described earlier. Current thoughts are challenging this tradition and bringing into focus views from a wider range of perspectives.

The belief and value components of the practice model form the foundation on which the whole of the rest of the model is built. They influence not only practice, but all aspects of our lives.

Goals of practice

Returning to the example of carpenters, their goals or what they expect to achieve are usually quite clear. For instance, at the start of their work, they will already have an idea about the size, design and finish of the chairs that they are trying to produce.

It is equally important in providing a service to patients that the overall purpose of the service is clearly understood by the practitioner, as well as the consumer of the service – in the case of nursing, the client or patient and, in a market-driven health care system, purchasers and policy-makers. This second component of the model therefore demands that the occupational group agrees on the common purpose towards which it is striving.

Again because there is so much variety among individuals, there may be some variation in the recognised goals. For instance, some teachers may see their goal as ensuring that the learner has sufficient knowledge to pass an examination. Others may identify a broader goal of helping learners to solve their own problems and to develop skills for a particular work situation. This of course is often overcome by educational institutes opting to aim for 'learning to take place' and leaving it to individual practitioners to decide on how to achieve that goal.

The goals of human service occupations are strongly influenced by social expectations and they rarely remain static. The traditional goals of health care have been to cure or control disease, and there is evidence that this is still true. This is exemplified by, for example, the content of many audit tools, but it must be added that in a market-driven arena cost and throughput issues are also apparent in identifying desired goals. However, practitioners and consumers alike are now increasingly calling for a wider view of the goals of health care, and there is a steady increase in the involvement of users in planning health care (Copperman and Morrison, 1995).

Knowledge and skills for practice

Just as the goals of practice arise from the beliefs and values adopted by the occupation, the knowledge and skills needed by practitioners are determined by the stated goals of the model. Once a discipline which involves practice has identified its beliefs and values, and what it is trying to achieve, it becomes relatively easy to identify the knowledge and skills required for practice.

Returning to the carpenter, if there is a belief that wood is a material which can be changed, and that through carving and fitting it can be made into a chair, then the carpenter must have knowledge about the properties of wood, and he must have skill in using the tools required to make a chair. To find out what knowledge and skills are required for a practice discipline (an occupation which gives a service to people), it is useful to consider the discipline's beliefs about humans and the goals of the discipline. In traditional health care, the basic views have been related to the belief in people as biological creatures who can be affected by disease, and the goals have been grounded in a desire to cure. This has therefore led to a need for knowledge based on the biological sciences and disease, supported by technical skills to administer treatment. If it is recognised that there are alternatives to these beliefs and goals, then inevitably there must be alternative or additional knowledge and skills related to other aspects of human behaviour which are required for practice.

Any model for practice must contain these three basic components – beliefs and values, goals of practice, and the knowledge and skills needed to reach those goals. By the very fact that we practice, all of us actually possess a personal model of this kind, although in many instances this has not been made explicit. A nursing model provides a framework through which the application of this structure to nursing itself can be brought to light, drawing on both personal views and those expressed by others. It enables us, as nurses, to make explicit to both patients/clients and colleagues the way in which we work and what we are trying to achieve.

THE NURSING PROCESS AND NURSING MODELS

A nursing model is a picture or representation of what nursing actually is. In fact it represents the actual 'goods' which are delivered to the client. All goods, however, need some vehicle through which they are delivered and the nursing process serves this function. The process itself says nothing about the content and is not specific to nursing. It is merely a sequence of steps passed through in order to achieve a desired end, and it can be seen in use by many other occupational groups. Furthermore, as practice becomes more expert these steps are moved through so rapidly that it is sometimes difficult to discern them (Benner and Wrubel, 1989; MacLeod, 1990), yet the shifting of information, assessment of options, desired goals and evaluation of outcomes does still occur.

Nursing can be likened to a package of goods which is to be delivered. The process of assessment, planning, implementation and evaluation is merely the means of ensuring that the package arrives safely. The package, or nursing itself, is the model which guides the process and contains the components of which nursing is made.

SYSTEMS OF CARE DELIVERY

A word must also be said here about care delivery systems, the choice of which is also influenced by the model of practice. Traditionally nursing work was allocated by task, a method of work organisation that reflected the bureaucratic, reductionist way in which health care was managed. It was also said to protect nurses from forming meaningful relationships with patients, which it was believed were hard to handle (Menzies, 1960), although with current thinking this view could be challenged. Task allocation also reflected the way in which scientific knowledge had been developed, dominated by the positivist regime described above, as well as the ever-increasing specialisation in health care.

Over the past 3 decades nurses and others have become more and more dissatisfied with this approach to work, and have gradually moved along a continuum from patient allocation through team nursing to primary nursing (Vaughan and Pillmoor, 1989; Pontin, 1999). In some ways this shift in the way in which nursing work is organised demonstrates a more fundamental shift in the values and beliefs on which practice is based. If there is to be respect for the person, viewed as more than a biological creature,

Figure 4.3 Models will influence day-to-day work.

then continuity of care and relationships between recipients and givers of care become important. If these beliefs are made apparent, then it becomes critical that a method of work organisation which facilitates rather than inhibits goal achievement is chosen, not only to provide more consistent care but also to enhance job satisfaction.

The interest in primary nursing, as a means of fulfilling these requirements, has been widespread and endorsed at a national level (Department of Health, 1991). While some people suggest that it is both a philosophy and a system of work organisation (Ersser and Tutton, 1991), Manthey (1992) suggests that it is primarily the latter. Hence much like the nursing process it is an adjunct to care delivery, inextricably linked with a practice model rather than a model in its own right.

This chapter has explored the notion of models for practice and expanded some of the underlying issues. The influences that beliefs and values have on practice, and the relationship of theories and concepts to practice, have been discussed. The manner in which these underlying issues affect the components of the model have also been highlighted, alongside what are considered to be the basic components of any model of an occupation which gives a service to people. While it is recognised that some of these things are not normally discussed by nurses, it is hoped that their relevance has become clear. Being explicit about the model on which nursing practice is based in a particular setting directly affects the delivery of nursing care to patients. Its importance cannot be denied.

Learning exercises

1. Reflect on the knowledge you use in practice and consider the paradigmatic stance adopted in the production of this knowledge.
2. Identify a theory from another discipline (for example, psychological theory on the stages of child development) and identify the concepts that make up that theory.
3. Think further on exercise 2 and try to identify a model that is used by practitioners that relates to the theory you selected.

Study questions

1. Define concept, theory and paradigm.
2. Discuss the three dominant paradigms and relate them to nursing knowledge.
3. List the components of a nursing model.
4. Identify the role of nursing models in relation to the nursing process.

Chapter 5

The Traditional Model for Nursing Practice

LEARNING OBJECTIVES

On completion of this chapter, the reader will be able to:

1. Define the biomedical model
2. Trace the historical basis for nursing's allegiance to the biomedical model
3. Identify and discuss the advantages and disadvantages of the biomedical model

NURSING AND THE SO-CALLED MEDICAL MODEL

All nurses – all people – have personal theories of nursing and all nursing teams work from a basis of local theory and a locally acceptable model for practice. Thus, although the term 'model' may be new, basing practice on a model has occurred since nursing began.

It is argued by many that the basic model which guided nursing has traditionally been the medical model. This 'biomedical' model has also traditionally been the basis for the practice of medicine in the Western world for the past few hundred years, exemplified by the structure of health care services which reflect medical specialties as well as the way in which roles are defined. Before describing this long-standing model, it is important to emphasise that it has been the subject of some criticism over the years, and is now rejected in part by many doctors, a number of whom practice from a much broader base. However, the medical establishment and the majority of medical schools still see the biomedical model as an accurate representation of the reality of doctoring. Brown and Seddon (1996) suggest that the body is viewed in conflicting ways in the health professions – as a biomechanical phenomena and a social phenomena – and that this results in an incomplete account of the 'causes' of illness and inadequate health care responses. This view is elaborated on by Pauli *et al.* (2000), who argue that nurses directly confront a growing body of data and that the extraordinarily productive contemporary biomedical model should be expanded beyond the physical and biological to incorporate meaningful information about how each patient's experiences impinge on health status. This 'expanded' biomedical model is referred to as a biocultural model by Morris (2000), who argues that the biocultural model respects the complications arising at the crossroads of biology and culture as deeply as the biomedical model respects the complexities of cellular processes. A biocultural model, while it takes seriously the reciprocal relations between culture and illness, does not imply that crystals will cure cancer or that consciousness will restore a missing limb. A biocultural model means that beliefs shape perception and alter bodily processes. It means that cultures shape beliefs. It means that illnesses occur in people who live in cultures that affect illnesses.

Following the outline of the model presented in Chapter 6, the biomedical model can be summarised into three basic components – namely beliefs and values, the goals of practice, and the knowledge needed to achieve these goals.

The beliefs and values which underlie the biomedical model

In this model people are seen as biological beings, made up of cells, which then make tissues, which then make organs, which then make systems. All of these interact and communicate with each other to achieve harmony or balance, a state called homeostasis. Biological homeostasis is seen as health, and is a state which is achievable but can be disturbed by trauma, malfunction or malformation. Such disturbance leads to disease or 'medical conditions'. Although this is the core belief of the model, and human beings are in part regarded almost like machines, development of the model in recent years has led to some acknowledgement of social and psychological disturbances of homeostasis. Indeed, stress-related ill health has been a common phenomenon of the 1990s. However, the emphasis remains on biological homeostasis and the physical signs and manifestations of it. The physical working parts of the person are of prime importance.

The goals of the biomedical model

Medical practice ultimately aims for biological homeostasis, the curing or control of disease, or the repair of trauma or malformation. The goal can be achieved by diagnosing the cause of disturbed homeostasis and treating it. When cure is impossible, the goal can be modified either to alleviate the manifestations of the disturbance, in other words treat the symptoms, or to postpone death.

However straightforward such a view may seem, it can, in itself, create some confusion for care-givers. For example, there has been recent court action to clarify the point at which feeding can be withdrawn from a patient who has been assessed as 'brain dead', causing major debate among health care workers (Shamash, 1995). Similarly, with limited resources some methods of prioritising health care have to be made, giving rise to exploration of predictor factors in intensive care units (Knaus *et al.*, 1985) and means of assessing the quality of life (Harris, 1987).

The knowledge needed to achieve the goals of the biomedical model

In order to diagnose and treat disease or trauma by administering specific treatments, the practitioner needs knowledge about the physical sciences and skills to recognise physical signs and symptoms. Such knowledge would therefore arise primarily from concepts and theories related to the physical sciences, for example:

- anatomy
- physiology
- biochemistry
- pharmacology
- pathology
- microbiology

The knowledge and skills focus on the physical being, and the gamut of 'faults' which may arise in the continuous functioning of the body must be included. There is however widespread concern that the application of evidence based practice from these scientific sources is not widespread in health care, leading to initiatives such as the Cochrane Collaboration (1993), a multinational service which overviews research to make it more readily available to practitioners. Thus, despite the heavy emphasis on these subjects during training, their use in practice is not always evident.

NURSING AND THE BIOMEDICAL MODEL

There is a great deal of evidence to suggest that the biomedical model is the model on which many nurses base their practice. Studies in nursing frequently report on how nurses continue to view patients as physical beings and pay little attention to the wider characteristics of human nature. Some still consider that the goals of nursing are frequently perceived as being cure orientated and that feelings of failure often arise in nurses when cure is not achieved. Anecdotal and formal evidence both support these suggestions, and discuss the very common atmosphere of routines, standardised activity and nurses' obsession with giving physical care.

Routinisation

Nursing in most Westernised countries, and countries influenced by the West in the colonial era, was, in the past, often based on a prescribed routine which was frequently laid down in the policy or procedure books which were strategically placed in each ward. These rules had traditionally been created by a hierarchy of nurses who saw it as their responsibility to ensure that the rules were adhered to. The end result of such an approach was standardised routines for patient care. The patient was seen as someone who should comply with a predictable pattern and follow the routine laid down by the regulations. Such routines were usually related to the medical diagnosis of the patient.

While procedure books as such have largely gone 'under cover', such routinisation can still be seen. For example, in many instances there is still an expectation that all people undergoing abdominal hysterectomy will walk to the bathroom on the first day postoperatively and will not require intramuscular analgesia after the second day. Indeed, with the advent of critical pathways (Hale, 1995), which make predictions for specific clinical conditions, there is an increasing interest in this approach to practice. Such routines focus primarily on the diagnostic label. While such practices do have some value, when used without skilled assessment there is a risk that they may depersonalise patients and discourage any close involvement between them and nurses, because the patients are identified as the possessors of a disease process rather than as individuals. They become known as 'the appendix in bed 6' who should be pain free by now, rather than Mrs James, a wife and mother and a woman with a life of her own.

A further modern example of this type of objective categorisation of people is the diagnostic related groupings used for costing in hospitals (Bardsley *et al.*, 1989). Indeed, many of the current practices such as standard setting (Royal College of Nursing, 1990) and clinical audit (NHS Management Executive, 1993) can, if misused, become masters to routinised care rather than diagnostic tools, as was the intention. It must be emphasised that this does not decry their use, but rather raises a word of caution about their potential abuse.

The classic biomedical model focuses on correctly diagnosing disease – the nurse's role being to accurately carry out medical prescriptions. Establishing routines to ensure that this happens is a natural result of adherence to the medical model. For instance, administration of analgesia at the same time each day, regardless of individual preferences, would be seen as good practice in these circumstances.

While some routines can be valuable and necessary – such as the safety measures to be followed preoperatively – their wider use can not only depersonalise care but also be potentially dangerous and wasteful of time. The unnecessary recording of observations, or the two-hourly turning of all bedridden patients, are examples of a waste of the precious resource of nursing time. Similarly a routinised approach to hygiene care or meeting nutritional needs may not only be time wasting but also lacking in sensitivity to personal concerns related to, for example, culture, ethnicity or personal preference.

Physical care

Routinisation is often accompanied by an obsession with physical care. Because the biomedical model focuses on people as physical beings, nurses who base their practice on it concentrate on the person's physical needs. Value is placed on those visible aspects of care such as cleanliness, prompt fulfilment of treatment and prescriptions, and tidy beds, cupboards and ward areas. Technical skills such as recording of electrocardiograms or taking intravenous blood are given more status than the ability to comfort distressed people or to share information with those who have little understanding of their own situation. Much of this concern is reflected in current debates around what is and is not legitimate nursing work, highlighted in recent times by the shortage of junior doctors and the increasing interest in clinical nurse specialists, nurse practitioners and physicians' assistants (Pickersgill, 1995). It also raises some concern about the growing interest in 'substitution' of one health care worker for another, most often a nurse for a doctor, which focuses on the fulfilment of tasks and fails to recognise that the skills which nurses bring to these new roles lead to a different and much fuller type of service (Richardson and Maynard, 1995).

The priority of care based on the biomedical model is always towards excellence in physical care, and other components are either left unrecognised or not seen as being important. However, both an obsession with physical care and routinisation have been said to be useful strategies in protecting nurses against the stress inherent in their work. Together they mean that nurses can maintain a distance from patients and not concern themselves with anything other than the disease process, physical care and the maintenance of a routine.

Getting the work done

'Getting through the work' is usually the major goal of nursing teams in the health service, which can be directly related to the emphasis of the biomedical model. There is little attention paid to the meeting of needs of people as individuals. High value is placed on nurses who are able to complete certain defined tasks before handing over to the next nurse on duty. The emphasis is again placed on completion of the visible tasks associated with physical care and routines. Since this is the mechanism used for setting priorities within the work environment, little or no time is left at the end of the day for the personalised aspects of care. With uncertainty in the current job market, being seen to conform has, it can be suggested, also become more prevalent.

Care versus cure

The overriding goal of the biomedical model is cure, and therefore nurses who base their practice on it also aim for this outcome. Such a view can cause confusion and problems for nurses who work in fields where a 'cure' is not possible. For example, uncertainty as to whether curing or caring is the goal of practice has been observed in long-stay psychiatric wards, young disabled units, mental handicap units and in the institutional and community care of the elderly – all areas where the patients cannot 'recover' or get 'completely better'. Nurses adhering to the medical model and working in these units are consistently faced with an inability to achieve the outcome of care that they believe to be appropriate, that is to cure. Thus death, or failure to cure, represents a failure in itself and the nurses as a consequence may become dissatisfied in their work.

If the orientation of the care-giver is towards cure, the manner in which care is provided will reflect this, laying stress on activities which relate to this end, rather than on providing an environment in which individualised care can be delivered. Risk taking for patients in, for example, mobilisation may be minimised as the right to free choice and personal autonomy would not be recognised and quality of life would be based on an assessment of physical safety and stability rather than personal goals.

The emphasis of cure as a general goal of nursing is still reflected today in the difficulties experienced in staffing units which care for chronically dependent people, although this is less evident than a decade ago. It is also seen in continuing education, where competition is intense for places on courses associated with complex technical care directed at cure, such as the intensive care or accident and emergency courses, whereas places on courses concerned with care of the elderly are more easily attained.

If it is believed that nursing should be available to anyone who is in need of nursing care, then it can be suggested that the biomedical model is no longer an appropriate basis for practice. It is limiting because it confines nursing to those who have a health care problem which can achieve cure, and it can create a dilemma for nurses who work with those people for whom such an outcome is unattainable.

The knowledge and skills given to nurses in their professional training a decade ago was structured around the beliefs inherent in the medical model. The curriculum revolved around anatomy, physiology, pathology and other physical sciences, although at a less detailed academic level than medical training. It included very little, if any, specified learning about the social, environmental and psychological components of human beings, let alone about theories of nursing. This meant that, just as in practice, doctors based their assessment, planning, care-giving and evaluation on a framework structured around the systems of the body, so did nurses. Although this pattern of nursing still prevails in some curricula, the tide is gradually turning.

Professional training and experience are not the only factors that determine the models of practice held by nurses. Nurses are individuals and will therefore always incorporate additional beliefs, goals and knowledge specific to themselves. However, the essence of each person's own model is profoundly influenced by the commonly shared model held by the professional group. While it is reasonable for us to assume that many nurses do operate from the perspective of the biomedical model, most nurses also expand it to include other beliefs and some use a very different approach. Nurses who strongly identify with the biological–physical view of human beings and the goal of cure in their work may also take into account the individual differences between people. Nevertheless, the focus may be on physical aspects and this will take precedence over other aspects of the person.

EVOLUTION OF THE BIOMEDICAL MODEL

The most influential model for practice in health care over the last century has been this so-called 'biomedical model', and it is both interesting and relevant to look briefly at its development as an understanding of what has gone before is invaluable for planning what is to come. Pietroni (1984), in writing of his commitment to holistic medicine, gives a succinct account of its evolution.

> It was with the explosion of knowledge that took place in the Renaissance that the major split between religion and science occurred – prior to that time thinking had been strongly influenced by the belief that all actions were divinely controlled. Rene Descartes, a great philosopher of the Renaissance, put forward the concept of dualism, of a mind free from external forces and able to think logically and independently. Thus he separated the body from the mind. He viewed the body as a machine capable of malfunction if some of the parts were not working, and suggested that the most effective way of studying this body or machine was to break it down into its component parts in order that the malfunctioning of each part could be identified and corrected.

Figure 5.1 Some people view the body as a machine capable of malfunction.

This philosophical view was to influence the way in which science, and in particular the science of heath care, progressed over the next 300 years. The mind and soul became the province of the clerics, while the body became the province of the doctor. As knowledge progressed, the body was split into smaller parts: first systems, then organs, then tissues, then cells and so on. This approach, known as the reductionist approach, has been invaluable in the achievement of scientific knowledge and has led to enormous knowledge about the management of disorders that affect the body. It is easily recognised in our current society by the innumerable specialties in both medicine and nursing concerned with only a small part of the whole person. The contribution of specialists must never be underestimated, since their knowledge and skills have led to the alleviation of immeasurable suffering in human beings. But it is out of these views that the biomedical model grew, viewing people as being made up of many parts, each of which was studied independently. The fight to cure or control disease is easily recognised as the goal. The ever more complex technical knowledge must also be recognised and valued within this framework.

The biomedical view remained largely unchallenged until recent times, and its influence can be seen not only in medicine but also in the way in which nursing has evolved. The dictionary definition of nursing says that it is concerned not only with nourishment but also with care for the decrepit or sick. Western society has long recognised the need for such a service, and nurses have always existed in one form or another. In early days the nursing role was largely carried out in the community by lay people, but nursing was also to be found in religious institutions. Bevis (1978) describes the underlying value of these religious institutions as asceticism, the dedicated individual committing his or her life to the care of others and providing the basic needs of food, shelter and comfort. Asceticism is associated with denial of one's own needs in order to serve others. It was demonstrated by a total commitment; the person lived within the institution where care was provided, dissociated from the outside world. Remnants of such an approach are still visible in old hospital buildings, where the matron's living quarters were within the hospital building and the sisters' rooms still provide a convenient meeting place for some staff within the confines of the ward itself.

It must also be acknowledged that a review of the popular literature concerned with life in the eighteenth and nineteenth centuries also reveals another kind of nurse, the Sarah Camps of this world, so vividly described by Dickens, with a greater love of the gin bottle than the patient. Nursing took on the cloak of refuge for many who were near destitution themselves.

It was the influence of Florence Nightingale, and some of her contemporaries such as Ethel Bedford Fenwick and Mary Seacole of the late nineteenth century, that was to change much of this. It can be argued that these 'activists' of their time sought to make nursing 'respectable', and one way in which they achieved this was to firmly attach it to medicine, describing the function of nursing as carrying out what doctors said was required for the care of the patient.

The inevitable result of this was a strong influence on the value systems, goals and knowledge of nursing. While the ascetic value of early days persisted, new values were taken on board. Bevis again describes this, first as romanticism, with a hero worship of the leaders, or doctors, and a subservient relationship to them. With the huge popularity of the Mills and Boon novels throughout the Western world, it would seem that the attraction of this view still holds strongly with a wide proportion of the population. However, with the burst of technology of the 1940s and 1950s, romanticism lost favour and she suggests that the overruling value became pragmatism, skilled technical nurses extending their role to cope with the direct effects of new technical knowledge.

Pragmatism is associated with a practical approach to assessing situations and acting on them. It tests things by their practical consequences. Since the underlying value system of nursing at this time was associated with disease and cure, the skills that were developed were also linked to them. The special courses that were developed, for example by the post-basic hospital schools, helped nurses to attain the specific practical skills associated with increased medical technology. Some acknowledgement was given to other aspects of care, but the emphasis lay on deepening the understanding of disease processes, their physical effects and their technical management.

While the importance of such technical skills is in no way underestimated, many people are now asking whether some of the essence of nursing has been lost through an overemphasis on them. Others, however, will suggest that the acquisition of technical skills as such is relatively easy and should not be viewed with such concern (Vaughan, 1990). Of far greater importance is what you do with those skills within a framework of nursing rather than as a mini doctor. Thus Watson (1979), for example, would call those technical skills the 'trim' of nursing, a necessary adjunct which serves to support the 'core nursing values'.

The reductionist approach that so strongly influenced medicine has played its part in nursing too. An understanding of the origins of many of the complementary paramedical groups such as physiotherapy, occupational therapy and social work clearly demonstrates that their roots lie in nursing. The splits have also occurred within nursing itself and many 'specialist' nurses have emerged with detailed and expert knowledge about particular aspects of their subject. The value of such people is immense, but as in so many situations, there is always a price to pay for such skills. The risks in this case are twofold. First, it has led to a loss of some skills by the 'ordinary' nurse. Somewhere the task of helping a patient to dress independently has been lost to occupational therapists, of encouraging mobility to physiotherapists, and of stoma care to stoma therapists. The patient has been split into many parts, his or her needs for each separate function being met by either specialist nurses who have extended their role in one particular direction or by relatively new occupational groups who have taken over some functions previously carried out by nurses. The notion of multi-skilling, where care-givers develop the skills relevant to the client group with whom they work, has been viewed very cautiously by many nurses. Maybe in the light of the ideas

Figure 5.2 The consequences of the reductionist approach.

outlined here it should be welcomed more openly, since the advantages to patients and clients could be considerable.

The trend towards specialisation complies with the original thoughts of Descartes many hundreds of years ago. It has led to considerable advantages, particularly a deeper knowledge and understanding of specific areas of care and the availability of expert knowledge. Yet in some areas the biomedical model and the divisions and specialisations it leads to are now being challenged. Many people from both nursing and medicine are asking whether alternative approaches may be more appropriate and are seeking ways of meeting people's health care needs more effectively. There is less talk of role extension, confined to learning new tasks, and more talk of role expansion, where nursing values and functions can be enhanced by the development of new skills. Indeed, directives from the United Kingdom Central Council (UKCC, 1992a) have opened up the opportunity for practitioners themselves to identify and develop the skills required to enhance their work without redress to central approval. Hence the emergence of alternative models of nursing, described by nurses for nursing. These models show nursing to have a distinct function in its own right, which is goal-directed rather than defined by task.

INFLUENCES OF THE BIOMEDICAL MODEL ON PRACTICE

There is no doubt that the biomedical model has, and still does, influence the practice of nursing, and we can observe how its ideas have actually affected nursing as a service as well as the structure of health care and the classification of knowledge and the boundaries of services.

A model is based on values and attitudes; in turn, a model influences what will be valued and what will be seen as being of more or less status or worth. The biomedical model values knowledge about the physical sciences and the performance of treatment activities that will lead to diagnosis or cure. This is reflected strongly in nursing today. At the ward or community level, nursing activities associated with diagnosis and treatment, which are also very often of a technical nature, are frequently seen as being of a higher status than those which relate to comfort and cleanliness. There is still a risk that those concerned with emotion and pleasure are of even less status. Importantly, this hierarchy of valued activities also extends to a hierarchy of roles in nursing.

Scenarios still exist where the 'higher-up nurse' is expected to perform cure-directed acts such as giving drugs, performing surgical dressings and so on. The 'lower-down nurse' will give the physical care activities, such as bathing or giving bedpans. The psychosocial care is given by anyone at all – if there is time to do it. Furthermore, if there is no time for the psychosocial care, it can be safely left undone because not only is it invisible but it is also perceived as being of less importance. With the increasing number of people working as care assistants and attaining recognition of their skills through National Vocational Qualifications, there is an increasing risk that the 'wholeness' of some so-called 'basic tasks' will be lost and bathing will be seen as merely an opportunity to attain cleanliness rather than one where a multitude of other activities such as assessment, counselling and teaching can occur. Such a hierarchy of tasks and roles is one of the reasons why the method of work organisation we often call task assignment or allocation was so popular, and why remnants of this system are still obvious in many clinical areas.

On a broader level, types of nursing that are valued are determined by the priorities set by the biomedical model. Nurses who work in high-technology units or acute hospital wards have traditionally been afforded higher status. Furthermore, until very recently, these areas tended to attract the 'best' nurses, and nurses working in these areas were assured of good career progression. Nursing in an elderly care unit, in a long-stay psychiatric hospital, in district nursing and in other non-cure areas was regarded with lower esteem, and these areas were thought of as the places where the less-bright nurse who could not cope or had blotted her copybook ended up. Although they are less common and trends are changing, with the advent of nurse-led services, such attitudes still exist and with the introduction of local pay bargaining, a situation can be seen where the areas where specialist skills can be more readily defined, such as accident and emergency departments or intensive care units, will also gain financial leads.

The biomedical model, therefore, has led to an emphasis on the technical, medically related aspects of the nursing role and to a resulting devaluation of acts related to how individuals experience their own illnesses or disabilities, such as listening, comforting or offering choices. It also creates confusion and dissatisfaction about nursing roles, such as that of the health visitor, which are not involved with diagnosing and treating disease, and can lead to divisions and separatist movements within the occupation of nursing itself. Confusion can also arise about what is and is not a legitimate nursing service, an overt example

Figure 5.3 The hierarchy of tasks and roles in nursing.

concerning continuing care. Quite where the responsibility lay for these traditional nursing services in the 1990s was uncertain, as there has been no clear directive about the boundaries of responsibility between health and social services. Indeed, certainly in the UK there is wide local variation in what is seen as health care, and hence provided by health care workers, and what is seen as social care, and hence often self-funded by the people concerned (Department of Health, 1990). Thus, while there is a strong feeling that it is nurses who should be providing services of nourishment and care for the sick, current interpretations leave this debate open.

The biomedical model is a well-developed one, and undoubtedly it at least gives direction to practice that is, in itself, useful. Its concentration on objectivity and efficiency was instrumental in developing nursing from a body of relatively unskilled and uneducated women, to an army of highly efficient workers who are crucial to any effective health care service. If the biomedical model is accepted by a nursing team as the appropriate framework on which to base practice, and all agree to pursue it, then it will, as any other model, give direction to the care given, ensure that the care is consistent and outline the requirements for effective care.

However, the biomedical model is reductionist and dualistic in approach – it both reduces the human body to a set of related parts and separates the mind from the body – hence it can be suggested that its common use in nursing is no longer appropriate. It is not geared to the needs of individuals and its dominant effect on health care has led to it being used in the interest of health professionals rather than those who seek, need or are directed to health care. Therefore it can no longer be acknowledged as a favoured choice when nursing teams are selecting a model for their practice.

Making the choice about what model to use depends on two major considerations: the feelings of the individuals involved and the advantages and disadvantages of the model. It is therefore useful to end this discussion of the biomedical model by looking at its advantages and disadvantages.

ADVANTAGES AND DISADVANTAGES OF THE BIOMEDICAL MODEL

Many people will argue that the biomedical model is the most efficient and effective one for use by health care workers. Some of the arguments that are put forward include the following.

1. The overriding concern of the patient is for cure and control of his or her disease, and this model gives clear direction in this respect.
2. The knowledge base it uses is developed from scientific experiment and in many instances is objective and proved beyond reasonable doubt.
3. Since the focus of the model is disease, there is no question but that it is the doctor who should ultimately be responsible for controlling all health care. Thus any confusion or disagreement over management, whether arising from the patient/client or other health care workers, can be overruled by the doctor.
4. Its value has been proved over the years and because of this it is non-threatening and understood by both patients and health care workers alike.
5. Since it limits itself to the physical domain, the less objective psycho-social areas can be ignored.

Regardless of the fact that these arguments have withstood the test of time, alternative views are now being raised more and more frequently. It is not only health care workers but patients themselves who are raising objections to the biomedical model. Some of these are as follows.

1. There is an expectation with the biomedical model that nurses will be the humanisers of care, an expectation which is often unmet.
2. The biomedical model leads to patients being labelled with a diagnosis rather than being known as a person. Many patients dislike this.
3. The biomedical model's emphasis on high technology leads to the loss of human care. Both health care workers and patients are becoming more and more dissatisfied with this.
4. The biomedical model concentrates information and decision-making in the hands of doctors and, to a lesser extent, other health professionals. Patients should have the right to information about their own health and some degree of choice in its management.
5. There is growing evidence that nurturing holistic care is healing in its own right and can have a very positive impact on health outcomes (cf. Griffiths and Evans, 1995), leading to a need to review the structures and priorities of the current health care system.

Capra (1982) suggests that the biomedical model demands that doctors hold the power in all decision-making and, as a result, 'the important role that nurses play in the healing process through their healing contacts with the patient is not fully recognised'. In other words, the human side of health care is devalued.

It is not our intention either to recommend or condemn this model to you. We present it as the traditional model on which practice has been based for many years and commend it for the contribution it has made in the past. However, there is a growing view amongst nurses that, as a basis for nursing practice it can no longer be considered appropriate. Both pressure from society and increased understanding of human nature have highlighted the restrictive nature of the biomedical model in terms of nursing practice, and alternative approaches are crucial to the provision of a satisfactory nursing service for patients.

Learning exercises

1. Examine the nursing notes in a clinical area and identify the degree to which the biomedical model is reflected in them.
2. Take care at a 'handover' to note down how much of the information shared is biomedically related and how much is non-biomedical.

Study questions

1. Define the biomedical model and discuss its advantages and disadvantages for (a) nurses and (b) patients/clients.
2. Identify the role of the biomedical model in contemporary nursing.

Chapter 6

Common Characteristics of Nursing Models – the Patient or Client

LEARNING OBJECTIVES

On completion of this chapter, the reader will be able to:

1 List the common features of nursing models in relation to views on the patient or client
2 Describe the main features of the following theories: systems theory, developmental theory and symbolic interaction theory
3 Discuss conceptualisations of human nature in relation to nursing practice
4 Explain how conceptualisations of the environment relate to nursing
5 Relate the concepts of patient autonomy and nurse/patient partnership from experience

Many models for practice have been developed specifically for nursing, mainly by American writers, and a large number have been published. All models have a different focus, but equally they all have many ideas in common. This chapter explores the three major theories on which nursing models are based. It also examines one of the features common to models of nursing, namely views of the patient or client. Considering basic theories and common features in this way will enable readers to recognise them as they appear in nursing theories presented in later chapters.

As we have already mentioned, theory can appear a little tedious and inaccessible for some at first sight and its relevance to real, live, practical nursing is not always immediately apparent. Much of this next chapter is made up of theory and may therefore need to be read more than once. Certainly we had great difficulty when first facing this kind of material. However, over the years we have personally come to find it very meaningful to the real nursing care given. The theories and concepts we are about to discuss are, we feel, knowledge which is fundamental to the eventual practical application of nursing models, whether in a ward or community nursing setting. Learning about them is not easy and many nurses, including us, have found this prelude to learning about models difficult. We do apologise for this, but urge you to press on with these chapters, re-reading them until they are meaningful.

All models for any discipline draw on theories and concepts. Three major theories have come to be recognised as having relevance to nursing – systems theory, developmental theory and interactionist theory. Some models focus mainly on one of the theories, some combine two of them or all three, but all models include the essence of all of them in some way or another. Despite their apparent complexity, it is worthwhile becoming familiar with the core of these three theories.

SYSTEMS THEORY

The idea of systems is one that is familiar to most nurses. The gastrointestinal system or the cardiovascular system are frequently talked about. Systems are also recognised in other walks of life – a filing system, a system of government or a computer system. People can also be described as systems.

There are particular characteristics that have been ascribed to things in order that they can be called systems. They usually have a common purpose. For example, the common purpose of the filing system may be seen as storage of documents. The parts of a system are interrelated and interdependent. Thus in the case of the cardiovascular system, the rate and pressure at which the blood is circulated are dependent on the strength of the muscular activity of the heart. Similarly, the force of contraction of the heart is dependent on the flow of blood through that organ. Both responses aim to maintain homeostasis.

All systems have boundaries that can be defined, in some cases more clearly than in others. Thus the boundary of a filing system can be clearly seen as the exterior cabinet, while the boundary of a government system is less easily defined. In all systems theory there is an emphasis on the interaction of the parts to form the whole. Each part can and should be studied separately, but functionally what is most important is the interaction of the parts and the eventual output or end result.

Two types of systems have traditionally been described. A closed system is one where the boundary does not allow for any interaction of the parts of the system with stimuli from the environment in which it exists. In reality some people suggest that there is no such thing as a closed system, since everything interacts with its environment.

An open system is one that can constantly interact with its environment through its boundary. There is an input to the system, an internal rearrangement of the system and feedback. Thus in the filing system the input may be a new document. This in turn will lead to some movement of the files to make room for it. The output or end result will be a retrievable document. Some people have described the cardiovascular system as a 'closed system', but in fact it is constantly interacting with its environment, responding to hormonal changes within the body, temperature changes in the immediate environment and emotional changes.

The characteristics of systems theory can be summarised as follows.

1. Systems seek to exist in a steady state, in a state of equilibrium where the parts of the system are in balance.
2. The parts of a system continually interrelate and interact with one another.
3. Each system has a boundary that is more clearly defined in some cases than in others.
4. A system can be affected by stresses occurring either within the whole system or external to the system but crossing its boundaries.
5. A stress will lead to a feedback in the system causing a change in the balance. This may be temporary or require a permanent change.
6. Systems can be described as 'closed' or 'open'. In closed systems the boundary is tight and cannot be crossed. In open systems the boundary is easily crossed or affected by external stimuli (see Fig. 6.1).

The majority of health care models are in fact based on systems theory, and the variations that occur between models are in the perceived boundaries of the system. The biomedical model is inclined to take each body system as an entity in its own right. However, in models of nursing, the whole system that is most usually taken is of human beings in their entirety. Thus people themselves are systems made up of subsystems and living in a suprasystem. The influence of systems theory is evident across health care. For example, its use as a basis for practice is described in psychosomatic rehabilitation (Paar and Grohmann, 2000), as an approach to patient safety (Eisenberg, 2000), chronic wound care (Beitz, 2001), the development of patient classification systems and staffing systems (Van Slyck, 2000), in joint replacement and in managed

Figure 6.1

WHOLE SYSTEM

A whole system
-has parts which are interdependent
-has a clear boundary
-is affected by internal/external stresses
-seeks to maintain a balance

care (Benham, 1999). Hancock (2000) also demonstrates its influence in nursing model development.

If a change occurs in one subsystem it will mean that the balance between all subsystems will be disrupted and this will have an impact on the whole organisation. The response to such a disruption or stress will be to seek to return to the previous state in order to restore the balance or equilibrium. If this is not possible then a new state of equilibrium must be sought. For instance, a broken leg will not only cause changes in the musculoskeletal subsystem but will have an effect on all the other subsystems that make up the person. However, it is likely to heal and the previous state of equilibrium will be restored. If the leg is amputated, there will be no opportunity to seek to return to the previous state of balance, and a new one must be found.

Just as changes in the subsystems of people will influence them as a whole, so changes in the suprasystem, those systems that make up the immediate and distant environment, will also have their effect. A change in the social circumstances surrounding the individual will cause 'stresses' which will cross the boundaries of the whole system – that is the whole person. Again the changes may be temporary, causing a transient imbalance in the whole system. For instance, an acute episode of illness will mean a temporary change in an individual's ability to earn a living. However, if the illness or disorder is of a permanent nature, as with the person who has had an amputation, a permanent change in the way in which the individual reacts to the environment will have to be found. The influence of systems theory is evident in the majority of nursing models. The whole system is usually seen as the human being. There is, however, considerable variation in the way in which the systems are described. Roper *et al.* (1990) use the activities of living as their framework. Roy (1984) uses the concept of stress or stimuli and the way in which humans adapt to them in four different modes, namely the physical, self-concept, role function and interdependence. The influence of systems theory can also be seen in the traditional medical model.

DEVELOPMENTAL THEORY

A second major organising theory that can be found in some nursing models is that of development. Developmental models centre around growth and change. The growth and change occur in recognised stages, are caused by identifiable variables and move in a predictable direction. While developmental theory may focus on growth, the theory can also be applied to a movement towards illness or death since this can be seen as a progressive, staged process.

Some proposals based on developmental theory are already well known to nurses. For example, Piaget (1932) clearly describes the stages through which he considers that a child progresses during development. He sees these stages as steps with fairly sudden transitions from one to another, rather than as a gentle slope. Thus at the initial sensori-motor stage, a child will only be aware of those things he can see or feel. The day will come when s/he will realise that objects suddenly hidden from sight are in fact still present but out of view, and s/he will start to seek them out. S/he has reached the concrete stage. Ultimately s/he will progress to a third stage of formal operations, able to perceive distant objects accurately and understand their consistency. S/he has attained insight about the abstract world.

Other developmental theories identify concepts different from those of Piaget, but all are similar in that development is described as a series of stages, interspersed by visible transitions, rather than as a gradual unfolding. Each stage is superseded, in an orderly manner, by the next stage, which may occur relatively promptly or over a more protracted period.

We also use the term development very widely in our everyday life: the development of a film, in a predictable staged direction; the failure to develop of a hyacinth bulb; the development of the signs and symptoms of an illness. Five aspects of developmental models have been identified (Chin, 1980). They can be summarised as follows.

Direction: The assumption that 'the system under observation is progressing somewhere'. As with systems theory, the thing which is under scrutiny may be very small, such as a cell or body organ; it may be a social system, such as a community; it may be a psychological system, such as an interpersonal relationship; or it may be the growth and development of people. It is assumed, however, that there is some implicit goal or end state that is being worked towards.

Identifiable states: The most obvious examples of identifiable states in developmental theory are those described by Piaget. There are distinct characteristics which mark each stage, level or phase. An everyday example of stages would be the progress of frog spawn to tadpole and then the transition to a frog. Stages can also be seen in Maslow's Hierarchy of Needs (1954). According to his theory, higher level needs such as love, self-esteem and self-actualisation are only met when lower level ones such as physiological and safety needs have been met. The movement from one identifiable state to another may be a sudden jump, as of a child moving from primary to secondary school. Alternatively, the transition may be more prolonged, as in the metamorphosis from tadpole to frog. Clinically a changing state may occur suddenly, as it would following an unexpected bereavement, or more slowly, as it would in the episodic nature of a disease process such as multiple sclerosis.

Form of progression: While change is inevitable, the course of the change may have certain characteristics. Four typical types of progression have been identified – linear, spiral, cyclical and branching.

A typical example of linear progression would be that of the movement from conception to death. It moves in one direction and unless there is an interruption, it will not regress.

Spiral progression can be seen when there is a return to the same subject at a higher level. This can be seen in the progress from simple sums to complex mathematics.

Cyclical progression is typically seen in problem-solving, when the same process is applied to different situations (e.g. the nursing process of assessment, planning, implementation and evaluation).

Finally, branching progression is seen when there is a choice and the system can move in two or more directions. For instance, it may be the

Figure 6.2 Forms of progression: linear, spiral, cyclical and branching.

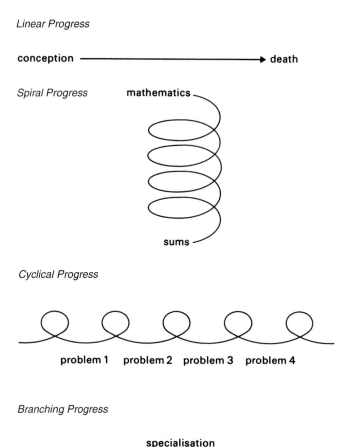

Linear Progress

conception ⟶ death

Spiral Progress

mathematics

sums

Cyclical Progress

problem 1   problem 2   problem 3   problem 4

Branching Progress

specialisation

marriage

career choice

choice of occupation, the management of an illness or the selection of a partner for life. Branching progression also leads to more and more specialisation within an organisation. The point at which a choice may be made can potentially lead to a developmental crisis (see Fig. 6.2).

Forces: Forces are seen as the factors which energise development. They have also been called stressors or stimuli and are the things that lead to change. There are many forces that lead to the development of people. These include hereditary factors, the environment, the interaction between the two, and the desire for self-actualisation. In day-to-day life we can sometimes recognise a particular force which has led to a change. It may be an individual who has inspired us, a trauma or disease, an alteration in social circumstances, or the acquisition of new knowledge. Alternatively, the force may be less conspicuous, a maturation process inherent in all of us which may be triggered by some external factor.

Potentiality: Potentiality refers to the conditions for growth and development, the 'potential', built into the present state. Thus in Piaget's theory, the child has the potential to mature to adulthood. There is some variation in opinion about how much this potential is in fact influenced by surrounding circumstances.

While not all models use developmental theory as their major focus for construction, its influence can be seen in many of them. Peplau's (1952) model takes developmental theory as the major organising theme. Roper *et al.* (1990) give developmental theory less conspicuous attention than the life continuum features as impacting on dependence or independence in the activities of living. If part of nursing is seen as helping individuals to develop and grow, the application of developmental theory is obvious since it explains the direction and manner in which changes may occur.

SYMBOLIC INTERACTION

The essence of this theory is the interaction that occurs between people and their environment. The control does not lie with either one or the other, with either the person or his or her environment. Interaction theories focus on the relationships that people form with each other in their day-to-day lives, and on the way those relationships develop through a series of interactions. Rose (1980) lists some basic assumptions that underlie the symbolic interaction theory. They can be summarised as follows.

A person lives in a symbolic as well as a physical world. In the physical world the individual receives stimuli through the senses of seeing, hearing, smelling, touching and tasting, and will respond to these stimuli. However, over a period of time, the symbols that are perceived will take on particular values and meaning for the person. For example, the word or symbol 'ward' does not just mean the physical environment of beds, curtains, patients and staff. It may also mean caring and loving, or pain and suffering. Thus, while in concrete terms the word 'ward' will have a similar meaning to most people, symbolically it may have many different meanings that have developed through previous interactions with other people in that environment. The meaning of the word has resulted from the response of the one person to the symbol that has been received. Rose suggests this ability is highly developed in human beings.

Through symbols people can evoke meanings and values other than their own in another person. This assumption is associated with a person's ability to be aware of the values and meanings of others. It implies that one has empathy, can understand the perspective of others, and take on a particular role. In interactions of this kind, where significant symbols are used, the communicator can only influence, rather than control, the observer. Thus the process is social in nature, observers putting their own meanings and values on the interaction. However, for the interaction to be meaningful, both participants must share similar meanings for words and movements. This raises issues about the many variations that occur in the use of both words and movements by people from different cultures and classes.

Figure 6.3   People view things differently.

People learn symbolic meanings and values through interacting with others. Each individual builds up an elaborate store of meanings and values through interaction with others. Similarly the way in which individuals interact will influence those around them. In time people can become skilled in knowing how others will react to them and adjust their behaviour accordingly. They can 'take on' specific roles in given situations which they have experienced previously in order to predict the responses.

Significant symbols usually occur in 'clusters', which dictate other values and meanings related to a cluster. In this assumption it is suggested that there is a group of meanings and values which can be recognised by a particular society. It is linked with the idea of the way we interpret particular roles. There is a normally accepted pattern of behaviour by all members of a particular society in relationship to that role. For instance, the role of parent is linked with caring and providing for children. If a father deviates from that role and, for instance, rejects a child, it will affect his interaction with other people in the society in which he lives.

Davis (1975) describes the socialisation of nurses, where student nurses 'learn' to take on a pattern of behaviour acceptable to experienced nurses and often different from their original view, as an example of this process. It can also be seen in individuals who take on the 'patient role', which is seen to be acceptable to the hospital staff as they respond to interactions with others in that setting.

Most people have a number of roles they take on according to the group of people with whom they are interacting at a given time. They usually accept symbols for each of these roles according to the society in which they live. They will, however, also have a 'whole person' role linked with the value and meaning they place on themselves as individuals.

It is possible to assess future courses of action through a thinking process rather than resorting to behaviour based on trial and error.

Since the logical conclusion of the process of symbolic interaction is that responses to a given situation can be predicted, trial and error behaviour is unnecessary. The way an individual predicts the future is based on past and present experience. It also influences present interaction. A person's ability for symbolic interaction heightens his or her awareness of the values and meanings of others.

While this theory may sound complex on first reading, its relevance to nursing is undeniable. Empathy, a quality inherent in symbolic interaction, is a characteristic often cited as essential to nursing. Similarly an understanding of the variety of roles we all play and the way in which they have developed can only help to enhance nursing. Threads of this theory are seen in most models. For instance, Roy (1984) talks about self-concept and interdependence as important areas of assessment. Symbolic interaction is the major focus of King's model (1981).

As we have already said, there is an element of all these theories in most of the early models of nursing. In more recent times, however, nursing theory has moved away from these guiding theories. Indeed, the authors of the additional models included in this second edition are more influenced by the philosophical ideas of existentialism and phenomenology (schools of thought which we will explain later). Despite this trend we still recognise the contribution these ideas make to most of the models of nursing. While these theories do not make for easy reading, we hope that we have been able to represent them in relatively simple terms without losing too much of their meaning.

Models based on these theories, to a large extent, all agree on a number of concepts about patients and nursing. The most important of these concepts are:

- health
- the holistic view of people
- the humanistic view of people
- the environment
- the autonomy of patients and clients
- the need to develop a productive or therapeutic relationship between those who nurse, and those who are nursed

HUMAN NATURE

It has already been suggested that the basis of the practice of any service-orientated group lies in the beliefs and values that are held by that group. In outlining the biomedical model of practice on which most health care has been based until recent times, the dualistic approach – the division of mind and body – proposed by Descartes was described. The result of such an approach has been an enormous increase in both knowledge and skills. However, over the last century other views of people have emerged which are now starting to influence our thoughts about the way in which nurses practice. The two most influential ones are those of holism and humanism. They are common features of the majority of models of nursing which will be described in this book, and therefore they warrant further discussion.

Holism

The word 'holism' was first introduced by Jan Christian Smuts (1926), a South African philosopher, in the early part of this century. Holism relates to the study of the whole organism or of whole systems, its spelling arising from the Greek word 'holos'. (The English spelling with a 'w' is a relatively recent fourteenth-century innovation!)

Underlying a holistic view of people are two basic assumptions or beliefs.

1. The individual always responds as a unified whole.
2. Individuals as a whole are different from and more than the sum of their parts.

Both these assumptions mean that there is now movement away from the ideas proposed by Descartes, who claimed that, in order to study the body as a machine, it could be broken down into its component parts. If the assumptions of holism are accepted, it indicates that there is a need to study the whole being, and the manner in which the body and mind interact.

Byrne and Thompson (1978) used the analogy of water to describe this phenomenon. Water as a whole is made up of two components, namely hydrogen and oxygen. Similarly, when considering people, there are at least two major components, namely the body and the mind; some people may choose to include a third, spiritual component. If the properties of the components of water are considered separately, they each have distinct characteristics. Oxygen will support combustion. Hydrogen is potentially explosive. However, when they are put together in the particular combination that makes up water, a completely different property, that of extinguishing fire, arises. Thus the whole is different from the sum of the parts. If the parts are studied independently rather than in unity, an inaccurate picture of water will emerge.

The underlying belief in a holistic view of people follows a similar view. By considering the functioning of the body without taking into consideration the response of the mind and spirit, an inaccurate picture of that person will emerge. Such inaccuracy will lead to difficulty in helping people solve problems and hence, in the long run, lead to extra cost both in terms of human suffering and money.

This view is not entirely unsupported by scientific evidence. As a young medical student, Hans Selye observed what he later described as a 'syndrome of just being sick' (1978). Unable in his early medical career to distinguish between the specific signs or symptoms of many diseases, he was aware of the similarities in many cases. Much later he was to reconsider this early observation and, through a series of experiments, conclude that there was in fact a syndrome, the general adaptation syndrome (GAS) occurring in the body when it was exposed to stress, whether the stress was physical or psychological in origin. Pietroni (1984) describes Selye as the 'father of modem stress work' and acknowledges his contribution in 'the difficult and painstaking job of putting body and mind back together again'. Selye's influence can also be seen quite clearly in many of the models of nursing described. The importance of stress, as an influence in development as well as a cause of ill

Figure 6.4 It's the ingredients that make the difference.

health when occurring in excess, is recognised in many models. Since the word 'stress' has become so widely used both professionally and by lay people, there are variations in its interpretation; some people only think of the physical side and others only consider psychological factors. Furthermore, it is often only considered in a negative manner as something that is harmful, whereas in fact it is also the stimulus for development and growth. The notion of stress is a common feature of many models, although it is not always referred to by the actual word 'stress'.

Humanism

The second underlying value that can frequently be recognised in nursing models is that of humanism. Humanism is often linked with a second school of thought known as existentialism. There is also a growing interest in phenomenology as both a philosophy and a research method, which has influenced more recent nursing theorists.

Humanism is based on the value of being human, of existing and of the quality of that existence. It places great emphasis on the nature of people. The emphasis of existentialism is also on people, but stresses the individual human being. Stevenson (1974) describes three main characteristics of existentialism. The first is the uniqueness of the individual person. He suggests that general theories about people are secondary to the importance of the individual. The second part is related to the 'meaning and purpose of human lives rather than … truths about the whole universe and how it works'. The third point that Stevenson makes, and maybe the one that is most relevant to us, is the freedom of individuals to choose. This is seen as the most valued human characteristic. Thus there is freedom for an individual to direct his own life, choose his own attitudes and behaviours.

The principles of humanistic existentialism have been subsumed by both Christian and atheist philosophers. For instance, Stevenson describes the view suggested by Kierkegaard that there are three main ways of life between which an individual could choose. These were the aesthetic way concerned with beauty, the ethical way concerned with right and wrong, and the religious way relating to God's direction and will. In Kierkegaard's view the religious way of life was the highest choice that an individual could make, but he suggested that 'it can only be reached by a free leap into the arms of God'.

Alternatively, Jean-Paul Sartre was an existentialist atheist denying the existence of God. In his opinion, humans are condemned to be free. We have no choice but to be free and cannot blame the course of our lives on the will of a higher being. Such freedom is, in his view, not a happy state. He feels we are responsible for our emotions and reactions. Thus, a statement such as 'I am stupid' is not to assert a fact already in existence, since we control what we make of our lives ourselves, but to anticipate how society will react to the resulting behaviour. We have the choice ourselves of changing the behaviour which leads us to attribute such characteristics to ourselves.

Bevis (1978) sees humanistic existentialism as the 'natural maturational philosophy for nursing'. Indeed, within the philosophy of humanistic existentialism are many of the ideas which are being discussed by nurses today, such as the value of human beings, their uniqueness as individuals, the quality of life and the freedom to choose – all topical subjects that are now widely debated within nursing. The application of humanism to health care would suggest that individuals should be able to make choices about how their health is managed and to explore methods that are complementary to either traditional medicine or traditional nursing. It also emphasises the responsibility of the individual in such circumstances.

Phenomenology

Phenomenology refers to a school of thought suggesting that it is the meaning of an experience which is important and that meaning will vary from person to person. It rejects the idea that we can explore truth by measuring outputs or products in concrete terms, as has been the case with the scientifically dominated medical model (see Chapter 3) but that, in order to help people, we must come to understand that person's own lived experience or, as Watson (1988) says, really knowing feeling. The ideas behind phenomenology have been attributed to philosophers such as Heidegger (1962) and Husserl (1970), and have been very influential in the design of nursing research in recent times. Most notably this was the guiding philosophy behind the work of nurse theorists such as Parse (1981), Benner (1984) and Watson (1988) in the mid-1980s.

Holism and humanism are not only reflected in many of the nursing models, they can also be recognised in society's changing attitudes to health and medicine. For example, there is an upsurge of interest in holistic medicine. Community Health Councils and Patients' Associations have been established. Doctors are being publicly challenged about the right to control and direct all health care by both patients and other health care workers alike. As Bevis says: 'The current philosophy that is swaying nursing thought and action is humanistic existentialism'.

THE ENVIRONMENT

Florence Nightingale paid a great deal of attention to the provision of an environment that was conducive to healing. She wrote of cleanliness, fresh air and calm as preconditions for recovery from illness (Nightingale, 1970). Later nursing theorists continued to include the environment in which people were nursed as an important consideration for nurses and enlarged the concept. In particular, people's interaction with and responses to their immediate and broader environment were integral parts of the work of Rogers (1970) and Neuman (1995). Environment, together with health, nursing and the person, are domain concepts, which are considered to be integral parts of any model that purports to give a general overview of nursing.

PATIENT/CLIENT AUTONOMY

Characteristic of most nursing models is the belief that the clients or patients are individuals who have the right to be involved in making informed choices about themselves and their future. This belief is often referred to as 'patient autonomy', and autonomy is defined as the freedom to make decisions within the limits of competence of the individual; the opposite of autonomy is having to comply with dictates from people who are in a superior position. The belief in autonomy suggests that we value patients and their contribution to their own health care.

Some models give more emphasis to the concept of autonomy than others. The model described by Orem (1991), which focuses on self-care, gives considerable emphasis to autonomy. As expounded in Orem's work, self-care is a good example of the notion of autonomy applied to a model for practice, and may serve to demonstrate its implications. Levin *et al.* (1979) define self-care as 'a process whereby a lay person function on his/her own behalf in health promotion and prevention, and in disease detection and treatment'. It therefore relies on the belief that the person who is the subject of nursing has both the ability and the right to be involved in choosing what happens to him or her. This belief arose from health care consumers, customers or patients in the 1960s, and began with anti-professional and anti-intellectual feelings that were popular at the time. There was a general desire by many people to return to a way of life that emphasised humanity, respect and sharing. This can be seen as a reaction to materialism and mechanistic practices in the world as a whole, as well as in the practice of nurses and other health workers. Health workers and 'professional people' in other disciplines still pursue practice which views the client as being dependent on them and therefore needing to be placed in a role whereby they seek help and are told what to do. Many nursing models concentrate on perceiving people's individual identities and rights, and are therefore moving away from practice that directs people and towards practice that supports and enables them to learn and use this learning to make their own decisions. Illich (1975) describes how increased professionalism in health care, and therefore a focus on a view of the patient that places a person in a position inferior to the practitioner, have led to the point where significant levels of human suffering are the very result of

Figure 6.5 Patient autonomy.

I'LL DO THAT

the professional practice of medicine, something he calls 'iatrogenesis'. He says that

> ... once society is so organised that medicine can transform people into patients because they are unborn, newborn, menopausal or some other 'at risk age', the population inevitably loses some of its autonomy to its healers.

Many other writers on health care stress how the professional worker can effectively remove the individual's right to autonomous decision-making for highly tenuous reasons, and that professional power can be exerted to make clients comply with professional values.

The belief in patient/client autonomy inherent in many nursing models assumes that, if responsibility for healthy living and health care is vested in the individual concerned and not a professional, health and recovery is more likely to occur. All patients should have the freedom to identify their own needs, and to decide on how these needs should be met. In practical terms, for example, the sick people being cared for by nurses should be given the power to make their own decisions about how they will be nursed. This may entail either selecting particular ways of carrying out a daily living activity or choosing to give the responsibility for the decisions to the nurse, because they feel unwell and are unable to decide for themselves. As Waterworth and Luker (1990) suggest, it is equally as coercive to force people into 'reluctant collaboration' as to deny them the right of choice. This latter option is an important one to stress because autonomy for patients does not necessarily mean that they must constantly make decisions – it simply means that they have enough power to choose whether to decide for themselves or to allow others to decide for them. Such a belief gives rise to another major concept which underlies many nursing models – that of the central importance of the relationship between helper and helped – the nurse and the patient.

PARTNERSHIP IN THE NURSE/PATIENT RELATIONSHIP

In models where the autonomy of the individual client is recognised, the practice of the discipline, its goals and the knowledge needed to achieve them are fundamentally different from those where the model focuses on a client who needs the expert intervention of the practitioner. The practitioner operates as a partner in practice with the client rather than a director of practice to, for, or at the client. In order to do this the practitioner has to share what he or she knows with the patient, rather than withholding this knowledge and telling the patient what is best. In this way patients become as knowledgeable about the various options which can be chosen to overcome their specific problems and are able to make their own choices. Partnership also demands that the practitioner complements the patient's own uniqueness, adapts knowledge to the patient's abilities and needs, and passes it on so that both can work out a plan of action instead of the practitioner 'plying a trade' on a take-it-or-leave-it basis.

In nursing, developing a relationship with a patient based on partnership conflicts with the popular biomedical model and assumes a different role for nurses and a different knowledge base. It suggests that the individual who needs nursing actually needs a practitioner who establishes a close relationship based on equality, and it emphasises patient learning to enable individuals to make informed choices. The majority of nursing models advocate partnership, and therefore the ability to facilitate learning, motivate and communicate. An understanding of psychology and sociology are included in the skills and knowledge that nurses need in order to nurse according to these models. These views also have major implications for the choice of methods of work organisation, favouring models of work organisation where each patient relates to one nurse for the coordination of his or her care.

Traditional practice based on the biomedical model has concentrated on telling patients what to do. Health care workers asked the patients 'would you like to get up now', but they expected compliance. Non-compliance was not approved of and sometimes sanctions were and still are applied. For example, the elderly obese lady who needs to lose weight if the soreness under her breast is to subside may only be offered non-fattening food even if she would prefer to tolerate the sore skin rather than the longing she feels for food when she is given no choice but to eat a low-fat diet. Although the values held by nurses may mean that they see dieting as the only choice, partnership demands that the elderly lady should be made fully aware, through teaching, of the value of losing weight. However, on the basis of partnership she should still have the power to choose to eat fattening foods without the nurse showing disapproval or applying sanctions.

A spin-off of this is the sanctions being applied in some areas to people who live 'non-healthy lifestyles' with a consequent withholding of some treatment regimes, the obvious example being the reluctance by some professionals to undertake cardiac surgery if the patient still smokes. While there is no doubt that decisions do have to be made in relation to using limited resources in the most effective way, it is questionable when the decisions about allocation of treatments lie solely in the hands of the professionals rather than the public at large.

All of these issues, which relate to patients or clients, are represented to a greater or lesser degree in the majority of nursing models. All models also express views on nursing and the nurse, and the common characteristics associated with these are considered in the next chapter.

Learning exercises

1. Consider the care of a patient that you have been involved in. Identify the way that care was organised and delivered to this patient and try to pinpoint the view of the patient, as perceived by: yourself, other nurses, the doctors, the physiotherapist, the social worker, other members of the team.
2. Still focusing on the patient you considered in exercise 1, try to imagine how each of the major theories discussed in this chapter could present a different perspective on planning and delivering her/his care.

Study questions

1. Write an explanatory paragraph on:
   systems theory
   developmental theory
   symbolic interaction theory
   human nature
   the environment
   patient autonomy
   nurse/patient partnership

Chapter 7

Common Characteristics of Nursing Models – the Nurse and Nursing

LEARNING OBJECTIVES

The issues discussed in Chapter 6 have been mainly related to patients or clients themselves. Those discussed in this chapter concern patients and clients, nurses and how nursing takes place.

They include views on health, views on nurses as part of the health care team and accountability for nursing practice.

HEALTH AS THE FOCUS OF NURSING

All models for health care workers include views about what health is, with the biomedical model viewing health as the absence of disease or disorder. Nursing models on the whole perceive health as a much wider concept relating to wellness and the achievement of potential but, like the biomedical model, they see the goal of practice revolving round the achievement and maintenance of this thing called health.

The biomedical model view of health or wellness is based on the concept of physiological homeostasis. Many years ago the World Health Organisation (1948) definition broadened the biomedical view of health out to a state of 'complete physical, mental and social well-being and not merely the absence of disease or infirmity'. This can be loosely seen to mean physiological, psychological and sociological homeostasis. However, both of these biomedical views – the more restricted one and the broader one – have been criticised. In particular, the definition of the WHO is said to be utopian and its very broadness may mean that few people, if any, can be considered healthy. It proposes a static state of complete well-being and opposes ideas about the dynamic nature of healthiness. Furthermore, many people, particularly medical sociologists, argue that the absence of disease is not an accurate description of the healthy state.

To be fair to those who currently practice according to the supposedly 'objective' biomedical model, the physiological concept of homeostasis is often expanded beyond the realms of biology and may encompass:

- body balance
- psychological and emotional balance
- cultural, social and political balance
- spiritual and philosophical balance

Nevertheless, the biomedical model sees disease, no matter how it defines the term, as something which can be resolved by the application of scientific knowledge, thus applying science as a means to achieve a state of health.

Some people see health as a different concept from wellness, while others suggest that both terms are interchangeable. It seems health states are frequently explained by either/or propositions – that is, one is either ill or well, diseased or healthy. In order for people to know that they are ill, they must have some concept of what is 'normal' against which to measure their current physical or mental condition. Those who support a rigid biomedical model regard illness as a deviation from a biological norm, and health or wellness as the maintenance of homeostasis in a physiological sense.

This view does not answer an important question: is health or wellness an objective state defined by doctors? Or, is it a subjective state perceived by individuals about themselves, and influenced by what the community they live in think about what is normal? In Ham's (1992) view there are significant differences between individual and collective views of health, with the efficacy of a health service often being judged by mortality rates that may not have real meaning to individual people.

Wellness and illness are universal phenomena. Everybody, everywhere has ideas about what 'being healthy' is. As yet there is no universal definition, but generally people do not want health rather than health care.

What is health or wellness also differs markedly between groups. For example, in Western society scabies is seen as unacceptable and unhealthy, whereas because of its endemic nature in some developing countries and the limited treatment provisions available, it is seen there as merely an irritating fact of life. Sociological theorists see illness as a deviation from social norms, that is something which is not regarded as a normal way of social living. Health and illness are therefore related to problems of deviance, conformity and social control. Friedson (1975) sees this social deviance as conduct that violates sufficiently valued norms. In concrete terms, this may mean lying in bed all day and being unable to do normal everyday things like shopping, talking and keeping clean and tidy.

In communities where being independent in these activities is normal, this sort of behaviour would be a deviance, a behaviour seen as abnormal. Most sociologists tend to define what is not health or wellness in order to then describe what it is. Parsons (1951), however, defined health as 'the state of optimum capacity for effective performance of valued tasks'. In effect, therefore, a person is well if he or she is able to conform to society's views of what is normal in terms of behaviour and carrying

Figure 7.1 The sick role carries privileges (for some!).

out certain tasks. The person who behaves in a way which society approves of, works in such a way and plays in such a way, can be regarded as being healthy and well. On the other hand, the person who shouts obscenities to people who wear red hats, or who is unable to get on and off the bus without help, may be seen in some societies (certainly our own) as being unwell or ill.

Field (1972) has put forward yet another view; he differentiates between illness and disease. Illness is, he says, the person's subjective experience of ill health, whereas disease is the medical conception of pathological abnormality. Figure 7.2 shows a schema to describe the relationship between disease and illness.

Following this schema, illness may be present or absent in disease, and people may feel ill even if there is no evidence of disease. This idea of disease and illness suggests therefore that health is merely the opposite of disease and wellness the opposite of illness.

Many nursing models consider that nursing should concern itself with wellness and health.

Common characteristics of nursing models – the nurse and nursing those who are said to be ill by medical diagnosis but also those who feel ill

If, on the other hand, we see health as the state in which people function well enough to conform with what is expected of them from the community they live in, then it is obvious that 'health' will vary from society to society. What is considered to be well in a poor region of South America may be very different from that of an affluent area of London. For example, the presence of minor aches in the back may be regarded as a perfectly natural, normal state in the former but may be seen as a reason for a prosperous Londoner to take to his or her bed.

Illness has to be legitimised or seen as valid by the societal group we live in before the position of being well and healthy ceases to exist. If the society sees a runny nose and headaches as being merely minor

Figure 7.2   Perceptions of health, disease, wellness and illness.

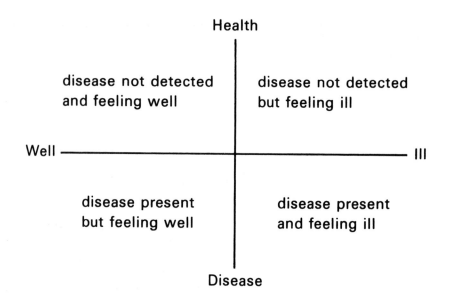

irritations, the person with a common cold will still be seen as being relatively healthy and will not be allowed to be regarded as a sick person. The concept of health is therefore determined in the sociological view by the society. Those of us who live in Western society may, according to Parsons (1951), be ascribed a sick role when we feel ill by the non-sick others. If this happens, certain privileges are given, but we have to fulfil certain obligations. The privileges are such things as being allowed to stay in bed, to stay off work and to have things done for us. The obligations are such things as having to have the sick role legitimised or made acceptable by a doctor stating a specific diagnosis. Neither are we allowed to do things which appear to be healthy. For example, looking ill and being able to say that the doctor said you had influenza may give you the privileges of time off from work and of having breakfast brought to bed. But if you jog around the park, go to the pub or disco, or dig in the garden you would not be meeting the obligations of the sick role and therefore the privileges may be withdrawn.

The values of society influence lay perceptions of illness and health. Apple (1960) describes two criteria by which people in Western society judge themselves to be ill.

1. The recency and novelty of the experience (when it has just happened and has not happened before).
2. The degree to which it interferes with ordinary activities.

To judge wellness, Bauman (1961) says that we use three criteria.

1. The subjective feeling of well-being.
2. The absence of any symptoms.
3. Being able to perform activities which those in good health can perform.

The sociological view of health sees illness as a form of deviance, determined by society itself, and certain rules or criteria seem to exist in each

Figure 7.3   The three continuums along which health can be defined (after Stacey, 1977).

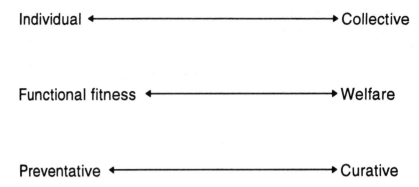

society to enable this to occur. Health or wellness is based on being able to behave in certain ways and carry out the tasks that are expected for a person to conform with what is seen as normal. Health care systems, and therefore nursing, are seen as mechanisms of social control to ensure isolation and treatment of ill members of society.

Drawing on the work of Stacey (1977), Ham (1992) suggests that concepts of health can be seen along a continuum with three distinct dimensions: the individual or collective; the functional fitness or welfare; and the preventative or curative (Figure 7.3). Within most Western societies it is the individual perspective demonstrated by fitness and cure rather than the collective model concerning the health of a whole nation and preventative measures which is dominant, a situation that can be attributed to the relative power of medicine. It must however be noted that changes are occurring, with an increasing interest in public health as well as a concern for some aspects of welfare such as hospice care and pain management.

Both the biomedical and sociological views of health and wellness are relevant to the discussion on health as a focus of nursing, but in isolation they do not match up to the common features of nursing models.

Nursing theorists attempt in many models to outline health or wellness from a holistic stance, which incorporates social and biological views, but includes other concepts. They frequently emphasise the 'reaching of potential' as the central concept in defining health.

Common characteristics of nursing models – the nurse and nursing concept in defining health

Rogers (1970) says that wellness is a feeling of wholeness and uniqueness. She describes it as:

1. 'A state of homeodynamic balance of energy.'
2. 'A continually evolving direction of growth.'
3. 'A sense of predictability, pattern and organisation of life.'
4. 'A sense of satisfaction with one's ability to conceptualise, think, imagine, communicate and experience sensations and feelings.'

Such sentiments and beliefs, although rather poetic, are common to practically all models for nursing practice. They come from the current linking of nursing to the beliefs in such things as holism, humanistic existentialism and the right to autonomy, which has been emphasised in this book. How we think about health is of course determined by our beliefs about human nature and, since nursing increasingly sees the human race as being made up of individuals who must be regarded in a whole way, the belief that health must be regarded holistically and from the perspective of the individual concerned is a logical basis for practice. The goals of models for nursing practice all, in some way, relate to the achievement of health, and health is almost always seen as the individual achieving his or her maximum potential. This incorporates the concepts of biological, sociological, psychological and spiritual balance or homeostasis. The knowledge and skill base required in nursing models includes those elements that will enable the nurse to promote health in individuals.

NURSING IN RELATION TO THE MULTIDISCIPLINARY CLINICAL TEAM

'The term multidisciplinary team is used to describe the group of National Health Service and other workers who are contributing to a patient's (or client's) health or care.' So says the secretariat of the Royal Commission on the National Health Service (1978). A whole range of disciplines work together to provide health care, including physiotherapists, occupational therapists, doctors, dieticians, domestic staff, care assistants, porters and many more. It must be added, however, that there is a strong move at the moment to shift the traditional role boundaries with the advent of such initiatives as patient-focused care (Morgan, 1993), re-engineering of health services and the increasing number of nurse practitioners who carry independent case loads (cf. Stilwell, 1987; Read *et al.*, 1992). Similarly, there is a growing interest in generic training for all health care workers (Chant, 1989), with specialisation arising at a later stage.

Nevertheless, all of these occupational groups hold a model to picture their work and the work of others. Health care workers by their very definition all broadly aim for health or wellness of the client, but each occupational and professional group will hold different perspectives on specific aspects of the nature of people and will have particular goals that are different from other groups and that many will fiercely defend. They will therefore require different knowledge, skills and attitudes.

Because of their common interest in the promotion of health, most of them will share common beliefs as well as beliefs specific to their discipline. For example, nurses, physiotherapists and occupational therapists may all see independence in daily living as a right of the client and would include that as one of the goals of practice. Similarly, all three would acknowledge a need for knowledge of anatomy and physiology, skills in patient teaching and motivation, and attitudes that include valuing the patient as an individual. Each, however, would have a different focus within these areas. A model for physiotherapy practice, for example, may focus on independence in body movement and on knowledge of the anatomy and physiology of muscles and soft tissues.

Alternatively, the occupational therapist may place more emphasis on specific and complete acts of living such as cooking or washing up, and may concentrate more on being knowledgeable about fine movements and the design of aids to support daily living acts than the physiotherapist. Nursing, too, has a different focus. If it didn't, then why have nurses at all? Although models for practice of all health workers are bound to overlap and share many similarities, the whole basis of multidisciplinary teamwork is the bringing together of people who are able to practice from different model bases acquired through professional training.

This may sound like 'common sense' and hardly worthy of much discussion. For multidisciplinary teams to work together, however, it is advisable that each other's role and basis for practice is understood and accepted by each discipline. Each member of the team can justify membership only if he or she has something to contribute that cannot be done as well by other members of the team.

Although a major function of nurses is to coordinate the contributions of the team members (because it is primarily nurses who provide a service which spans 24 hours in both hospitals and the community), there must be some specific contributions to patient care which are clearly 'nursing' if nurses are needed at all. The development of models to describe nursing's contribution to patient care is therefore essential if patients are to receive a service that is acceptable. Such an end can only be achieved if the teamwork it requires is unmarred by conflict between members or individual people working in isolation. This can arise if the different disciplines are unable to be clear about what they believe in, aim for and know about. Therefore cooperation will only be possible if each of these disciplines can offer such a picture of their practice to each other. Nursing has been particularly disadvantaged in playing a full part in teamwork because of its inability or reluctance to be clear about its contribution. The need to be clear increases as time progresses because of the acceleration of specialisation in health care discussed earlier and the relatively new development of service centres where nurses form a triumvirate with doctors and administrators to lead a clinical service.

Nursing teams are members of a much bigger multidisciplinary clinical team, but their contribution to care can, and should, be equal to that of the contributions of others. Sometimes the contribution of a specific discipline will inevitably be greater because of the needs of the patient, but this will change as the patient's needs change. For example, the person with a severe headache that has an obvious physiological

WITHDRAWN FROM STOCK

Figure 7.4   Without explicit models for practice, conflict can occur.

Education Centre Library
Southend Hospital, Prittlewell Chase
sex SS0 0RY
Tel: 01702 435555 ext. 2618

cause and is resolvable by taking a certain drug will clearly need the contribution of the medical member of the multidisciplinary clinical team in primary health care and will need little from other members. However, if the headache makes him dizzy and unable to meet his daily living needs, the district nurse may have to contribute just as much to his care, and sometimes far more than, the general practitioner. Furthermore it is now recognised that many patients occupy acute hospital beds beyond the point when they have become medically stable because of their continuing need for acute care from other health care workers. There are now examples where their care is formally being handed over to nurses who have the authority to manage both admission and discharge, calling on medical services in much the same way as a general practitioner's advice would be sought in the community (Pearson *et al.*, 1992; Evans and Griffiths, 1994).

There is much argument about the nature of the multidisciplinary teamwork between disciplines, particularly in relation to leadership. Many doctors argue that they have the greatest contribution to make to care and therefore should always lead the other health care disciplines. On the other hand, some nurses dispute this and suggest that leadership should be determined for each individual patient on the basis of which professional worker is best suited to lead the care exemplified by the increasing number of autonomous independent practitioners in many areas of nursing (cf. Stilwell, 1987; Read *et al.*, 1992). Many nurses who have started looking at their work from the basis of a model for practice consider that some patients primarily need medical care with the help of others – so the doctor should lead the care; some primarily need physiotherapy with the help of others – so the physiotherapist should lead the care; and some primarily need nursing with the help of others – so the nurse should lead the care. Such a view could, they argue, be applied to all professional health care workers. Although disputed by medical colleagues at the time, as far back as 1978 McFarlane suggested:

> It is no longer appropriate that doctors should assume primacy over other professions, taking the major responsibility for care. I suggest that medical leadership of the team often restricts the full assessment of health needs, particularly in cases where the medical model of care is inappropriate to the problem, e.g. in terminal care.

It can be suggested that the radical nature of this statement still held true in the 1990s, since her suggestions require an attitudinal change of far greater magnitude than may first be apparent. Nevertheless, many changes along the recommendations she made are occurring in service delivery and early evaluations are proving very positive (e.g. Griffiths and Evans, 1995).

It is not possible, in this discussion, to consider the argument about the nature of multidisciplinary teams in depth, because the background is complex and would need a book in itself. However, it is clear that only a limited contribution can be made until nurses in any team are able to describe their particular contribution with clarity. Agreeing on a model for practice is an important foundation of knowledge for nurses wishing to contribute equally in health care multidisciplinary teamwork.

ACCOUNTABILITY FOR PRACTICE

There has been a great deal of discussion about whether or not nurses can, or should, be held accountable for their own practice. The answer to such a question is the single most important factor in the development of nursing. If nurses are not prepared as an occupational group to stand accountable for their own decision-making and actions, then they cannot expect either patients/clients or other colleagues working in health care to value or respect their opinions, a view which is reflected in some codes of professional practice (UKCC, 1992a).

So what is this thing called 'accountability' and how does it relate to models for practice? According to Lewis and Batey (1982), accountability implies 'formal obligation to disclose'. You must be able to say:

1. What it is you are trying to achieve (your goal).
2. How you are trying to achieve it (your actions).
3. The justification for your actions (your knowledge base).
4. The outcome of your actions (your evaluation).

In other words, nursing actions must be explainable, defendable and based on knowledge rather than tradition or myth, a notion supported by the much wider drive for an increase in the use of evidence based medicine (Department of Health, 1995). We have found it a salutary exercise to ask ourselves whether we are in a position to respond accurately to some of the questions posed above. Without a clear statement of intent, it is impossible to justify why certain actions have been taken. Without evaluation, it is difficult to decide whether or not our actions have been effective in helping a patient or client to either maintain or move towards his or her desired goal. Many nursing actions today are based on traditional myths, for instance the routine observations carried out in so many circumstances which can be both time-consuming for nurses and disruptive for the patient. Why are they being taken? What are the criteria on which a decision is made for them to start or stop? Another commonly given example of a nursing tradition is the addition of salt to the bath. When there is no evidence of its therapeutic effect, how can there be justification for continuing a practice which is largely based on folklore?

We (Pearson and Vaughan, 1984) suggest that there are three major criteria that have to be met in order for a nurse to be accountable. First, there must be a statement about the expected outcome or the goal which it is hoped will be achieved. Second, the rationale on which practice is based must be made clear. Third, there must be an established system of evaluation in order to see whether or not the goal has been achieved.

One of the functions of a model of nursing is to identify the broad goal of practice, although it may be as broad or as unspecific as to cure disease or to strive towards self-care and independence. Once this broad philosophically based goal has been agreed upon within a team, it becomes much easier to identify goals in day-to-day practice. Not only will it give guidance to the identification of goals, but also to the part to be played by all concerned as well as the range of knowledge and skills

Figure 7.5 Some practice is based on folklore.

required to fulfil this function. A very simple example is the difference in action of two nurses working with a patient with a colostomy. One will attend to the colostomy for the patient, perhaps with a goal of keeping the patient clean. The second will assist the patient in caring for his or her own colostomy, requiring teaching as well as technical skills, possibly in this case with a goal based on the belief in self-care or independence. If these two nurses are working in the same area, the result for the patient can only be confusion. However, if the team of nurses agrees upon the model of nursing on which they base their practice, such confusion can be avoided.

Accountability and responsibility

There is a considerable lack of clarity about the two notions of account-ability and responsibility, different authorities interpreting them in dif-ferent ways. Some people use the words interchangeably, while others clearly differentiate between them. Because interpretation of these words is unclear, it is important to try to clarify the underlying issues.

While the two ideas are inextricably linked, there is a clear difference between them. Accountability concerns being answerable and implies that a situation has been assessed, a plan has been made and carried out, and the results evaluated. Responsibility refers to the task or 'charge'. Thus nurses can be offered the 'charge' or responsibility for carrying out a particular action. In agreeing to accept the responsibility for that action, they become accountable for fulfilling it. Implicit in this statement is the need for the person concerned to have the authority to act since it is unreasonable to hold people to account for actions over which they have no authority.

A job description usually itemises the 'tasks' for which an individual is responsible. In agreeing to fulfil that job description, the individual becomes accountable for carrying them out. In this instance, the body to whom he or she is accountable will be the employing authority. However, at a clinical level, the agreement will be that the nurse will accept the responsibility for delivering nursing care. It becomes obvious then, that the nurse must be accountable to the recipient of the service that is offered, that is the patient or client, an issue which is gaining more and more public acknowledgement and rightly so. This line of account-ability, between the giver of care or the nurse and the recipient of care or the patient or client is, we would suggest, the most important one. Nurses should be in a position to explain and defend their actions either to the patients or the bodies that protect them.

The major function of the nursing registration bodies is to protect the public. These authorities were usually established in response to legisla-tion, their remit being to ensure that safe standards of practice are offered by nurses. In order to achieve this aim, they have to establish the criteria they recognise as the minimal level of achievement which an individual must attain in order to be called a nurse. In other words, they must be able to identify what nursing is, the purpose of nursing or the goals it is trying to achieve, and the knowledge and skills that are necessary to achieve these goals. In many instances such organisations have drawn up a Code of Conduct (UKCC, 1992b) as a means of making this purpose explicit. Without this background, they would not be able to fulfil their function of protecting the public.

Central authorities have also been given the 'charge' or responsibility of approving the educational programmes for nurses. For many years most curricula were largely based on the biomedical model already described. However, this emphasis is now changing, evidenced by changes in curriculum approach increasingly adopted across the Western World from the 1990s and the linking of continuing education to contin-uing registration (UKCC, 1993).

Contemporary curricula invariably concentrate on developing an individual nurse's skill in order to practice as an advocate and a teacher as well as to deliver the traditional nurturing care of nursing. The resulting courses emphasise helping student nurses to develop insight into their own needs as people in order that they may develop relationships with people with, for example, learning disabilities as valued individuals.

It could be argued that ideally a single unified model of nursing should be agreed upon in order to bring uniformity into practice. However, we feel that clinical nurses should have the right to choose the detailed model on which they base their practice. Nevertheless the influence of the value systems, the goals of practice and the knowledge and skills required are reflected within a syllabus. This is one way in which the central controlling bodies of nursing can demonstrate to the public their accountability for protecting patients.

Use of an explicit model for practice is an essential beginning to accountability and responsibility in nursing. It will clarify what nursing is, helping individual practitioners to decide what work they will agree to accept. It will identify for all nurses the knowledge they require to practice. In day-to-day work the model will be the guiding force that will help them to decide what to assess, how to plan and set goals, what part they will take in the action and what to evaluate.

EXISTING NURSING MODELS

Having explored the 'hard core' of nursing models in these first chapters, we can now look at specific models described by nurses, for nurses, in the literature. In the next chapters, we describe specific models for practice, using the following structures already introduced.

1. The beliefs and values on which the model is based, related to:
   (a) the person;
   (b) health; and
   (c) the environment.
2. The goals of nursing practice.
3. The knowledge and skills the nurse needs to develop in order to achieve these goals.

In order to show how they may be applied practically, the introductory chapters include an assessment framework and a brief care plan derived from the model described. They are not intended to be 'ideal' examples but are merely used to demonstrate how each model can be used in practice. The concluding chapters introduce the models of Paterson and Zderad, Watson and Parse; whilst the concluding part of these chapters demonstrate the clinical applicability of the work, care plans have not been included. We chose to make this change in format, not only to introduce models which have arisen from an interpretive paradigm, but also because we appreciate that there are other quite acceptable means of organising and documenting nursing care.

We have deliberately limited the following chapters to an account of the specific concepts of each model on the assumption that the common issues already discussed in earlier chapters will be linked to them. We would strongly recommend that once the reader has gained a broad overview and a 'feel' for some of the models available she or he explores the writings of the original authors for a more detailed account.

RELATING NURSING MODELS TO THE ASSESSMENT PHASE OF THE NURSING PROCESS

The nursing process is currently seen as an effective way of delivering nursing – a method of carrying it through. But the nursing itself has to be made clear through agreeing on a model. One model may be selected; an amalgamation of a number of them; or a framework developed by the nursing team itself. The 'process' cannot happen without an agreement on nursing.

The most concrete example of how a model affects practice is the structure it gives to assessment. For example, the biomedical model sees the patient as being made up of body systems, and those who practice according to this model would logically structure assessment according to these systems. Some doctors use a structured assessment form reflecting this belief, which would follow the type of outline below.

- Complains of …
- History of present condition …
- Past medical history …

- Social history ...
- Functional enquiry ...
- Drugs ...
- Allergies ...
- O/E central nervous system ...
- Respiratory system ..., etc.

This is obviously based on body systems and on the goal of practice being related to the diagnosis and treatment of disease or illness.

Specific nursing models give clear direction to the structure of the nursing assessment as well as to identifying patient problems amenable to nursing actions, to goal setting, to care planning, to implementation and to evaluation. To demonstrate this practical application of each model, an assessment of a patient, based on the model under discussion, is included in some chapters. It must however be added that the models are not intended as a rigid structure which must, at all times, be adhered to. In the early days of practice most of us needed some sort of framework to help us make sense of nursing. As clinical expertise in nursing develops we learn to prioritise, being, for example, selective in the assessment process in relation to both content and timing. Thus, with experience, an assessment tool becomes a guideline or aide-mémoire, and skilled clinical decisions can be made about what is included or excluded. However, bearing in mind the discussion on accountability given above, it must also be remembered that it is necessary to account for omission as well as action.

Some of the nursing models we describe may 'ring a bell' immediately and mean something to you personally and to the sort of practice you are currently engaged in. Others may have less meaning for you or be less relevant to your interest. All of them, however, are serious attempts by nurses to use concepts and theories to represent the reality of nursing practice.

Throughout the following chapters we describe some aspects of nursing for one specific patient and show how the approaches to care vary according to the model. While there are similarities in the basic difficulty identified as being experienced by the patient, the approach, recording, goal setting and management are all slightly different and are dependent on the specific beliefs and goals of the model.

The patient concerned is Mr Gordon Smith, a 67-year-old man who has rheumatoid arthritis. He has lived alone since his dearly loved wife died. Although he is lonely he values his independence and ability to manage for himself without relying on others for support. Recently his physical condition has deteriorated and he has been referred for review of his care to a nurse.

One of Mr Smith's problems relates to an inadequate dietary intake and consideration of this specific problem will be pursued from the different perspectives of each model described. An assessment of his needs is given in each case, followed by problem identification, goal setting, planning of action (showing the involvement of both the nurse and the patient) and evaluation. We hope that this will allow a comparison of the various models for nursing and help individual readers to consider which model is closest to his or her own views of nursing.

Learning exercises

1. Pick up the records of any patient and analyse the contributions made by members of the multidisciplinary team.
2. Compare the language used by medicine with that of nursing and determine whether these two groups are working from a wellness perspective or an illness perspective.

Study questions

1. Write notes on health and wellness.
2. Explain the practical implications of each perspective.
3. List the benefits to the patient of multidisciplinary teamwork.

Chapter 8

The Activities of Living Model for Nursing

LEARNING OBJECTIVES

On completion of this chapter, the reader will be able to:

1. Assess patients with complex needs using the activities of living
2. Discuss the factors that influence the activities of living
3. Explain how the model promotes patient individuality
4. Estimate the degree to which the model might enhance practice

The 'activities of living' model for nursing was developed by Nancy Roper, Winifred Logan and Alison Tierney (Roper *et al.*, 1980). Their initial work arose from the findings of a research project on the clinical experience of student nurses (Roper, 1976). The authors are all graduates of the University of Edinburgh and have an impressive range of nursing experience. This model was the first attempt by British nurses to develop a conceptual model for nursing; it is used widely in the United Kingdom and is becoming increasingly well known internationally.

The model is appreciated for its clarity. Most practitioners and students who use the model are able to refer directly to the original texts rather than rely, as many do when studying, on some of the more complex American works, or secondary sources. The authors have encouraged criticism of their work, that has appeared in four editions (Roper *et al.*, 1980, 1985, 1990, 1996). In these new works they have responded to readers' comments and to the changing climate surrounding the discipline of nursing. In the third edition the link between nursing and health is accentuated, chapters on biology, psychology and sociology have been omitted and more attention given to consideration of the factors which influence 'activities of living' and the individualisation of care. In their final publication (Roper *et al.*, 2000) they leave an enduring account of the model with an invitation to nurses to take the work forward. They include a critique of the work and defend its position as a model.

Tierney (1998) claims the contribution that the model has made to nursing is that it has encouraged nurses to refocus on health rather than ill health, appreciate the complexity of nursing, reconsider their professional relationship with medicine, individualise nursing and make practising nurses aware of the use of theory. Fraser (1990, 1996) contends the model is overly physically/physiologically oriented, a factor that has more to do with interpretation than the intent of the authors. However, it has been addressed in later editions but also it is this orientation that is one of the reasons for the model's acceptance in acute areas.

Although the activities of living model specifically relates to practice, Web (1997) demonstrates the use of the model as a theoretical framework for a care plan audit within an evaluative study of primary nursing.

LIVING ACTIVITIES

Although the activities of living model incorporates most of the issues discussed in earlier chapters, such as holism, partnership and health, the crux of the model is that all individuals are involved in certain activities which enable them to live and grow. They quote Virginia Henderson's definition of nursing (1966):

> The unique function of the nurse is to assist the individual, sick or well, in the performance of those activities contributing to health or its recovery (or to a peaceful death) that he [sic] would perform unaided if he had the necessary strength, will or knowledge, and to do this in such a way as to help him to gain independence as rapidly as possible.

Henderson described what nursing does by listing 14 'activities of daily living'. She suggests that nursing is:

> Helping the patient with these activities or providing conditions under which he can perform them unaided.

Roper, Logan and Tierney have developed Henderson's ideas into a model which focuses on the activities people engage in to live, and linking lifestyle with health and ill health. People's need for nursing is relatively short and therefore the resumption of normality is to be promoted.

BELIEFS AND VALUES

The person

The model focuses on the client as an individual engaged in living throughout his or her lifespan, and moving from dependence to independence, according to age, circumstances and environment. The important ideas underlying the model are: the progression of a person along a lifespan; a dependence/independence continuum; the activities of living and influencing factors; and lastly individuality.

Lifespan

An individual is seen to begin living at conception, and to end the process at death – a somewhat obvious fact perhaps, but an important part of the model. As people engage in the process of living, their position on the lifespan influences their capacity for independence; progress in the lifespan is of course unidirectional.

The dependence/independence continuum

This continuum is moved along dynamically and is affected by a whole range of factors, both predictable and sometimes surprising. For example, newborn babies will naturally be at the dependent end of the continuum

---

Box 8.1   A model for living (from Roper *et al.*, 1990, with permission)

Activities of living	Lifespan Conception → Death
Preventing	**Continuum**
Comforting	Totally dependent ↔ Totally
Seeking	independent
Maintaining a safe environment	_____
Communicating	_____
Breathing	_____
Eating and drinking	_____
Eliminating	_____
Personal cleansing and dressing	_____
Controlling body temperature	_____
Mobilising	_____
Working and playing	_____
Expressing sexuality	_____
Sleeping	_____
Dying	_____

because they are not mature enough to be self-sufficient in many activities of living; mature adults of 30 years may be at the independent end in virtually all of the activities of living, but may become dependent if illness or trauma occurs or if they are placed in an environment with which they are unfamiliar, for example, the middle of the Amazon jungle.

The activities of living In the model, individuals are seen as engaging in 12 basic activities of living. However, there are stages in the lifespan when the individual cannot yet, or no longer can, perform one or more of the activities. Specific circumstances may also restrict performance in one or more of the activities.

The 12 activities are:

1. Maintaining a safe environment
2. Communicating
3. Breathing
4. Eating and drinking
5. Eliminating
6. Personal cleansing and dressing
7. Controlling body temperature
8. Working and playing
9. Mobilising
10. Sleeping
11. Expressing sexuality
12. Dying

Factors influencing activities of living Each activity is seen to have five components – physical, physiological, sociocultural, environmental and politico-economic. For example, eating involves the passage of nutrients through various anatomical structures and being acted upon by various physiological processes. The nutrients themselves have a chemical basis and physiological purpose. Eating and nutrition are also affected by physiological factors, with some people eating to meet physiological needs and others not eating because of psychological influences. Eating is also a social act: for example, in Western society, people rarely eat with their fingers whereas this may be the accepted norm in some other societies. It can be associated with social functions that have little to do with physical hunger. Poverty is a prime cause of malnourishment, and religious beliefs often have rules associated with eating. Environmental factors such as the weather or pests may destroy whole crops of vital foods and have a major impact on people's nutrition.

Individuality in living

Each person will be affected by a unique range of influencing factors, and the result is that they will manifest differences in the way they live.

The model also identifies three types of activities, all of which are closely interrelated to each other and to the 12 activities of living.

Preventing activities: These are engaged in to prevent those things that will impair living, such as illness and accidents. Performing acts of personal hygiene to prevent infection, and looking right, left, then right again before crossing the road are examples of preventing activities.

Comforting activities: These are performed to give physical, psychological and social comfort. Resting in bed, having hot drinks and keeping warm when suffering from influenza are examples of comforting activities.

Seeking activities: These activities are those carried out in the pursuit of knowledge, new experiences and answers to new problems. Going to see the doctor or pharmacist when a symptom is experienced is an example of a seeking activity.

Roper (1976) emphasises the closeness and the overlapping nature of the three types of activities. If a person is suffering illness, she or he will, by carrying out certain activities of living, seek advice, look for comfort by seeing a doctor, and thus try to overcome the illness and prevent it from recurring.

The model of living represents the individual – the subject of nursing– engaged in the process of living. Roper (1976) describes the subject of nursing thus:

> *Basically, people are envisaged as carrying out various activities during a lifespan from conception to death. Their main objective is seen as attaining self-fulfilment and maximum independence in each activity of daily living within the limitations set by their particular circumstances. Many activities of a preventing, comforting and seeking nature are performed and people appropriately alter priorities among the activities of daily living. In these ways, the individual endeavours to be healthy and independent in the process of living.*

Health

As a concept, health is given more attention in the third edition, although everyday living has always been a focus of the model. The authors make the point that health, as a concept, changes as does society and current thought. They plot various notions of health over the ages, ranging from health as an ideal abstract notion that is unattainable to more modern notions of health as a subjective estimation of well-being. The idea that health is a state or a continuum (with health at one end and illness at the other) is regarded as outmoded. Rather, health 'is a dynamic process with many facets' (Roper *et al.*, 1990, p. 5).

Environment

The environment is defined as anything external to the person. It is deemed to be an essential component of 'living activities' and is one of the 'influencing factors' which impinge upon all the activities of living.

THE GOALS OF NURSING

When the individual is unable to be independent in any of the activities of living, and the family or social grouping is unable to ensure that the activities are performed, nursing is needed.

From the model of living developed to describe the individual, it follows that the goals of nursing relate to the activities of living. Nursing aims at the following.

1. The individual acquiring, maintaining or restoring maximum independence in the activities of living, or enabling him or her to cope with dependence on others if circumstances make this necessary.
2. Enabling the individual to carry out preventing activities independently to avoid ill health.
3. Providing comforting strategies to promote recovery and eventual independence.
4. Providing medically prescribed treatments to overcome illness or its symptoms, leading to recovery and eventual independence.

KNOWLEDGE AND SKILLS FOR PRACTICE

Roper *et al.* (1990) present a diagrammatic representation of a 'model for nursing' based on the model of living. Nurses therefore need knowledge concerning the physiological, sociocultural, environmental, politico-economic and psychological aspects of each of the 12 activities of living.

Box 8.2   A model for nursing (from Roper *et al*, 1990, with permission)

Nursing components

Patient's lifespan
Conception → Death

Totally dependent ↔ Totally independent
Circumstance

Activities of living
Preventing
Comforting
Dependent

Understanding and abilities are also required in the following areas: the human developmental progression along the lifespan; the appropriate skills and attitudes to enable nurses to comfort people, educate them and carry out medical prescriptions; in meeting 'seeking' and 'preventing' needs; and in carrying out the activities of living for those unable to do so while helping clients to cope with dependence in itself.

In order to promote independence in the activities of living, or actually to perform them for others when needed, the model outlines the problem-solving process it is recommended that nurses should follow:

- assessment of the patient
- identification of the patient's problems and statement of expected outcomes
- planning of care
- implementation of care
- evaluation of the outcomes of care

Roper *et al.* (1980, 1985, 1990) suggest that their text is a useful introduction to nursing. Initial nursing education may be based on knowledge of each activity of living, and on the use of the problem-solving process. Students should be encouraged to apply this knowledge to promote independence appropriate to the individual client's circumstances and position on the lifespan and the dependence/independence continuum.

ASSESSMENT USING THE ACTIVITIES OF LIVING MODEL

At assessment the nurse aims at establishing what the patient can and cannot do in each of the activities of living, bearing in mind physical, sociocultural, psychological, environmental and politico-economic factors which may influence the person. The 12 activities of living provide the framework for assessment. The patient and nurse discuss each one and identify the usual routine and any obstacles to the accomplishment of the usual routine and therefore to independence.

Maintaining a safe environment

This refers to seeking and preventing activities, and to the safety of carrying out the activities of living. It may include environmental factors, such as housing and furnishing; sensory factors, such as the ability to hear oncoming traffic or to smell gas; personal health-related behaviour, such as smoking; and psychosocial factors, such as the presence of inappropriate fears or irrational behaviour.

Communicating

Through communication itself – between the nurse, the patient and the family – the patient's usual forms of communication and social interaction are established and any difficulties identified. These could include the sensory obstacles of bad hearing or sight.

Breathing

Baseline measurements, e.g. respiration count or peak flow measurement, may be recorded, along with the observation of the colour of mucous membranes and breathing characteristics. Any difficulties related to breathing are identified, as are potentially harmful factors such as smoking or the general pollution of the air or the effects of stress factors.

Eating and drinking

This activity embraces cultural attitudes towards food and drink, personal preference and an assessment of the state of nutrition. Usual eating and drinking patterns are explored, and physical actions such as the ability to cook unaided and to chew food are included, and maybe the person's ability to pay for food.

Eliminating

Bowel and bladder functions are discussed under this heading. A record is made of how the patient usually maintains normal function of the bowels and bladder, what type of facilities the patient has at home and possible cultural influences. *different ways - Benefits cultra* :

Personal cleansing and dressing

Again, usual patterns are discussed, such as frequency of baths. Any difficulties in maintaining independence are identified. The condition of the skin, nails and hair would be included in this section.

Controlling body temperature

As well as baseline measurement of temperature where appropriate, what the patient usually does to stay warm or become cool would be recorded. For example, if the patient has a coal fire at home, it would be noted, as would the patient's preference for iced drinks when he or she is feeling too hot.

Mobilising

The degree of activity and mobility are ascertained, and usual daily activity is recorded. If the patient appears apathetic and reluctant to mobilise, this would be recorded under this heading, as would their usual mode of transport, e.g. bus or car.

Working and playing

The nature of the patient's present or past occupation is recorded, and recreational and relaxational pursuits discussed.

Expressing sexuality

Those aspects of sexuality relevant to the current need for nursing are explored. This may include sexual activity in patients with certain medical conditions or disability, and the expression of masculinity and femininity in such things as dress, make-up or perfumes.

Sleeping

The patient's usual sleeping patterns, where they sleep and the strategies employed by the patient to induce sleep are recorded.

Dying

Where appropriate, feelings and views on dying are explored.

Throughout assessment, the activities usually performed independently are recorded, as well as those activities which cannot be performed without assistance. The assessment thus allows the nurse to enable the patient to pursue his or her usual daily life patterns as well as to identify activities which cannot be performed independently. All activities that cannot be carried out independently are treated as problems during assessment. Thus, the organisation of information gathered during assessment using this model is structured around the 12 activities of living described by Roper *et al.* (1990). Figure 8.1 is an example of an assessment form developed in a small community unit.

An outline concerning Mr Smith was given on page 85 and we will be returning to him throughout the following chapters. From the perspective of the activities of living model, the assessing nurse noted that Mr Smith 'looked thin', his clothes were too big for him and he had lost 5 kg in weight. On asking the patient about his usual activities, it was discovered that he did not eat breakfast and that he had lunch from the Meals-on-Wheels service on Tuesdays and Thursdays, and from a home help on every other day of the week. He said, however, that he did not eat these lunches and instead had cake and biscuits for tea and only drank cold

	COMMUNITY	
HOSPITAL/UNIT:	HOSPITAL	
	DAY UNIT	

PATIENT ASSESSMENT FORM : BASIC DATA

DATE OF ADMISSION	DATE OF ASSESSMENT	NURSE

MALE ☐ AGE ☐   SURNAME _____   FORENAMES _____

FEMALE ☐ DATE OF BIRTH _____   Prefers to be addressed as _____

SINGLE/MARRIED/WIDOWED/OTHER

ADDRESS OF USUAL RESIDENCE _____

TYPE OF ACCOMMODATION _____

FAMILY/OTHERS AT THIS RESIDENCE _____

NEXT OF KIN   NAME _____   ADDRESS _____
               RELATIONSHIP _____   TEL. NO. _____

SIGNIFICANT OTHERS
(incl. relatives/dependants
visitors/helpers/neighbours) _____

SUPPORT SERVICES _____

OCCUPATION _____

RELIGIOUS BELIEFS & RELEVANT PRACTICES _____

SIGNIFICANT LIFE CRISIS

PATIENT'S PERCEPTION OF CURRENT HEALTH STATUS _____

FAMILY'S PERCEPTION OF PATIENT'S HEALTH STATUS _____

REASON FOR ADMISSION

MEDICAL INFORMATION (e.g. diagnosis, past history, allergies)

WEIGHT _____
URINE _____
                SG. _____   ALB _____
TEMP _____   PULSE _____
B.P. _____   RESP _____

DISCHARGE ARRANGEMENTS:
(to be completed on referral)

MAIN SOURCE FOR ASSESSMENT: PROJECTED DATE OF DISCHARGE

SIGNIFICANT OTHERS INTERVIEWED : YES/NO   ARRANGEMENTS DISCUSSED WITH:

IF YES, DETAILS OF INTERVIEW

RELATIVES _____   OTHERS _____
                    HOME HELP _____

D/N _____
H/V _____
SOC. WORKER

Figure 8.1   An assessment form.

ASSESSMENT OF ACTIVITIES OF LIVING   DATE

AL	USUAL ROUTINES: WHAT HE/SHE CAN AND CANNOT DO INDEPENDENTLY	PATIENT'S PROBLEMS (ACTUAL/POTENTIAL) (P) = POTENTIAL
MAINTAINING A SAFE ENVIRONMENT		
COMMUNICATING		
BREATHING		
EATING AND DRINKING		
ELIMINATING		
PERSONAL CLEANSING AND DRESSING		
CONTROLLING BODY TEMPERATURE		
MOBILISING		
WORKING AND PLAYING		
EXPRESSING SEXUALITY		
SLEEPING		
DYING		

Figure 8.1   An assessment form *(cont.)*.

ASSESSMENT		ASSESSMENT	
DATE	OUTSTANDING PROBLEMS	DATE	OUTSTANDING PROBLEMS

Figure 8.1   An assessment form *(cont.)*.

drinks. He was unable to cook, to make tea safely or to make sandwiches. The assessment therefore showed that Mr Smith was dependent on others for an adequate dietary intake, and that he was unable to cope with this dependence, as suggested by his behaviour in not eating food prepared by others. The other two activities (comforting and seeking) are used to promote exploration to determine factors on which to base nursing care.

CARE PLANNING

Patient problems relating to the activities of living are identified during assessment and transferred to the plan of care. The goals agreed on by the nurse and patient, when using this model, must relate realistically to those implicit in the model. In other words, the goals must centre around the patient achieving independence in the activities of living or coping with any dependencies he or she may have.

The overriding requirement is for the patient to agree to the way in which goals are to be achieved and to the schedule for achieving them in as full a way as possible. The model focuses on the behaviour of the individual, and this must be reflected in the problem and goal statements in the care plan. Such an approach is seen as essential to the evaluation of the appropriateness and effectiveness of the nursing intervention.

Box 8.3 shows how Mr Smith's problems and goals would be recorded following this model.

In this example, nursing care is aimed at preventing further deterioration in health status, at an adequate intake of food, and at independence in the activity of living concerned – that is eating and drinking. Such independence should, in fact, achieve the other two aims of increasing daily calorie intake and maintaining weight.

The activities of living model for nursing

The effects of the nursing action taken can be evaluated by comparing the goals with both progress made and the eventual outcome.

The nursing action is what the nurse and patient will do to overcome the problem and achieve the goal. It is a clear description of what the

---

Box 8.3   The problem and goal statements

Problem (i.e. lack of independence in activity of living)	Goal (i.e. outcome which will indicate independence or a coping with dependence)
1. Loss of 5 kg in weight	Weight will remain at same level or rise
2. Intake of less than 1000 calories per day	Will eat at least 1500 calories per day
3. Unable to prepare own meals	Will be able to prepare a meal of his own choice without assistance

Box 8.4   The nursing action

Nursing Action
(i.e. how the nurse will promote the patient's independence in the activities of living *or* help the patient to cope with dependence in the process of living)
1. Weigh Mr Smith weekly at 9 a.m. He should be wearing his pyjamas.
2. a. Offer choices of food at breakfast, lunch and dinner.
   b. Check how much food is eaten at each meal: estimate calorific value; record; and inform Mr Smith each morning of his estimated calorific intake on the preceding day.
   c. Refer to OT for assessment, provision of aids, and teaching on food preparation.
   d. Ask Mr Smith to make pot of tea at breakfast and tea time in ward kitchen, everyday, with the help of aids.

nurse will do to promote independence in the activities of living by carrying out the activities of living, comforting, preventing and dependent components of nursing (see Box 8.4).

Evaluation focuses on movement towards, or away from, the goals of care, and since they are stated in measurable terms the effectiveness of the care can easily be seen.

A PATIENT CARE STUDY

Mrs Maude Fitzpatrick, aged 87, was referred to the district nursing sister by the general practitioner. On her initial, and two subsequent, visits, the nurse attempted to assess Mrs Fitzpatrick from the basis of the activities of living model for nursing. In addition to the basic biographical information, the patient's usual patterns of living were assessed with the involvement of her daughter, who was responsible for the performance of some of her mother's activities of living. Problems in the activities of living were identified by the nurse through systematically reviewing all of them. Figure 8.2 shows the written assessment arrived at. The problems identified were used to formulate a plan of care, as shown in Figure 8.3.

The focus of the care plan, planned collaboratively with the patient and her daughter, is on the performance of the activities of living – in this case, elimination (problems 1 and 3), personal cleansing and dressing (problem 2), sleeping (problem 3) and communication (problem 4). Those activities of living which were currently being performed independently or being met by the daughter in a way acceptable to her and Mrs Fitzpatrick were not included in the district nurse's plan. It concentrates the patient's energy on the process of living as independently as possible, and on coping with dependence in instances where this is the only realistic alternative. Throughout this account of Mrs Fitzpatrick's care, the emphasis is on the behaviour which people need to engage in to live, within the context of their position on the lifespan, and

COMMUNITY	✓
HOSPITAL	
DAY UNIT	

HOSPITAL/UNIT:

PATIENT ASSESSMENT FORM : BASIC DATA

DATE OF ~~ADMISSION~~ *First visit*   DATE OF ASSESSMENT *2.2.96*   NURSE *Anne Wood*

MALE [ ]   AGE [86]   SURNAME *Fitzpatrick*   FORENAMES *Maude Elizabeth*

FEMALE [X]   DATE OF BIRTH *1.8.09*   Prefers to be addressed as

SINGLE/MARRIED/WIDOWED/OTHER   *Mrs. Fitzpatrick*

ADDRESS OF USUAL RESIDENCE   *1, The Bungalows, South Milton*

TYPE OF ACCOMMODATION   *2 bedroomed council bungalow. Central heating. No stairs.*

FAMILY/OTHERS AT THIS RESIDENCE   *Daughter*

NEXT OF KIN   NAME *Miss Mary Fitzpatrick*   ADDRESS *as above*
RELATIONSHIP *daughter*   TEL. NO. *None*

SIGNIFICANT OTHERS   *Son - John and family, live in Dorset.*
(incl. relatives/dependants visitors/helpers/neighbours)   *Mr + Mrs Hardy — next door neighbours.*

SUPPORT SERVICES   *Social worker (Nick Hall) Home help (June Timpson) Mon. + Fri.*

OCCUPATION   *Retired from " doing housework for toffs" when 68.*

RELIGIOUS BELIEFS & RELEVANT PRACTICES   *RC priest visits weekly.*

SIGNIFICANT LIFE CRISIS *Loss of husband. "I still mourn for him after 15 years."*

PATIENT'S PERCEPTION OF CURRENT HEALTH STATUS *Has weak bladder + arthritis but "well in herself".*
FAMILY'S PERCEPTION OF PATIENT'S HEALTH STATUS *Daughter says she is worse: senile with poor mobility.*
REASON FOR ~~ADMISSION~~ *Referral   Night-time incontinence. Sore under breasts. Help in bath.*

MEDICAL INFORMATION (e.g. diagnosis, past history, allergies)

No apparent medical reason for incontinence - ? due to immobility?

Osteoarthritis of hips and knees for last nine years.

MAIN SOURCE FOR ASSESSMENT: *patient and daughter*

WEIGHT	*13 stone*
URINE	*NAD*
	SG. ALB
TEMP *37°C*	PULSE *82*
B.P. *140/90*	RESP *20*

DISCHARGE ARRANGEMENTS:
(to be completed on referral)
Probably needs long-term support.
PROJECTED DATE OF DISCHARGE   *Not known.*

SIGNIFICANT OTHERS INTERVIEWED : (YES) NO   ARRANGEMENTS DISCUSSED WITH:

IF YES, DETAILS OF INTERVIEW   RELATIVES _____   OTHERS _____
Daughter anxious about continuing   HOME HELP _____
to care for her mother.

D/N _____
H/V _____
SOC. WORKER

Figure 8.2   The assessment

ASSESSMENT OF ACTIVITIES OF LIVING   DATE 2.2.96

AL	USUAL ROUTINES: WHAT HE/SHE CAN AND CANNOT DO INDEPENDENTLY	PATIENT'S PROBLEMS (ACTUAL/POTENTIAL) (P) = POTENTIAL
MAINTAINING A SAFE ENVIRONMENT	Hangs on To furniture To get around.	
COMMUNICATING	Hears well. Wears glasses.	
BREATHING	Breathes easily and noiselessly.	
EATING AND DRINKING	Wears dentures. Likes toast for breakfast, a cooked lunch, sandwiches for supper. Can't manage tough meat and hard foods. Likes tea and stout.	
ELIMINATING	Opens bowels every other day. Takes Senokot x 2 daily. Dry during the day. Incontinent of urine at night. Can't get up quickly enough at night and usually wets bed x 1.	
PERSONAL CLEANSING AND DRESSING	Can dress herself apart from stockings. Unable To bathe independently - unable To get into bath. Washes own face and hands. Daughter gives wash down weekly.	
CONTROLLING BODY TEMPERATURE	Body temperature normal. House warm - Central heating.	
MOBILISING	Walks around house using furniture. Cannot get out alone. Very slow, especially in morning. Difficulty in walking to toilet.	
WORKING AND PLAYING	TV and daily paper. Does no housework.	
EXPRESSING SEXUALITY	Misses husband still.	
SLEEPING	Dozes in afternoon. Bed at 9 p.m. Difficulty in sleeping because of incontinence. Wakes around 2 a.m. and wets bed. Can get back to sleep if daughter changes bed.	
DYING	Wishes she was dead because she is a burden To her daughter, especially since the bed-wetting started.	

Figure 8.2   The assessment (cont.).

DATE	NO.	PROBLEM	GOAL	NURSING ACTION	REVIEW DATE
2.2.96	1	Incontinence of urine at night because of difficulty in walking.	Will remain dry throughout the night.	1. Change bedtime to 11 p.m. 2. Have her go to toilet before bed. 3. Set alarm for 2 a.m. to wake for toilet. 4. Provide commode at bedside.	9.2.96
	2	Unable to bathe unaided.	Skin will be clean and fresh.	Weekly general bath, using bath seat and step on Thursdays with help of nurse + daughter.	9.2.96
	3	Disturbed sleep because of incontinence.	Will sleep a minimum of 5 hours per night.	Report daily.	9.2.96
	4	Feels she is a burden on her daughter.	Facial expression will be relaxed and she will not mention such feelings in conversation.	Observe and report on moods and conversation.	9.2.96

NAME	NO.	PRIMARY NURSE
Mrs Maude Fitzpatrick	48	Anne Wood

Figure 8.3   The care plan.

the dependence/independence continuum. This is the emphasis of the activities of living model, which incorporates the physical, social, politico-economic and psychological components of behaviour.

Learning exercises

1. Choose a suitable patient that you are currently looking after. Rewrite their assessment notes using the Roper, Logan and Tierney model as an assessment framework.
2. Compare the assessment that you have written with the one that already exists.

Study questions

1. Write a one-page discussion on the use of the Roper, Logan and Tierney model in the assessment of patients.
2. Consider the patient you have just assessed and write an introduction of this person for a member of the Allied Health Team to which s/he might need to be referred.

Chapter 9

The Self–Care Model for Nursing

LEARNING OBJECTIVES

On completion of this chapter, the reader will be able to:

1. Argue the pros and cons of self-care as a means of health consumer empowerment
2. Identify the theories underpinning the self-care model
3. Relate the theory of self-care deficit to the identification of client problems requiring nursing support

The 'self-care' model was developed by Dorothea Orem, a well-known and respected nursing theorist from the USA. Her ideas were conceived and developed during the 1960s, 1970s and 1980s, a period in America which saw the growth of consumer awareness and the celebration of the individual. She disseminated her work through consultation, conferences and publications, and the theory is described in her book *Nursing Concepts of Practice*, first published in 1971 and revised in the new editions of 1980, 1985 and 1991. It is a popular model in American and British nursing circles, and one that is used widely by practitioners.

Based on the issues discussed in Chapters 3–7, the model focuses on the concept of 'self-care' and, contends Meleis (1991), derives from and expands the theory of human needs. Although the idea of self-care seems, at first sight, to be common sense, it is in fact complex with social, economic, moral and political ramifications. Initially it was a radical shift from the prevailing notion of nursing, where nursing care was considered to be 'care for' the patient and when 'bedside nurses', let alone patients, made few decisions regarding nursing therapy. Taylor *et al.* (2000) provide a useful overview of the theoretical underpinning of Orem's work. They identify three theories: theory of nursing systems, theory of self-care deficit, theory of self-care.

Although the model provides for care for people at all levels of dependency, the model is particularly appreciated in the area of disease prevention and health promotion because of the emphasis on individual responsibility. Moore and Pichler (2000) have recently taken Orem's work to identify and measure factors that affect people's ability to self-care. Lauder (2001) has used the model as a theoretical basis for self-neglect, proposing to investigate the deficiencies in self-care agency explained in Orem's model.

Before concentrating on the three parts of the model, a brief examination of the concept of 'self-care' is in order.

THE CONCEPT OF SELF-CARE

Levin *et al.* (1979) define self-care as:

> *a process whereby a lay person functions on his/her own behalf in health promotion and prevention, and in disease detection and treatment.*

Evidently self-care is associated therefore with a general desire to enable and allow people to take the initiative in being responsible for their own health care, when this is possible. There is an underlying assumption in this theory that ordinary people in contemporary society want to be more in control of their lives.

Norris (1979) suggests that the idea of self-care first arose in consumer groups in the 1960s, with anti-professional and anti-intellectual feelings, and an urge for people to return to the kind of life which emphasises 'being human, respecting, and giving'. Norris suggests that the changes were of course far more interesting and complex than just an anti-intellectual backlash, and he cites the rising disquiet brought about by the increases in materialism and mechanism in Western society, which appeared to have a de-humanising effect with world-wide repercussions.

Many writers from all spheres, not only health care, support the notion of self-care. In health care, self-care fundamentally affirms that people and families should be allowed to take initiative and responsibility and to develop their own potential in matters regarding their health. Bennett (1980) says:

> *When nurses discuss self-care, they need to remember that individuals, healthy and ill, are demanding increased control of their health care. They want to be active in the decision-making process: that is, they want to be able to identify their self-care needs, to establish their learning goals, and to evaluate their self-care behaviour. Patients are rejecting the passive recipient role whereby decisions are made by the nurse, independent of their input. Individuals want to assume responsibility for all aspects of care.*

Whilst bearing this in mind, the reader should remember that many consumers of health care have traditionally regarded medicine as the gate-keeper of the service and viewed medical knowledge with awe; a specialist knowledge which lay persons did not feel equipped to grasp and for which they expected to defer to professionals. In return for their high regard, clients of the health service expected, and in some instances still do today, to be cared for by professionally competent hearts, hands and minds with little contribution on their part besides suffering and accepting. Whilst public opinion has changed enormously with the explosion of information technology, there is still a significant minority with such views. These people may well be confused and in some instances made indignant by nurses who encourage them actively to participate in and accept responsibility for their own care and therapy.

Orem (1991) describes self-care as: 'care that is performed by oneself for oneself when one has reached a state of maturity that is enabling for consistent, controlled, effective, and purposeful action'.

It is learned behaviour, aided by intellectual curiosity, instruction and supervision from others and experience in performing self-care measures. Nurses who accept the concept of self-care as a basis for practice consequently value the patient's right to be regarded as an individual with unique needs, and the ability to meet their own self-care needs. If one thinks about this carefully, it becomes apparent that promoting self-care is indeed a radical approach to health care. It means that instead of telling patients or clients what to do, and doing things for them, the nurse actually works towards enabling them to make decisions and do things for themselves except when this is impossible. Norris (1979) points out that the structures of the health service are sometimes obstacles to self-care.

The hospital environment itself may be hostile to the goal of reducing patient dependency; nurses dispensing medication by dose and physicians refusing to provide medical records to patients are examples (Norris, 1979).

Some may comment that these examples are dated now, since the introduction of self-medication schemes and the 'Freedom of Information' Act have increased the opportunities for patients to participate in their care and treatment. However, readers are challenged to consider in how many hospitals and health care institutions patients/clients are allowed access to their own medications or encouraged to hold or read their medical or nursing records.

Predictably, some opposition towards promoting self-care is voiced. One political view sees self-care as a way of pushing responsibility for care back on individuals themselves in an attempt to reduce the need for state provision. Advocates for self-care counter this argument by suggesting that, in fact, the self-care model actually requires as much state resources as the traditional health-care system – but that such provisions be used differently. Professionally, handing back enough knowledge to allow informed decision-making by the patient threatens the health care professionals themselves, and Levin *et al.* (1979) say that 'resistance by some health professionals to increased employment of self-care modes is to be expected'.

One feminist writer (Webster, 1991) cautions that dependent care involves the help of family and relatives. In most cases, family and relatives mean women. This shift in responsibility may be regarded as another burden for the already over-taxed women carers in our society. The resources and support required for carers in the community are an example of how self-care means a shift in resources rather than a reduction in expenditure on health care. Webster (1991) criticises the self-care theorists for concentrating too much on the responsibilities of the individual within society and not enough upon the social structures that contribute to health.

On the other hand, some customers or potential patients logically argue that when the responsibility for healthy living and health care is vested in the individual and not the professional, the hoped-for healthy society is more likely to become part of our reality. There is a rising realisation among American nurses of the enormous potential of developing the self-care concept in nursing. Mullin (1981) described Orem's self-care nursing model as 'the most liberating and dynamic idea that has been introduced into the practice of medical/surgical nursing for at least 20 years', and proposed that it heralded positive and profound reform in nursing practice. The reforms that have occurred could perhaps be related more accurately to technological advances and a shorter length of stay than an ideological shift. However, the changes have resulted in responsibility shifting to patients/consumers and there is evidence of self-care being adopted in many practice situations. Meleis (1991) comments that most of the literature relates to self-care as a guide to practice rather than addressing the knotty question of evaluation, such as whether it makes a significant difference in terms of outcomes.

BELIEFS AND VALUES

The person

The beliefs about humanity in the self-care model of nursing include all those discussed in the introductory chapters, but emphasis is placed on the notion that all individuals have self-care needs, and that they have the right and ability to meet these needs themselves, except when their ability is in some way compromised.

The person who meets the self-care needs is the self-care agent; in the normal, healthy, mature adult this agency is best vested in individuals themselves. However, the parent is the self-care agent for a newborn infant and the relative or nurse is the self-care agent for an unconscious person. Joseph (1980) has presented six basic premises on which the self-care model for nursing is founded, and these in themselves summarise the view of people in relation to self-care.

1. Self-care is based on voluntary actions that humans are capable of undertaking.
2. Self-care is based on deliberate and thoughtful judgement that leads to appropriate acts.
3. Self-care is required of every person and is a universal requisite for meeting basic human needs.
4. Adults have the right and responsibility to care for themselves in order to maintain their health, life and well-being. Sometimes they may have these responsibilities for others as well, including the children and elderly in a family.
5. Self-care is behaviour that evolves through a combination of social and cognitive experience and is learned through one's interpersonal relationships, communications and culture.
6. Self-care contributes to the self-esteem and self-image of a person and is directly affected by self-concept.

Some self-care needs, or in Orem's model self-care requisites, are universal. That is, they are common to all human beings and are associated with human functioning and life processes. Often referred to as 'basic human needs', the universal self-care requisites are:

- the maintenance of a sufficient intake of air
- the maintenance of a sufficient intake of water
- the maintenance of a sufficient intake of food
- the provision of care associated with elimination processes and excrements
- the maintenance of a balance between activity and rest
- the maintenance of a balance between solitude and social interaction
- the prevention of hazards to human life, human functioning and human well-being
- the promotion of human functioning and development within social groups in accordance with human potential, known human limitations and the human desire to be normal

Orem describes two further categories of self-care requisites that arise out of the influence of events on the universal self-care requisites.

Developmental self-care requisites

These occur according to the stage of development of the individual, and for the environment in which he or she lives, in terms of its effects on development. They are related either to life changes in the individual or lifecycle stages (see Figure 9.1).

Health deviation self-care requisites

These arise out of ill health and are needs which become apparent because illness or disability demands a change in self-care behaviour.

When there is a demand to care for oneself and the individual is able to meet that demand, self-care is possible. If, on the other hand, the demand is greater than the individual's capacity or ability to meet it, an imbalance occurs and this is called a self-care deficit (see Figure 9.2).

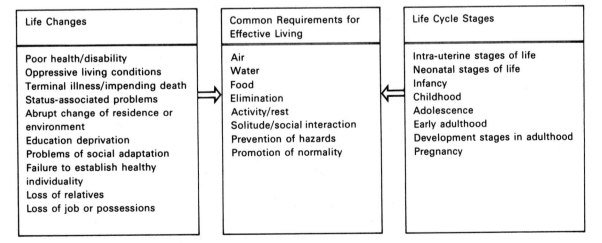

Life Changes	Common Requirements for Effective Living	Life Cycle Stages
Poor health/disability	Air	Intra-uterine stages of life
Oppressive living conditions	Water	Neonatal stages of life
Terminal illness/impending death	Food	Infancy
Status-associated problems	Elimination	Childhood
Abrupt change of residence or environment	Activity/rest	Adolescence
Education deprivation	Solitude/social interaction	Early adulthood
Problems of social adaptation	Prevention of hazards	Development stages in adulthood
Failure to establish healthy individuality	Promotion of normality	Pregnancy
Loss of relatives		
Loss of job or possessions		

Figure 9.1   Development influences on self-care in relation to the requirements for effective living (after Pearson and Vaughan, 1984). Source: Pearson A, Vaughan B 1984 Module 1: Nursing Practice and the Nursing Process. In: A Systematic Approach to Nursing Care – an introduction. Milton Keynes Open University, with permission.

Figure 9.2 Demand versus ability in self-care.

D = Demand
A = Ability to meet demand

The view of the individual within this model revolves around the fundamental belief that a need for self-care always exists and that ideally one has the right and ability to meet this need. When the self-care demand is greater than the individual's ability to meet it, the resulting self-care deficit needs to be met. With a newborn baby, the parent acts as the self-care agent and Orem calls this 'dependent care'. Dependent care is that which is given to someone by a relative, guardian or friend; that is, a meaningful other. If the self-care deficit creates a demand which is more than can be met by self-care and dependent care, nursing in one form or another is required.

Orem's consideration of infants and children is sketchy. However, she does refer to them and clearly her work is used in the paediatric sphere (While, 1991), where family involvement in care has long been an integral component of practice. Likewise, her consideration of psychiatric clients is cursory, yet the framework of concepts and theories accommodates the mental health client well, as demonstrated by Buckwalter and Kerfoot (1982) and Compton (1989). Orem (1991) states that her theory is a general one and pertains to all people who require a nursing service.

THE SELF-CARE MODEL FOR NURSING

Health

Orem's (1991) description of health is a state of personal integrity in terms of both function and structure. She relates this to a state of well-being in physical, social and psychological terms. A person's health status changes throughout the life span, and maintenance of heath is achieved through the process of self-care. Health is related to the individual's ability to self-care. When health is compromised interest is focused upon the effect this has upon the person's ability to self-care. The self-care theory concentrates predominantly on the person in a compromised health state although, as will be seen later in the chapter, the supportive educative nursing system is designed to ensure optimum independent well-being through actions that provide the client with health education and support.

Environment

The person and the environment are seen as systems that are in constant communication. The person adapts to the environment and uses technology in order to control it. The nurse needs to consider the patient's environment in terms of 'physical, chemical, biologic and social features' (Orem, 1991). Environmental conditions are significant and have both negative and positive effects on individuals, families and indeed communities. For example, a family atmosphere that is supportive and economically stable may be good for the health of its members, however a hurricane may have devastating effects on the health of a whole community.

THE GOALS OF NURSING

People require nursing when they, or their meaningful others, are unable to cope with self-care deficits occasioned by some health-related problem. In this case the nurse becomes a self-care agent, or as Orem (1985) terms it 'a nursing agency', for the patient and attempts to meet his or her self-care requisites. Following from her explanation of the person (p. 106), the goals for nursing logically appear, in Orem's (1985) theory, to be the meeting of self-care needs. This can be achieved by the following.

1. Reducing the self-care demand to a level which the patient or client is capable of meeting, that is, eliminating the self-care deficit.
2. Enabling the patients or clients to increase their ability to meet the self-care demand, and thus eliminating any self-care deficits.
3. Enabling the patient's or client's meaningful others to give dependent care when self-care is impossible, so that, again, any self-care deficits are eliminated.
4. When none of these can be achieved, by the nurse meeting the individual's self-care needs directly.

KNOWLEDGE AND SKILLS FOR PRACTICE

Nursing helps people to meet self-care needs by using one of three 'nursing systems', and through five 'helping methods'.

Nursing systems

Totally compensatory nursing system

In this system the nurse takes on responsibility for actually carrying out those activities which will meet self-care needs. For example, totally unconscious, acutely ill people will be unable to do many things for themselves and often relatives are unable to give the needed dependent care. Another example may be a dying patient/client who, whilst she or he and the family are able to meet physical needs, deliberately chooses to conserve her/his energies for communication and decides to allow the nurse to be the self-care agent in this area.

Partially compensatory nursing system

In this system the nurse is still needed to carry out some activities which contribute towards the meeting of self-care needs. However, the patient is able to meet some of the needs or a meaningful other can give dependent care. For example, elderly people living at home may be able to meet most of their self-care needs, but may receive some dependent care from their family, and need the help of a nurse to lift them in and out of the bath every week.

Educative/supportive nursing system

In this system patients are potentially capable of meeting self-care needs, and the nurse's activity relates to teaching and supporting them so that they will eventually be able to meet the self-care need. Alternatively, a relative or friend may be helped by a nurse to give dependent care to a person in need. For example, this approach may apply to the postoperative patient discharged home with a new colostomy who is physically capable of coping with the stoma appliances but who still needs information and advice regarding some changes in lifestyle.

Nurses help patients using a nursing system, and through five helping methods:

- acting for or doing for the patient/client
- teaching the patient/client
- guiding the patient/client
- supporting the patient/client
- providing an environment in which the patient/client can develop and grow

To do all this, five main areas for nursing practice are described.

1. Entering into and maintaining nurse–patient relationships with individuals, families or groups until patients can be legitimately discharged from nursing.
2. Determining if and how patients can be helped through nursing.
3. Responding to patients' requests, desires and needs for contact with the nurse and for assistance.
4. Prescribing, providing and regulating direct help to patients and their families and friends in the form of nursing.
5. Coordinating and integrating nursing with the patient's daily living, with other health care needed or being received, and with social and educational services needed or being received.

Given the view of the patient/client encompassed in this model, and the way nursing is delivered, it can be seen that a broad knowledge base is required if the goals of the model are to be achieved. The competent nurse needs knowledge about individuals and each self-care requisite; knowledge and skills related to identifying self-care deficits, prescribing and giving direct care when necessary; and appropriate knowledge, skills and attitudes to enable the nurse to work through the five helping methods.

ASSESSMENT USING THE SELF-CARE MODEL

Assessment from the self-care perspective focuses on the three categories of self-care requisites and aims at identifying self-care deficits. Following assessment, the nurse proceeds to work together with the patient and the family in planning strategies that will eliminate the deficit by either reducing the self-care demand, increasing the patient's ability to meet the demand, enabling a meaningful other to give dependent care or meeting the self-care demand directly.

The aim of assessment is to establish the individual's self-care needs and to identify whether or not there are any self-care deficits (see Figure 9.3). The three groups of self-care requisites can be used as a framework to guide assessment.

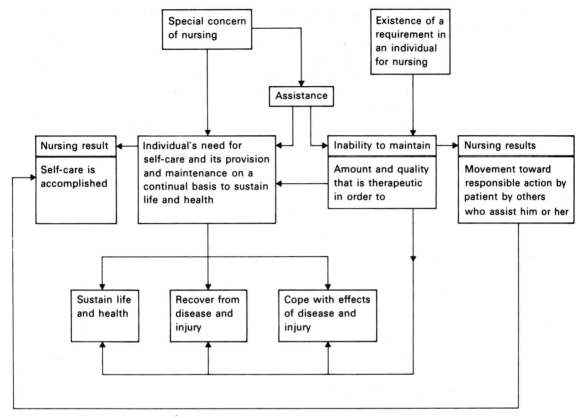

Figure 9.3 A diagrammatic representation of Orem's self-care model (after NDCG, 1973). Source: Nursing Development Conference Group (1973) Concept Formulization in Nursing. Boston: Little Brown & Co.

Universal self-care requisites

Using observation, measurement and dialogue between the patient and the nurse, normal patterns for the individual related to each of the universal requisites are discovered and any inabilities to perform self-care are identified and analysed. For example, during assessment of Mr Smith the nurse may note signs of weight loss in the patient such as clothes which are too big and loose abdominal skin. The patient himself may tell the nurse that because of the arthritis in his hands he is no longer able to prepare his own food and has to rely on assistance from the home help and the Meals-on-Wheels service for cooked meals. In the past, food preparation has always stimulated his appetite. Weighing the patient shows a loss of 5 kg.

Thus the assessment shows a self-care deficit in relation to the maintenance of sufficient intake of food which gives rise to the need for nursing action. Currently the home help and Meals-on-Wheels service are acting as 'self-care agents' and giving dependent care, but it may be possible through nursing to help the patient to meet his own demand and remove the self-care deficit.

Developmental self-care requisites

(In the same way, the nurse and patient together identify changes in the patient's lifestyle or lifecycle and the developmental needs which arise from these.) For example, the growing disability experienced through progressive rheumatoid arthritis leads to a need for acknowledgement on the patient's part that changes in lifestyle are needed. The patient also needs to acquire knowledge and skills to perform self-care acts in a different way and to modify the environment in order to develop new approaches to such acts.

Health deviation self-care requisites

Observations of behaviour that may lead to illness and the effects of illness and disease on the individual are considered in this part of the assessment. In this case, where a patient is suffering from rheumatoid arthritis, there may be a range of requisites that need consideration, such as taking appropriate medications and understanding their actions and side actions, taking a planned diet or supporting affected joints with splints. The organisation of the recording of the information gathered during assessment can be structured around the three areas of self-care requisites devised by Orem. Figure 9.4 is an example of such a form that was developed by a team of nurses working on a 36-bedded ward.

CARE PLANNING

Once the self-care deficits have been identified from the assessment they can be used as the problem statements on the care plan. The goals established between the nurse and the patient when focusing on self-care must relate realistically to those employed in the model, namely the following.

- To reduce self-care demand to a level which the patient/client is capable of meeting, for example arranging for a patient/client with pneumonia to rest in bed in order to decrease the demand for oxygen.
- To enable the patient/client to increase his or her ability to meet the self-care demand, for example providing facilities on a ward for a patient with a kidney stone to make whatever drinks s/he requires to maintain a fluid intake of at least 3 litres a day.
- To enable the patient's relatives or supporters to give dependent care when self-care is impossible, for example showing a husband how to help and tempt his wife to eat following a stroke.
- To meet the patient's self-care needs directly through nursing when none of the other three alternatives is realistic, for example, giving oral toilet to an unconscious patient.

Thus the overriding goal of this model is the elimination of self-care deficits. Orem (1980) recommends that both the problem statement and the goal statement should be formulated in such a way as to describe an observable behaviour or measurable entity to allow for evaluation. Box 9.1 shows how Mr Smith's problem would be recorded using this model.

In this example, nursing has aimed at increasing Mr Smith's own ability to meet the self-care demand through the nurse taking an educative/supportive role. Often, of course, this will not be realistic and

NAME: D.O.B.   M.S.W.   NOK: OTHER PERSONS   WHO IS TO BE
                                                          IMPORTANT TO   CONTACTED IN
ADDRESS: PATIENT   EMERGENCY
Prefers to be addressed
as:

Tel: ASSESSMENT – OF SELF-CARE DEFICITS

DOCTOR: 1. HEALTH DEVIATION SELF CARE REQUISITES   2. UNIVERSAL SELF CARE REQUISITES

PRIMARY NURSE: MEDICAL INFORMATION   BASE LINE FUNCTIONS

REASON FOR   RELEVANT PAST MEDICAL HISTORY   Rate   Rhythm   Cough
ADMISSION
                                                                 Breathing
                                                                 Circulation
                     MEDICAL DIAGNOSIS   Pulse Rate   Rhythm   B/P

                     DRUGS TAKEN AT HOME
                                                                 Colour   Skin Lips;
                     ALLERGIES

PATIENT'S   PATIENT'S FEELINGS & EXPECTATIONS   TEMPERATURE   WEIGHT
UNDERSTANDING OF   RELATED TO PRESENT ILLNESS   USUAL PATTERNS CONCERNING DAILY
ADMISSION   FLUID INTAKE

                                                                 ORAL   cc/mm
                                                                 LIKES
                     NURSE'S INITIAL IMPRESSION   DISLIKES
                     PHYSICAL AND SOCIAL   FOOD INTAKE – TYPE, TIME, REGULAR
                                                                 APPETITE, LIKES DISLIKES
FAMILY'S
UNDERSTANDING OF
ADMISSION

                     KNOWLEDGE/INFORMATION/SKILLS NEEDED   SPECIAL DIET (WHY?)
                     FOR CONTINUED SELF-CARE AFTER DISCHARGE   IS PATIENT THIN/OBESE/NORMAL
SOURCE OF ASSESSMENT   Teeth
                                                                 Mouth
SERVICES PROVIDED BEFORE
ADMISSION/SERVICES AFTER
DISCHARGE   HEALTH VISITOR –   SOCIAL WORKER –   HOME HELP –
DISTRICT NURSE –   MEALS ON WHEELS –   ANY OTHER –
CARE ASSISTANT –

Figure 9.4   The assessment form.

UNIVERSAL SELF-CARE REQUISITES CONT'D

ELIMINATION: CONTINENCE, FREQUENCY, TIMING, COLOUR, AMOUNT, REGULARITY, AIDS NEEDED.

URINE

FAECES

URINALYSIS

CONDITION OF SKIN, NAILS AND HAIR

USUAL PATTERNS OF HYGIENE

SLEEP AND REST, BEDTIME ROUTINE AIDS TO SLEEP

DAILY ACTIVITIES, RECREATION & BODY MOVEMENT

PERSONAL CHARACTERISTICS

BIOLOGICAL RHYTHM BEST TIME/WORST TIME OF DAY

WHAT PATIENT IS ABLE TO DO HIS/HERSELF, WANTS TO DO WITHOUT HELP

WHAT PATIENT WOULD EVENTUALLY LIKE TO DO INDEPENDENTLY

SELF-CONCEPT: BODY IMAGE AND SELF ESTEEM

PAINS OR OTHER SENSATIONS

BALANCE BETWEEN SOLITUDE AND SOCIALISING

COMMUNICATION

FAMILY, FRIENDS, RELATIONSHIPS AND RESPONSIBILITIES

SEXUALITY: INFORMATION ABOUT MARITAL STATUS, RELATIONSHIPS

OCCUPATION AND LIVING ACCOMMODATION

DEVELOPMENTAL SELF-CARE REQUISITES: NOTE THE MAJOR LIFE CHANGES, DEVIATION FROM GROWTH AND DEVELOPMENT NORMS: HOW THE PATIENT COPES WITH THEM, WHAT OR WHO HELPS HIM/HER (CULTURE, RELIGION, BELIEFS, VALUES)

Figure 9.4 The assessment form (cont.).

Box 9.1   The problem and goal statement

Problem (i.e. self-care deficit)	Goal (i.e. outcome which will indicate elimination of self-care deficit)
Inability to cook own food because of loss of fine movement in hands	Will be able to prepare a cooked meal of his own choice without help

other options will have to be selected. Of course, it may be the case that Mr Smith's other problems are such that the nurse will choose other nursing systems when planning care with him.

Evaluation of the care can be undertaken by comparing behaviour described in the problem statement with that described in the goal statement. In this case, the patient's initial behaviour was that he could not cook a meal; the goal was that he would be able to perform this action and at evaluation evidence of his ability to do so should be sought.

During the period between the initial assessment and the final assessment of the goal, continuous evaluation revolves around the degree of movement towards or away from the final goal. It may be necessary to modify the nursing action prescribed if movement towards the final goal is not being achieved.

The nursing action is written in a clear and unambiguous way and describes the type of act which the nurse will perform using one or more of the five helping methods:

- acting for
- teaching
- guiding
- supporting
- providing a suitable environment

The nurse's choice of action is influenced by the cause of the deficit. Orem (1991) identifies three types of causes of self-care deficits or problems; in this list they are related to the example of Mr Smith.

- Limited behaviour – loss of fine movement.
- Attitude – loss of motivation to eat which was stimulated previously by the process of cooking.
- Lack of knowledge – unaware of the range of utensils available and the foods essential for health and weight maintenance.

Evaluation

If it becomes apparent that there is no progress in Mr Smith's ability to prepare meals, the plan may need to be revised. For example, it could be changed from aiming to enable him to meet his own self-care needs to aiming to assist the home help in acting as the self-care agent, but still

Box 9.2   The nursing action

Nursing action (i.e. The act that the nurse will perform to lead to the elimination of the self-care deficit)	Type of nursing action
1. Refer to OT for	
a. provision of apparatus	Guiding
b. teaching the use of the aids	
2. Discuss possibility of weekly menus and drawing up menu plan	Teaching
3. Weight weekly on Friday at 9 a.m. in pyjamas	Supporting

including him in the planning and preparing of food. If, however, he succeeds in gaining the requisite skills, the self-care deficit will have been eliminated.

A PATIENT CARE STUDY

Graham Thompson is a 20-year-old man admitted to the trauma ward following a road traffic accident where he had sustained a fracture of the left femur. Since he was both physically shocked and in some degree of pain when first admitted, the full assessment was spread over 2 days using information obtained by both his primary nurse and the associate nurses involved in his care. The biographical information was recorded as well as the assessment of self-care abilities. Deficits in self-care were recognised by the nurse who systematically assessed all of the self-care requisites identified in the model. Figure 9.5 shows the recordings made during his assessment. From this information the nurse was able to identify Graham's deficits in self-care and thus formulate the care plan.

In this case a deviation in the health care demands, that is the fractured femur he had sustained, led to a deficit in Graham's self-care ability in meeting his universal needs, his development needs and his health deviation needs, as shown on the care plan in Figure 9.6.

The focus of the care plan was on teaching Graham to meet as many of his own self-care needs as possible, and only acting for him when there was no other alternative. For example, in relation to his restricted mobility, the nurse's actions concentrated on teaching him the need for movement and methods he could use to help himself, rather than changing Graham's position for him or acting on his behalf.

Health deviation requisites are also recognised. For example, in problems 6 and 7 on the care plan, a lack of knowledge about his own health and the risk of a recurrence of the incident which had led to his admission were identified as problems. In order to help Graham take care of his own health, the nurse's actions emphasised teaching him about his condition and the maintenance of health. his own health, the nurse's

NAME: *Graham Thompson*   D.O.B. *1.12.76*   M.S.W.   NOK: *Father*
Same address and phone

ADDRESS: *12 The Gassens*   Prefers to be addressed   OTHER PERSONS   WHO IS TO BE
Highview, Morpeth   as: *Graham*   IMPORTANT TO   CONTACTED IN
    PATIENT   EMERGENCY
    Girlfriend   *Father*
    May Prew

Tel: *Morpeth 76815*   ASSESSMENT – OF SELF-CARE DEFICITS

DOCTOR: *Dr AT Robinson*   1. HEALTH DEVIATION SELF CARE REQUISITES   2. UNIVERSAL SELF CARE REQUISITES

PRIMARY NURSE: MEDICAL INFORMATION   BASE LINE FUNCTIONS
Paul Peterson

REASON FOR ADMISSION   RELEVANT PAST MEDICAL HISTORY | | Rate | Rhythm | Cough |
Emergency admission   *Broken nose 2 years ago* | Breathing | 20 | Reg. | None |
following crash. Riding | Circulation | Toes – pink and warm |
motorbike. Skidded and   MEDICAL DIAGNOSIS *Fractured left femur* | | Rate | Rhythm | B/P |
hit lamppost. Fractured | Pulse Rate | 76 | Reg. | 120/70 |
left femur and multiple   DRUGS TAKEN AT HOME   *None*
abrasions to left arm.   Colour   Skin Lips:
PATIENT'S UNDERSTANDING OF   ALLERGIES   *None*   *Nailbeds and extremities – pink.*
ADMISSION   TEMPERATURE *38°C*   WEIGHT *lost 3/6*
"Can't remember much –   PATIENT'S FEELINGS & EXPECTATIONS   USUAL PATTERNS CONCERNING DAILY
I have a broken thigh   RELATED TO PRESENT ILLNESS   FLUID INTAKE
bone which will take   *Glad he is not worse – expects to*   ORAL *2500* cc/mm
about 3 months to knit   *be back to normal in about 4 months.*   LIKES *Tea, coffee, lemonade, bitter*
together."   *Expects to get bored.*   DISLIKES *Milk*
FAMILY'S UNDERSTANDING OF   NURSE'S INITIAL IMPRESSION   FOOD INTAKE – TYPE, TIME, REGULAR
ADMISSION   PHYSICAL AND SOCIAL   APPETITE, LIKES DISLIKES
"Broken leg, but every-   *Physically "fit" – has lots of friends.*   *Cooked breakfast – fried eggs*
thing else is alright."   *Says "I'll enjoy myself in here, even*   *Lunch – sandwiches*
    if it kills me.   *Dinner – meat & vegetables*
SOURCE OF ASSESSMENT *Graham*   KNOWLEDGE/INFORMATION/SKILLS NEEDED   SPECIAL DIET (WHY?) *No*
    FOR CONTINUED SELF-CARE AFTER DISCHARGE   IS PATIENT THIN/OBESE/NORMAL
SERVICES PROVIDED BEFORE   *1. Healing process of bone.*   Teeth *Own*
ADMISSION/SERVICES AFTER   *2. Exercises to maintain muscles.*   Mouth *clean, moist*
DISCHARGE   *3. Road safety.*
DISTRICT NURSE –   SOCIAL WORKER –   HOME HELP –
CARE ASSISTANT –   HEALTH VISITOR –   ANY OTHER –
    MEALS ON WHEELS –

Figure 9.5   The assessment.

UNIVERSAL SELF-CARE REQUISITES CONT'D

ELIMINATION: CONTINENCE, FREQUENCY, TIMING. COLOUR, AMOUNT, REGULARITY, AIDS NEEDED.

URINE

Says it's normal. Dislikes using urinal in bed.

FAECES

Opens bowels, usually daily, in evening.

URINALYSIS

No abnormalities

CONDITION OF SKIN, NAILS AND HAIR

Skin - healthy. Left arm lacerated. Tullle gras and crepe bandage applied in A+E from wrist to shoulder.

Nails - short + clean. Hair on collar. Washes it daily. Dries it with a hair drier.

USUAL PATTERNS OF HYGIENE

Bath - every week day on return from work. Doesn't usually bathe at weekend except if "going somewhere special".

SLEEP AND REST, BEDTIME ROUTINE AIDS TO SLEEP

Goes to bed about midnight. Up at 7 a.m. Mon - Fri, 10-11 a.m. weekends. Goes to sleep "as soon as head touches pillow".

DAILY ACTIVITIES, RECREATION & BODY MOVEMENT

Swims weekly. Football training 2 x week. Pub most nights with mates + girlfriend.

PERSONAL CHARACTERISTICS

BIOLOGICAL RHYTHM BEST TIME/WORST TIME OF DAY

"Hopeless and bad tempered in morning and late at night."

WHAT PATIENT IS ABLE TO DO HIS/HERSELF, WANTS TO DO WITHOUT HELP

Usually independent. While on Thomas Splint he needs all equipment brought to him. Can do everything himself.

WHAT PATIENT WOULD EVENTUALLY LIKE TO DO INDEPENDENTLY

"Everything"

SELF-CONCEPT: BODY IMAGE AND SELF ESTEEM

Appears to have high self esteem and sees himself as "a good looking bloke with a gammy leg."

PAINS OR OTHER SENSATIONS

Cramp in left foot. Otherwise no pain.

BALANCE BETWEEN SOLITUDE AND SOCIALISING

Likes to be with people most of the time. Some privacy when with girlfriend.

COMMUNICATION

Talks easily to people.

FAMILY, FRIENDS, RELATIONSHIPS AND RESPONSIBILITIES

Close to father. Dislikes sister. "Mum is okay." Lives with family.

SEXUALITY: INFORMATION ABOUT MARITAL STATUS, RELATIONSHIPS

Has had same girlfriend for 3 years. She is very important to him. Saving to get married.

OCCUPATION AND LIVING ACCOMMODATION Apprentice plumber - Morpeth District Council. Lives in 3 bedroomed house with upstairs toilet.

DEVELOPMENTAL SELF-CARE REQUISITES: NOTE THE MAJOR LIFE CHANGES, DEVIATION FROM GROWTH AND DEVELOPMENT NORMS: HOW THE PATIENT COPES WITH THEM, WHAT OR WHO HELPS HIM/HER (CULTURE, RELIGION, BELIEFS, VALUES) Wants "own place" as soon as he can marry - and to continue to develop relationship with Mary.

Figure 9.5 The assessment. (cont.).

DATE	NO.	PROBLEM	GOAL	NURSING ACTION	REVIEW DATE
	1.	Immobility due to fractured femur + pressure of Thomas splint leading to potential problems of –			
	a.	Breakdown of skin due to pressure + friction.	Intact, unreddened pressure areas.	Explain risks fully. To lift himself off bed using monkey pole for at least 2 min. every hour when awake. Check elbows, heels, sacrum and spinous pro-cesses daily at bedmaking. Apply oil to splint ring at 10 a.m. + 6 p.m.	
	b.	Wasting of quadri-ceps. Thigh girth = 52 cm.	Thigh girth not to fall below 50 cm.	Teach static quadriceps exercises. To exercise and maintain ankle 20 times/hour when awake. Mea-sure thigh at 10 a.m. on Mon. + Thurs.	
NAME			NO.	PRIMARY NURSE	

Figure 9.6   The care plan.

DATE	NO.	PROBLEM	GOAL	NURSING ACTION	REVIEW DATE
	c.	Deep vein thrombosis.	Calf soft and toes pink + warm.	Check calf and circulation to toes at bedmaking time.	
	d.	Constipation.	Daily bowel action.	Vegetables at main meal daily. Record bowel action. If none for 3 days, give aperients as charted.	
	2.	Inability to meet own toilet needs due to immobility.	Can pass urine and faeces when desired.	Leave urinal within easy reach. Give bedpan on request and screen bed. Is able to lift on and off without help. Leave air freshner on locker top.	
	3.	may become bored with restricted activities.	Will say he is reasonably occupied.	Suggest that family provides TV and tape recorder with ear attachment.	
NAME			NO.	PRIMARY NURSE	

Figure 9.6   The care plan *(cont.)*.

DATE	NO.	PROBLEM	GOAL	NURSING ACTION	REVIEW DATE
	4.	Cramp in left foot.	Any cramp will be relieved in 5 minutes.	Teach ankle exercises to be carried out when cramp occurs. (To circle ankle in full range of movement.) Massage foot when requested.	
	5.	May feel isolated from friends or a lack of privacy.	Will maintain contact with friends. Will have privacy when required.	Encourage friends to visit. Screen bed if desired when girlfriend visits.	
	6.	Lack of knowledge about condition.	Will be able to describe healing process of bone and process of muscle wasting when asked.	Teach, using diagrams – a. structure + healing process of bone. b. structure and function of muscle.	
	7.	Similar injury may occur.	Will not be involved in a similar accident in future.	Teach road safety rules. Give pamphet on road safety to read.	

NAME		NO.	PRIMARY NURSE	

Figure 9.6   The care plan (cont.).

actions emphasised teaching him about his condition and the maintenance of health.

In terms of developmental self-care requisites, the nurse recognised that Graham's injury had interrupted his normal lifestyle and prevented him from interacting with peers. The reaction he may have experienced from his friends and the lack of privacy for maintaining important relationships were taken into account in problem 5. Throughout the descriptions of Graham's care, the issue of encouraging him to function on his own behalf in health promotion, prevention and treatment was highlighted, since that is the central focus of the model.

Learning exercises

1. Prepare a two-minute debate arguing for the use of Orem's Self-Care Model in the Intensive Care Unit.
2. Select one of the patients you are currently looking after. Look in the notes and identify the patient's self care deficits.

Study questions

1. Write notes on the behaviours and things that might be observed in an area that uses the Orem Self-Care Model in practice.

Chapter 10

An Adaptation Model for Nursing

LEARNING OBJECTIVES

On completion of this chapter, the reader will be able to:

1. Assess clients to identify actual and potential behaviours that are maladaptive or inappropriate
2. Discuss the degree to which the model embraces ideals of humanism and holism
3. Recognise the potential of behaviours that are adaptive
4. Write a care plan that emphasises positive adaptation

The model for nursing described by Sister Callista Roy was developed in America throughout the 1960s and first put into use in a university nursing programme in California in 1970. Roy has been a prolific writer contributing to nursing literature in journals, conference proceedings and books. The model is described in her book *Introduction to Nursing: An Adaptation Model* published in 1976 with a second edition in 1984. In 1986 she combined with Andrews to write *Essentials of the Roy Adaptation Model*, and again in 1999 (Roy and Andrews, 1999) to focus particularly on humanism and veritivity – the common good, human meaning and the value of spirituality.

Throughout the years Roy has refined and developed the theory, progressively addressing and incorporating a humanistic and holistic view of the person. Evidence of Sister Roy's theological background is obvious in the constructs underlying the model. The influences of science and philosophy are reflected in the reconfigured philosophical and scientific assumptions for the model. The philosophical assumptions concentrate on the power of human meaning and person centred values.

Philosophical assumptions for the twenty-first century (Roy, 1997, p. 45)

1. Persons have mutual relationships with the world and with a God-figure.
2. Human meaning is rooted in an omega point convergence of the universe.
3. God is intimately revealed in the diversity of creation and is the common destiny of creation.
4. Persons use human creative abilities of awareness, enlightenment and faith.
5. Persons are accountable for the processes of deriving, sustaining and transforming the universe.

The scientific assumptions underpin the notion of adapation. They include modern ideas from systems theory and have been related to the '... ideas and language of cosmologists who look at evolution of the known universe' (Roy, 1997, p. 44).

Scientific assumptions for the twenty-first century

1. Systems of matter and energy progress to higher levels of complex self-organisation.
2. Consciousness and meaning are constitutive of person and environment integration.
3. Awareness of self and environment is rooted in thinking and feeling.
4. Human decisions are accountable for the integration of creative processes.
5. Thinking and feeling mediate human action.
6. System relationships include acceptance, protection and fostering of interdependence.
7. Persons and the earth have common patterns and integral relations.
8. Person and environment transformations are created in human consciousness.
9. Integration of human and environment means results in adaptation.

The model has been used in practice, as a framework for nursing and in particular as a theoretical framework for research (e.g. Jirovec et al., 1999 in a study to develop a urine control theory). Chiou (2000) has more recently undertaken a meta-analysis of the interrelationships between the modes in Roy's adaptation model. Considering the criticism that models generally are under-tested, this work is laudable.

The model is largely based on systems theory, although account is taken of some thoughts from interactionist theory. Roy related adaptation level theory, from the field of psychophysics, to the world of nursing. She drew on practice by classifying patient behaviours as they were described to her by nurses (Malinski, 2000). The view from which the model has been developed is of the individual, as a whole system, responding or adapting to changes or stimuli. These stimuli are within the individual or in the surrounding environment.

In her work Roy states the assumptions or beliefs on which the model is based, the goals she sees nurses trying to achieve and the knowledge they require in order to do so. In describing how the model may be put into use, she uses a problem-solving approach recommending a guide for assessment, problem identification, the setting of goals, and the planning, implementation and evaluation of care. She also gives some guidance on the setting of priorities. Her rationale for using this model is that it both enhances a client-centred nursing approach and supports the idea of professional accountability for nursing as a scientific, service-oriented discipline.

BELIEFS AND VALUES

Roy (1976) points out that the beliefs on which this model is based may not be scientifically proven but are generally accepted as being true.

The person

In her theory, Roy views people as individuals who are in constant interaction with the environment. Rambo (1984) describes a set of assumptions, an understanding of which is the key to the remainder of the model. These assumptions include the following.

1. Each person is seen as an integrated whole, with biological, psychological and social components and in constant interaction with the surrounding environment.
2. In order to maintain homeostasis or integrity, people must respond or adapt to any changes that occur, either from internal or external stimuli. Roy refers to two subsystems of adaptation, the regulator and cognator mechanisms. The regulator system refers to the reflex physiological regulatory systems such as the endocrine and the autonomic nervous system. The cognator system refers to thoughtful responses to stimuli.
3. Environment: all circumstances, conditions or changes which challenge the person as an adaptive system are considered as 'the environment'. These stimuli affect people's behaviour or development. The person is seen to be in constant interaction with the continuously changing environment. Both internal and external factors are identified as stimuli and they are categorised into three groups.

   - *Focal*: Those things that immediately affect them, such as a chest infection, a bereavement or a new baby.
   - *Contextual*: All the other stimuli present at the time which may influence a negative response to the focal stimulus, such as anaemia, poor housing or social isolation. They are the surrounding circumstances.
   - *Residual*: These are the beliefs, attitudes and traits of an individual, developed from the past but affecting the current response. For instance, one person's upbringing may teach him or her to tolerate low back pain without complaint, while another person might consider it abnormal and require treatment for it.

4. Every person has what is known as an individual adaptation zone that is concerned with his or her capacity to respond to stimuli. Provided that all the stimuli that affect an individual fall within that zone, the responses s/he makes to them will maintain that person's integrity and are seen as adaptive or positive. If, however, the stimuli are too great, the adaptations made in response will not be able to maintain integrity and are seen as maladaptive or negative. The size of an individual's adaptive zone varies from person to person. For instance, under the pressure of pending examinations, one individual may adapt by following a pre-planned revision schedule. This response is a positive adaptation within the personal zone. Another person may respond by sleeplessness, poor concentration and loss of appetite; a negative adaptation outside his or her personal zone.

5. All people have certain needs that they endeavour to meet in order to maintain integrity. Roy divides these needs into four different modes:

   - *Physiological* – associated with the structure of the body and the way it functions.
   - *Self-concept* – concerned with the way one perceives oneself, with mental activity and with the expression of feelings.
   - *Role function* – concerned with the psychosocial wholeness in fulfilling one's own role and society's expectations of various roles.
   - *Interdependence* – the balance between dependence on others and independence in achieving things for oneself.

6. Health: an individual's ability to remain healthy is dependent on having sufficient energy and ability to make positive adaptations to stimuli. Illness occurs when the responses made fall outside an individual's adaptation zone either because there is insufficient energy or the stimulus is too great. Health and illness are seen as lying on a continuum, and movement along this continuum is an inevitable part of life.

Some of the terms which Roy uses to describe the assumptions or beliefs of this model may not be familiar and may require two or three readings before they can be used with ease. Nevertheless, they are worth pursuing since, once mastered, they provide a meaningful base on which to build a model for practice. A word of warning should be proffered here though. Whilst nurses are capable of learning the exact meaning of these terms it is unlikely that all patients or clients will wish to study the syntax of the theory in quite the same way. Some may be surprised that their behaviour is termed 'maladaptive' and feel they are excluded from participating in care which is defined with such unfamiliar words. It could be suggested that whilst these words may convey precise meanings they do not necessarily communicate an ethos of caring concern.

THE GOALS OF NURSING

In Roy's view the purpose of nursing is to help people to adapt to stimuli in any of the four categories identified in order to help them free energy to respond to other stimuli. She suggests that a goal statement should include the behaviour that is to be changed and the direction of the change. She also emphasises that since it is the behaviour of the patient or client that is to be changed, he or she must be involved in identifying goals whenever possible. If Roy's assumptions are to be believed, then human behaviour is constantly directed towards an attempt to maintain integrity or homeostasis. In many instances, whether or not this has been achieved can be judged by a knowledge of norms. Such knowledge can also be used to help patients to identify their own goals.

It must, however, be pointed out that norms are only guidelines and may vary among individuals or in different societies. For instance, while some physiological norms are fairly constant for all people, such as the levels of potassium in the blood, others may vary widely, such as the frequency of elimination. Similarly, what is a socially acceptable way of behaving in one society may be unacceptable in another.

To summarise the goals of nursing according to Roy's model, they are:

- related to achieving adaptive responses in the physiological, self-concept, role function and interdependence modes
- stated in behavioural terms
- guided by a knowledge of 'norms'
- planned in conjunction with the patient

KNOWLEDGE AND SKILLS FOR PRACTICE

The knowledge base on which Roy's model is built obviously relates to her views about people and the goals of nursing. It can be divided into four main sections, associated with the four adaptive modes, namely the physiological, self-concept, role function and interdependence modes, each one derived from the theory of disciplines allied to nursing.

Roy examines the person in terms of parts. This reduction of the whole to parts for study is the traditional method employed for objective study. A view of holism described by Kramer (1990) is that the person cannot be regarded as an object composed of independently understandable parts; literally the whole is more than a conglomeration of its parts. While Roy believes in the holistic nature of people, particularly in her later work (Andrews and Roy, 1986; Roy and Andrews, 1999), she still exploits the old tradition of reduction to understand and explain human beings when appropriate.

Physical mode

Roy identifies six basic physiological needs that have to be met in order to maintain integrity:

- exercise and rest
- nutrition
- elimination
- fluid and electrolytes
- oxygenation and circulation
- regulation of temperature, senses and the endocrine system

In each area it is necessary to have knowledge of body structure and function, the standards or ranges which are accepted as normal, the stresses which can affect them, and the sort of maladaptive behaviour which may occur.

Self-concept

As Rambo (1984) points out, self-concept is a difficult thing to explain, but when related to adaptation nursing it 'consists of feelings and beliefs that permit an individual to know who he or she is and feel that the self is adequate in meeting needs and desires'.

Broadly, self-concept is divided into two parts. The physical self concerns how people actually perceive themselves in relation to their feelings, sensations, appearance and body image. Difficulties in this area are often experienced as a feeling of loss, such as might occur following mutilating surgery, or even the perceived loss of sexual ability following myocardial infarction. The personal self concerns the consistency of personal standards and behaviours, ideals and moral/ethical issues. Feelings of anxiety, powerlessness or guilt may point towards difficulties in this area.

Role function

Roy (1976) describes role as 'the title given to the individual – mother, son, student, carpenter – as well as the behaviours that society expects an individual to perform in order to maintain the title'.

The idea of a 'role tree' has been used by Rambo (1984) to clarify the subject (see Figure 10.1). The trunk of the tree represents the primary, relatively consistent, predetermined role of an individual; it is related to

Figure 10.1   The role tree.

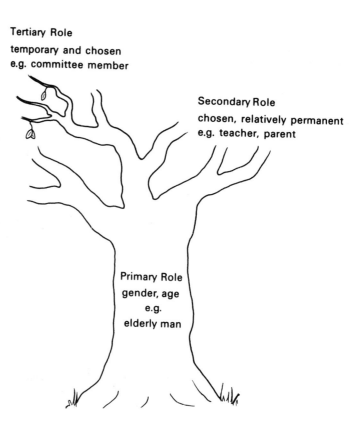

Tertiary Role
temporary and chosen
e.g. committee member

Secondary Role
chosen, relatively permanent
e.g. teacher, parent

Primary Role
gender, age
e.g.
elderly man

gender and age group, such as adolescent girl or elderly man. The branches represent the secondary roles that are relatively permanent, may be chosen, and are linked with stages of life such as parent, engineer, student or spouse. The leaves of the tree represent tertiary roles, which are usually temporary, freely chosen and relatively minor. Examples may include committee member, tennis player or club secretary.

It is often a sudden change in secondary roles that leads to difficulties, e.g. problems with a new job, a sudden bereavement or parenthood. Inability to master a role, conflict between two roles, or too many roles, are all things to be on the alert for as potentially problematic.

Interdependence

The final area of knowledge which is related to this model pertains to the mode of interdependence, the fine balance between dependence on others and independence. Dependence is demonstrated by a need for affiliation with others, for their care, support and approval. Independence is demonstrated by the ability to achieve, to make decisions and to initiate actions by oneself. Interdependence is seen as a balance between the two extremes of taking and giving, the ability to stand alone but not to be so fiercely independent that sharing with others becomes impossible. Figure 10.2 is a diagrammatic representation of Roy's adaptation model for nursing.

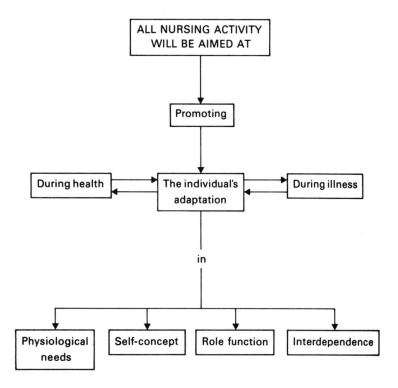

Figure 10.2   A diagrammatic representation of Roy's adaptation model (after NDCG, 1973). Source: Nursing Development Conference Group (1973) Concept Formulization in Nursing. Boston: Little Brown & Co.

ASSESSMENT USING AN ADAPTATION MODEL

The focus of this model is adaptation and the aim of assessment is twofold: to identify the actual and potential behaviours of the client which are seen as maladaptive or inappropriate, and to identify the stimuli or causes of the maladaptive behaviour.

The four adaptation modes can be used as the basic framework to guide assessment. To recap, these are the physiological, self-concept, role function and interdependence modes.

Roy recommends that assessment has two distinct parts. First level assessment is concerned with describing the current behaviour of the patient, while second level assessment is concerned with the factors or stimuli that have caused the behaviour.

First level assessment

This is the stage of the nursing process at which data are collected and a judgement is made as to whether the person's response to stressors is adaptive or maladaptive. Within each of the four modes, basic human needs are identified which can be affected by either deficits or excesses, for example, too little oxygen, too high a blood sugar or too much dependency. The nurse uses interview, observation and measurement skills to assess the current behaviour of the patient in each of the four modes and, based on this assessment, makes a tentative judgement as to whether the behaviour is adaptive, maladaptive or potentially maladaptive.

Second level assessment

This is the stage of assessment at which the cause of the behaviour is identified. It is an essential step since the nursing actions are based on the information gained. The stimuli affecting the patient's behaviour are identified in the three groups discussed earlier in this chapter, namely focal stimuli, contextual or surrounding stimuli, and residual stimuli. In some instances the focal stimulus of one of the patient's problems may be the contextual stimulus of another and this may initially lead to some confusion. For example, the focal stimulus of a problem of difficulty with breathing may be the presence of a chest infection and the contextual stimulus may be a broken leg causing restricted movement. However, the broken leg itself will be the focal stimulus or a direct cause of the behavioural problem of immobility (see Figure 10.3). However, as with any other assessment guide, the user overcomes this difficulty with ingenuity and common sense.

Information may be gathered from the patient, from friends or relatives, from other health care workers or from laboratory findings. Considering Mr Smith's assessment and his problem of weight loss, information was gathered from him about each of the four adaptive modes, using the adaptation framework.

Physiological

At first level assessment, the nurse may observe that Mr Smith appears thin and has loose fitting clothes. During the interview s/he may ascertain that his nutritional intake is low, that he has no appetite and that his weight has fallen by 5 kg. This will lead to the recognition that he has a behavioural problem which is maladaptive in relationship to his nutritional needs. Proceeding to second level assessment, the nurse will attempt to ascertain why the weight loss has occurred, since this will

Figure 10.3 A single stressor identified as both a focal and contextual stimulus.

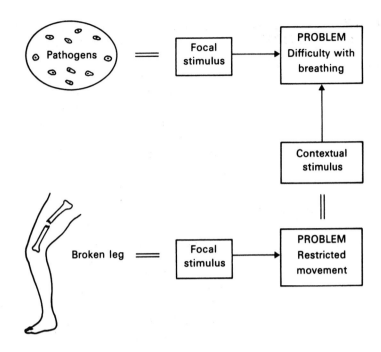

give him/her information about the focus of the nursing intervention. At this stage he/she may discover Mr Smith's inability to prepare his own food due to the limitations arising from his rheumatoid arthritis. This information is recorded as shown in Box 10.1.

Self-concept

During conversation the nurse may ascertain that Mr Smith has always enjoyed preparing his own meals and that his inability to do so at the moment has left a gap in his life. He describes feelings of loss about his ability to be able to cook for himself, which to him has always been important for developing an appetite for food. Using this information the nurse may perceive a problem related to self-concept, a feeling of loss of ability (see Box 10.2).

Role function

A secondary role function for Mr Smith has been that of cooking his own food, which is currently lost. The nurse observes that he has not been

---

Box 10.1   A care plan item – physiological

		Stimulus	
Patient behaviour	Focal	Contextual	Residual
Loss of 5 kg in weight over last 3 months	Inability to prepare own food	Loss of fine hand movement due to rheumatoid arthritis	

Box 10.2   A care plan item – self-concept

Patient behaviour	Stimulus		
	Focal	Contextual	Residual
Upset at not being able to cook own food	Loss of ability to cook	Cooking is an integral part of his normal lifestyle	

able to adjust to changes in his ability to maintain this role through alterations caused by his rheumatoid arthritis (see Box 10.3).

Interdependence   The focus of assessment in this area is the balance between giving and taking actions. Through discussion with Mr Smith, the nurse may perceive that all his life he has been independent of others and unwilling to accept help. The dependence caused by his reliance on others for help in preparing food has led to difficulty in his accepting any help (see Box 10.4).

It is fairly easy to structure a formal assessment form using the framework that Roy suggests. Following a section for biographical and medical information, the four adaptation modes that she has identified can be used as main headings with subsections of the components of each one. However, provided that the nurse is familiar with the content of the model, an alternative would be to use a freer format. In this way the emphasis of the assessment can be directed towards the major areas of concern of the patient without becoming too bulky or wasting space. Some people have also chosen to simplify the language, calling focal stimuli direct causes, contextual stimuli indirect causes and residual stimuli past causes, which may make the structure easier to understand. Figure 10.4 is an example of an assessment form which follows a more formal structure, demonstrating how information relating to both individual strengths and areas giving rise to difficulties can be gathered.

Box 10.3   A care plan item – role function

Patient behaviour	Stimulus		
	Focal	Contextual	Residual
Does not eat food prepared by other people	Has always seen himself as the 'best cook'	Dislikes accepting support from others	Has lived alone for 20 years

Box 10.4   A care plan item – interdependence

Patient behaviour	Stimulus		
	Focal	Contextual	Residual
Mr Smith says he dislikes accepting any help from the 'welfare'	Has always lived independently and dislikes help from others	No longer able to meet nutritional needs independently	

In this way the areas of strength can be drawn upon when formulating a plan of action. Information concerning biographical data follows a simple standard format (see Figure 10.4).

CARE PLANNING

Although both adaptive and maladaptive behaviour may be recorded during assessment, the identification of problems arises out of the actual or potential maladaptive behaviour. The goals focus on an adjustment of the maladaptive behaviour to lie within the norms, whether those norms are universal, as in such things as temperature, or individual, as may be the case in eating habits. Since the goal of nursing is aimed towards adjusting the patient's behaviour to be within these norms, great emphasis is placed on formulating them jointly with the patient. The overriding goal in this model is that the patient should move towards adaptive behaviour. The problem and goal statements are always stated in behavioural terms which can either be observed or measured in order that it is possible to readily evaluate the effectiveness of care (see Box 10.5).

In this example the goal is related to producing a demonstration of positive or adaptive behaviour. Evaluation was undertaken by measuring the weight at predetermined intervals to ascertain whether it had become stable and by recording the amount of food eaten.

The nursing action is aimed towards adjusting the stimuli, which have led to the maladaptive behaviour. This is why it is so essential to identify these causes during second level assessment. If the stimulus is unalterable, it may be necessary for the nurse to intervene on behalf of the patient (see Box 10.6).

Further problems would be identified from the information gathered at assessment in relation to Mr Smith's loss of independence, self-concept and role function and dealt with in a similar way.

A PATIENT CARE STUDY

Tracey Foster is a 21-year-old woman admitted from the waiting list to a busy acute general surgical ward. She has been attended by her general practitioner for episodes of biliary colic and has had an ultrasound which has confirmed the presence of gall stones.

Ward	Admission Date	House Officer	Consultant	
		Reason for Admission	G.P.	Tel. No.'s
			Social Worker	
		Surgery / Treatment	Relatives Staying	
Age	Marital Status			
D.O.B.	Occupation			
Religion	Baptised	Patient's Understanding of Admission	Dependants/Siblings	
Likes to be Referred to as				

NEXT OF KIN	Tel. No.'s	Family's Understanding of Admission	DISCHARGE ARRANGEMENTS	
Name				Needed	Ordered
Address			Out-Patients		
			District Nurse		
		Relevant Past Medical History	Convalescence		
Meaningful Others			Health Visitor		
			Home Help		
			Transport		
TYPE OF ADMISSION			Discharge Advice		
Emergency / Waiting List			TTO's		
Provisional Medical Diagnosis			Others		
		Allergies/Infectious Diseases	Drugs Taken At Home	
Actual Medical Diagnosis				
			Discharge Date	

Figure 10.4   The assessment form.

Modes	Behaviour	Stimuli		
		Focal	Contextural	Residual
SELF-CONCEPT 1. Physical self:				
2. Personal self:				
ROLE FUNCTION 1. Primary:				
2. Secondary				
3. Tertiary				
INTERDEPENDENCE 1.				
2.				

The amount of space in each section can be adjusted according to the particular needs of each unit.

Figure 10.4   The assessment form *(cont.)*.

Modes	Behaviour	Stimuli		
		Focal	Contextual	Residual
PHYSIOLOGICAL 1. Oxygen & Circulation:				
2. Fluid & Electrolytes:				
3. Elimination:				
4. Nutrition:				
5. Rest/Activity:				
6. Regulation:				

Figure 10.4   The assessment form *(cont.)*.

Box 10.5   Planning care

Problem (i.e. maladaptive behaviour)	Goal (i.e. adaptive behaviour)

Weight loss caused by
  a. inability to cook own food
  b. loss of appetite
	Able to eat sufficient food to maintain weight

Tracey's assessment was undertaken on the morning of admission. The amount of recording is relatively short as it is recognised that in this type of situation time is limited. However, even in this situation, it is possible to record all information essential to care in a relatively brief way. The biographical data are recorded in a format that can be used almost universally. However, the data related to adaptive and maladaptive behaviour are recorded using the format suggested by Roy for both first and second level assessment, recording both the behaviour and the cause of the behaviour. Figure 10.5 shows the recordings made during Tracey's assessment.

From the data collected the nurse is able to identify both actual and potential maladaptive behaviour or problems and continue to formulate the care plan. In this case maladaptive behaviour in all four modes is identified, although some of the problems overlapped as shown in the care plan in Figure 10.6. The nursing action is planned in accordance with the stimuli that have been identified as leading to the problems. For instance, problem 1 relates to the risk of chest infection, a physiological difficulty caused by smoking habits and impending anaesthesia. The action is aimed towards altering the smoking habits and providing preventative support to lessen the risks during anaesthesia. Problem 4 relates to difficulties ascertained through assessment of the role function and interdependence modes, and action is again planned around the identified courses.

The whole emphasis of this study has been on the identification of adaptive and maladaptive behaviour, on the stimuli leading to this behaviour and the way in which the nurse can help the patient to

Box 10.6   The nursing action

Nursing Action
(i.e. alteration of the stimuli which have led to the maladaptive behaviour)

1. Refer to occupational therapist for
   a. provision of appropriate aids
   b. teaching use of aids
2. Discuss possible weekly menus and draft a sample with Mr Smith
3. Weigh weekly on Fridays at 9.00 a.m. in pyjamas

Ward	Roy	Admission Date	12.7.94		House Officer	Dr Arnold		Consultant	Dr Deacon	

Tracey Foster
Flat 12
Hamlet House
22 South Street
Acton

Reason for Admission
Episodes of biliary colic caused by gall stones.
For cholecystectomy 13.7.84

G.P. Dr Smith   Tel. No.'s 82715

Social Worker None

Relatives Staying No

Surgery / Treatment

Age	21	Marital Status	Single

D.O.B. 23.4.73   Occupation Typist

Religion C of E   Baptised

Likes to be Referred to as Tracey

Patient's Understanding of Admission
"My gall bladder is blocked with stones
which keep giving me awful pains. I
need them out."

Dependants/Siblings None

Family's Understanding of Admission
As above.

DISCHARGE ARRANGEMENTS		
	Needed	Ordered
Out-Patients		
District Nurse		
Convalescence		
Health Visitor		
Home Help		
Transport		
Discharge Advice		
TTO's		
Others		

NEXT OF KIN	Parents	Tel. No.'s	None

Name Mr & Mrs Foster

Address 31 The High Street
Acton

Relevant Past Medical History
Nil relevant.
No previous hospital admission.

Meaningful Others
Barbara Smith, Sue Kelland (Flatmates)
Flat 2, Hamlet Hse, 22 South St. Tel 78326

TYPE OF ADMISSION

Emergency / Waiting List Waiting list

Provisional Medical Diagnosis

Allergies/Infectious Diseases	Drugs Taken At Home
None.	Paracetamol occa-sionally for headaches and pains. Had pethidine for biliary colic with effect

Actual Medical Diagnosis
Intermittent biliary colic from gall
stones. Confirmed by cholecystogram.

Discharge Date

Figure 10.5   The assessment form.

Modes	Behaviour	Stimuli		
		Focal	Contextual	Residual
PHYSIOLOGICAL 1. Oxygen & Circulation:	No current difficulty but smokes 10 cigarettes a day.	Cigarette smoke is an irritant to breathing.	For anaesthetic tomorrow. Breathing may be restricted by pain postoperatively.	Family all smoke.
2. Fluid & Electrolytes:	No observed difficulties.			
3. Elimination:	Opens bowels daily after breakfast. No difficulty with micturition. Urine testing-NAD.			
4. Nutrition:	Conscious of figure but enjoys food. Eats balanced diet. Pain and nausea if fatty foods eaten.	Bile flow to gut impaired. Limited knowledge of cause of pain.		
5. Rest/Activity:	Usually sleeps well but currently cannot get off to sleep.	Anxious about impending surgery.	Unfamiliar surroundings.	
6. Regulation:	No difficulties noted: T 36.8°C BP 120/70 P 72			

Figure 10.5   The assessment form (cont.).

Modes	Behaviour	Stimuli		
		Focal	Contextural	Residual
SELF-CONCEPT 1. Physical self:	Says she is concerned about appearance of scar.	Impending surgery will leave scar.	No previous surgical scars.	Mother has large scar from surgery 20 years ago.
2. Personal self:	Concerned that she "won't be brave".	No previous experience of surgery.	Cries easily.	
ROLE FUNCTION 1. Primary:	Young woman.			
2. Secondary	New job as a typist. Anxious about not being able to work for 4-6 weeks.	Requires sick leave following surgery.	Feels insecure in new job.	Father is unemployed at present.
3. Tertiary	Swims weekly. Likes pop music and discos.			
INTERDEPENDENCE 1.	Freedom restricted by hospitalisation.	Never been in hospital before.		Dislikes new surroundings.
2.	Plans to convalesce with family.	Has been living with 2 friends in flat for 6 months.	Family unhappy about moving out of home.	Sister did not move from home until married.

The amount of space in each section can be adjusted according to the particular needs of each unit.

Figure 10.5   The assessment form *(cont.)*.

NURSING RECORD

CARE PLAN_____   MR/MRS/(MISS) _Tracey Foster_____

Admissions Care Plan

Date	Problems — Actual (A) and Potential (P)	Desired Outcome	Nursing Action
12.7.94	1. (P) Chest infection due to smoking habit and impending surgery.	Respiratory rate not more than 18/min. No cough.	Refer to physiotherapist for deep breathing exercises. Supervise breathing exercises hourly when awake. Advise to restrict or, if possible, stop smoking.
	2. (P) Pain and nausea if fatty foods are eaten.	Will not complain of pain or nausea.	Fat free diet prior to surgery.
	3. (A) Unable to sleep due to anxiety and strange environment.	Will sleep minimum of 6 undisturbed hours at night.	Warm milk at bed time. Offer sedatives as charted if desired.
	Anxiety due to: a) surgical scar. b) ability to cope. c) security of job. d) temporary loss of independence.	Is able to discuss anxieties freely in a relaxed way.	a) Describe likely progress of surgical scar. Show photos of previous patients' scars. b) Discuss fears about surgery and explain postoperative management of pain etc. Offer her time to ask questions.

Figure 10.6   The care plan.

manage the stimuli in order to attain positive adaptation. The overall goal can be seen as maintaining integrity or homeostasis, and the actions are focused around manipulating the stimuli in such a way as to achieve this goal. The resultant plan is easy to follow, with clear guidance on the type of behaviour to be looked for during evaluation, thus enabling the nurse to make a judgement about both the accuracy of her assessment and the effectiveness of her planned intervention.

Learning exercises

1. Consider your own behaviours when stressed and identify the most adaptive.
2. Observe a newly admitted patient and with a first level of assessment identify whether the person's response to stressors is adaptive or maladaptive.

Study questions

1. Write notes on Self Concept, Role Function and Interdependence.
2. Prepare a 10-minute overview of the Roy Adaptation Model to present to a class of nursing students.

Chapter 11

The Health Care Systems Model for Nursing

LEARNING OBJECTIVES

On completion of this chapter, the reader will be able to:

1. Apply Neuman's assessment questions with patients
2. Plan a multidisciplinary strategy for patient care
3. Appreciate the systems approach to providing a patient-centred health service

Betty Neuman's concern for the need to develop a broad-based conceptual framework for curriculum design which would provide unity, co-ordination and integration of the nursing course content at UCIA was the original impetus for this model (Neuman and Young, 1972). She first described her theory in a paper (Neuman, 1970) and after a decade of more work published a book, *The Neuman Systems Model: Application to Nursing Education and Practice* in 1982, with a second edition in 1989 and a third in 1995. An American nurse, Betty Neuman had considerable experience in the mental health field of nursing. Her model has moved away from the traditional 'illness' model to one that encompasses a 'total person approach to patient care'. The strength of her model lies in the emphasis given to prevention, health education, wellness, the management of ill health and an interdisciplinary approach (Figure 11.1).

Neuman (1980) suggests that this model is not restricted to nursing but can be shared by anyone working in health care systems. Rather than fragmenting care, Neuman offers an interdisciplinary approach and pulls together the goals and emphasis of the disciplines concerned with health care. She appreciates the complementary work of doctors and nurses within society and suggests that nurses should broaden rather than restrict their input (Neuman, 1996). While Neuman is definite about seeing a unique role for nursing in the model (see Figure 11.2), Craddock and Stanhope (1980) suggest that her model is not clear in pointing out what that role is. However, they do find the model helpful in identifying clients' needs for health care and suggest that in using this approach, the nursing role has potential for developing more independently. Neuman and Wyatt (1981) do express some concern about the nursing role, recognising the danger of a split between what they call the 'technical' and the 'professional' nurse. They see the role of the nurse as caring, collaborating and co-ordinating with health care workers and feel that the model described here supports these functions. Neuman has drawn on several theories in developing the health care systems model. Systems theory and stress adaptation have been described in earlier chapters. There is also evidence of Gestalt and field theories. These theories emphasise how we normally live in a carefully balanced equilibrium. If a problem arises, tension occurs and disrupts the equilibrium. This disruption is the driving force which leads us to interact with our environment and adapt or change. Components of developmental theory can also be recognised in the work. Although originally devised for use in curriculum development, the model has been tried and tested in clinical settings and as a framework for management. Neuman (1996) has reviewed the extent to which her model has been used by researchers and reports that it is equally useful to researchers collecting qualitative and quantitative data.

BELIEFS AND VALUES

The person

Neuman (1980) describes the person as a whole system, with psychological, physiological, sociocultural, developmental and spiritual components. Meleis (1991) comments that consideration of the spiritual being was added in later years to Neuman's work. There is a very strong emphasis in this model on viewing the individual as a whole person, affected by all the variables that can impinge on human beings. People are seen as open systems in constant interaction with their environment.

Neuman (1980) recognises that there are common features in any species and a core of such features in people. This central core or central structure is a person's energy resource and if it is compromised that person is at risk. The core is made up of basic survival factors, such as physiological, anatomical and genetic features. There are however a range of unique variables within this common core, giving each person his or her own individual baseline. For example, while all human beings require sufficient pressure to circulate the blood, the actual degree of pressure may vary from person to person.

Surrounding this basic energy resource are lines of resistance which protect it in order that it can remain stable. The lines of resistance may be such things as immune defences, coping behaviours or physiological mechanisms. These defences can vary from person to person according to their stage of development, their lifestyle or past experience. They function to help individuals maintain a harmony between the internal and external factors in their environment. In total they form an individual's normal line of defence, which is a relatively stable state developed over a period of time. This line is partly acquired through the responses or adaptations that have been experienced previously. For example, someone who has suffered from measles in the past will have acquired immunity against the virus and be able to resist future exposures. Similarly, past experience of successfully preparing for examinations will lead to the ability to cope with future exposures to this type of situation.

Surrounding this normal line of defence is also a flexible line of defence, which Neuman likens to an accordion. It can vary from day to day and can be affected by such things as the amount of rest, the nutritional state or the number of interactions that are occurring at that particular point in time. For example, a mother who is tired following the birth of a second child may be less tolerant of the attention sought by her first child. Similarly, there is a known association between stressful life events such as divorce or a change of job and physical illness. At a simpler level, a late night may well lead to less tolerant behaviour the following day. The variables that can affect these lines of defence arise from physiological, psychological, sociocultural and developmental sources.

Environment

Throughout a lifespan each person is subject to environmental stressors which are seen as stimuli that produce tension within the system. The tension has potential to cause a disequilibrium or a disturbance in the harmony of the individual and requires a response. The lines of

Figure 11.1 The health care systems model.

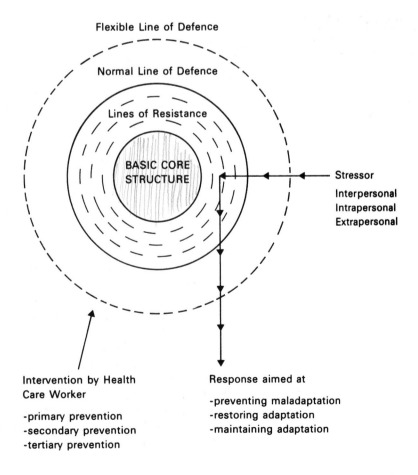

Flexible Line of Defence

Normal Line of Defence

Lines of Resistance

BASIC CORE STRUCTURE

Stressor
Interpersonal
Intrapersonal
Extrapersonal

Intervention by Health Care Worker

-primary prevention
-secondary prevention
-tertiary prevention

Response aimed at

-preventing maladaptation
-restoring adaptation
-maintaining adaptation

defence respond to the stressors to prevent them from reaching the central energy resource since, if this is impinged upon, life is threatened. Stressors can be divided into three categories as follows (Figure 11.1).

Intrapersonal These occur within the individual. As well as stressors related to disease, infection or trauma, conditioned responses to life events such as grief or developmental changes are included in this category.

Interpersonal These occur between one or more other people. Events such as conflict within a family, role changes and dependency may be included here.

Extrapersonal These occur outside the individual. World environmental health issues, poverty, pollution, deprivation, educational systems or cultural changes are classified as extrapersonal stressors.

Many stressors are universal and will always affect people. An example of such a stressor is loss, which can affect us all even if we have developed different lines of defence and respond differently. The response to a stressor varies from individual to individual according to how effective the lines of defence are in that particular situation, and how much disruption occurs within the system. The responses to stressors can also occur at intrapersonal, interpersonal or extrapersonal levels. For example, a family quarrel can lead to intrapersonal changes such as loss of sleep, interpersonal changes such as poor family communications, and extrapersonal changes such as loss of earnings from difficulty in concentrating at work.

Health

Neuman (1989) describes health or wellness as a point on a continuum between order and disorder; she uses the terms negentropy and entropy, which besides denoting respectively states of order and disorder, relate to amounts of available and unavailable energy in a system. Wellness is a reflection of the system's stability.

THE GOALS OF NURSING

Clients require nursing when they are unable to cope with environmental stressors. The broad goal that is sought in this model is the stability of the system – that is, the whole person. Once again there are three categories that goals can be placed in. These link with the situation and the foci of the intervention. They are related to preventing maladaptation, restoring adaptation and maintaining adaptation.

Primary prevention

If a stressor is suspected or identified before a reaction with the system occurs, the goal of care is either to reduce the possibility of an encounter with the stressor or to strengthen the line of defence in order that a reaction can be reduced or stopped. This area of care links strongly with current trends in environmental health, preventative care and health education. It would include such things as immunisation programmes and education about relaxation techniques and managing one's own health. The prime purpose is to prevent maladaptation occurring.

Secondary prevention

This type of intervention occurs after a stressor has crossed the line of defence and caused a reaction. In this instance the goal of care is aimed towards helping an individual to return to his or her own normal health state or, to use Neuman's terms, to reconstitute. She emphasises that what is seen as healthy for one person may not be the same for another. At this stage the focus of intervention is to restore adaptation and stability.

Tertiary prevention

The third type of intervention is generally started after the 'treatment stage'. The purpose of therapy at this stage is to help a person to maintain or stabilise his or her healthy state in order to avoid the possibility of a recurrence of the reaction that occurred previously. Thus help is directed towards maintenance and educational-type activities. Some of the interventions are similar to those that arise at the primary level but they occur after, rather than before, a reaction has occurred.

As Neuman points out, the normal line of defence, or the individual's ability to respond to stressors after they have been affected and have already begun to react to stress, may be different from the beginning stage. In some instances it may settle at a lower level if the lines of defence have been permanently damaged. However, in other cases, a 'higher level of wellness' can be achieved if the normal line of defence is strengthened and widened.

KNOWLEDGE AND SKILLS FOR PRACTICE

Since the emphasis of this model is on the interrelationship of all variables that affect human beings, the knowledge required is drawn from psychological, physiological, sociocultural and developmental theories, all of which can affect human behaviour. The focus is on identifying universal stressors (stressors which can affect anyone) and considering their impact in each of the four areas. Neuman and Young (1972) use loss as an example of a universal stressor that may lead to patient problems. They then clarify the knowledge required in each of the four areas mentioned above. For example, theories about role, cultural change and social structure may be related to sociocultural loss. Similarly, theories about sensory deprivation, immune response and pain may be associated with physiological loss. Nurse education in this instance relies heavily upon relating knowledge from allied disciplines to nursing practice.

Another feature of this model is its emphasis on health promotion and illness prevention, which leads to a necessity for knowledge and skills related to teaching and learning. If nurses wish to develop their ability as health educators, then this should be a component of the curriculum. Similarly, the health team approach advocated in the model leads to a requirement that nurses have an understanding of the structure and scope of the health care services and of the services that can be offered by different occupational groups.

ASSESSMENT USING THE HEALTH CARE SYSTEMS MODEL

Neuman suggests that there are three basic principles to be considered in relation to a nursing assessment.

- Good assessment requires knowledge of all the factors influencing a patient's perceptual field.
- The meaning that a stressor has to the patient is validated by the patient as well as by the care-giver.
- Factors in the care-giver's perceptual field that influence the assessor's review of the patient's situation should become apparent.

Unlike some of the other models that have been described, the assessment format in this instance is fairly unstructured. However, Neuman has identified a number of categories that must be included during assessment.

- Biographical data.
- Stressors from the patient's perception – those factors which the patient sees as causing the major difficulties.
- Stressors from the nurse's perception – those factors which the nurse sees as causing the major difficulties.
- Intrapersonal, interpersonal and extrapersonal factors affecting an individual and his or her personal relationships. These are the responses to the stressors and may be considered under four categories, namely physiological, psychological, sociocultural and developmental factors.
- A statement of the problems in rank order reconciling any variation between the perceptions of the nurse and the perceptions of the patient.

During assessment, Neuman suggests that a progressive approach is taken, moving from general points to more specific details. This is

Figure 11.2 A diagrammatic representation of the health care systems model.

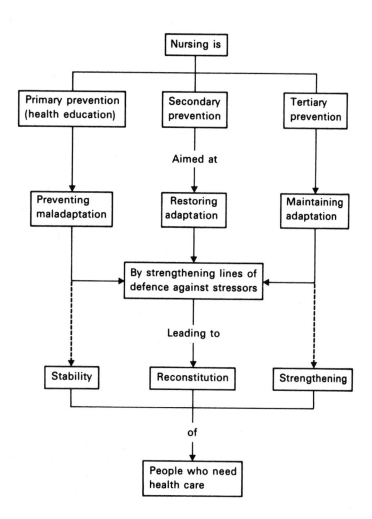

achieved through gaining initial information by general questions and observations and gradually progressing towards more specific assessment and categorisation of information.

In order to obtain the necessary information about stressors that are present, Neuman suggests that six basic questions should be posed and answered by both the patient and the nurse. In this way variations in perception can be identified so that they can be discussed and reconciled. The six questions, slightly modified for use in the United Kingdom, are as follows.

1. What do you consider to be your major problem, difficulty or area of concern?
2. How has this affected your usual pattern of living or lifestyle?
3. Have you ever experienced a similar problem previously? If so, what was that problem and how did you handle it? Was your handling of the problem successful?
4. What do you anticipate for yourself in the future as a consequence of your present situation?
5. What are you doing and what can you do to help yourself?
6. What do you expect care-givers, family, friends and others to do for you?

As information is gathered, more specific questions may need to be asked within each category in order to ascertain more detailed information. By recording both the patient's and the nurse's responses to each question area, any variation in response can be identified and, whenever possible, reconciled. It must be remembered, however, that the client's perceptions and values should always be respected. The categorisation of the data, once collected, does follow a more formal structure. It is classified into three major areas – intrapersonal, interpersonal and extrapersonal factors – and each case further subdivided into groups related to physiological, psychological and developmental factors. Neuman also emphasises that information may be gathered from other sources such as other health care workers or laboratory tests. A suggested format for recording data is shown in Figure 11.3.

Returning to Mr Smith (see Chapter 10) and concentrating on his nutritional state, the responses given by both the patient and the nurses included the following.

Question 1

What do you consider to be your major problem, difficulty or area of concern?

Patient's perception: Not able to look after myself and manage things how I like them.

Nurse's perception: Independence reduced by restricted movement. Joints of fingers, hands and wrists severely affected by rheumatoid arthritis. Thin with loose clothes indicating weight loss.

Question 2

How has this affected your usual pattern of living or lifestyle?

Patient's perception: It has affected the timing of my meals and what is available. The ability to prepare meals or drinks by myself has been lost.

Nurse's perception: Reduced food intake leading to weight loss. Dislike of food prepared by others.

Ward:	Admission Date:	Consultant:
		GP: Tel. No's:
		House Officer:
Age:	Marital Status:	Social Worker
DOB:	Occupation:	Relatives Staying:
Religion:	Baptised:	Relevant Past Medical History:
Likes to be Referred to as:		
NEXT OF KIN: Tel. No's: Name: Address:		
Meaningful Others:		
		Allergies/Infectious Diseases:
Dependents/Siblings:		
TYPE OF ADMISSION:		
Emergency/Waiting List:		
Medical Diagnosis:		
Reason for Admission:		Drugs Taken at Home:
Surgery/Treatment:		

Figure 11.3   The assessment form

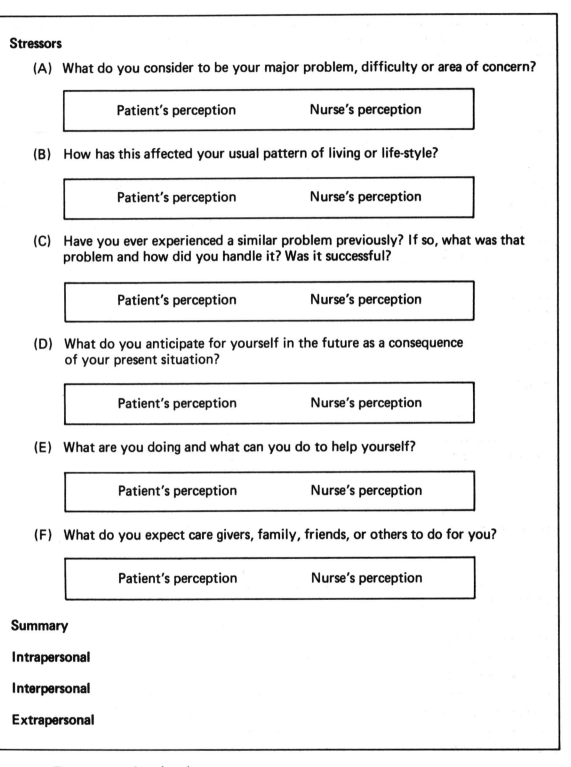

Stressors

(A)   What do you consider to be your major problem, difficulty or area of concern?

Patient's perception	Nurse's perception

(B)   How has this affected your usual pattern of living or life-style?

Patient's perception	Nurse's perception

(C)   Have you ever experienced a similar problem previously? If so, what was that problem and how did you handle it? Was it successful?

Patient's perception	Nurse's perception

(D)   What do you anticipate for yourself in the future as a consequence of your present situation?

Patient's perception	Nurse's perception

(E)   What are you doing and what can you do to help yourself?

Patient's perception	Nurse's perception

(F)   What do you expect care givers, family, friends, or others to do for you?

Patient's perception	Nurse's perception

Summary

Intrapersonal

Interpersonal

Extrapersonal

Figure 11.3   The assessment form *(cont.)*.

Question 3   Have you ever experienced a similar problem before? If so, what was that problem and how did you handle it? Was your handling of the problem successful?

Patient's perception: No previous experience, although this has been coming on for years.

Nurse's perception: Problem should have been identified earlier to prevent current situation.

Question 4   What do you anticipate for yourself in the future as a consequence of your present situation?

Patient's perception: I hope to gain strength in hands and arms so that I can cook my own meals. I think that the physiotherapist will be able to help me.

Nurse's perception: Hopes for full independence in preparing meals may be unrealistic. Occupational therapist may be able to advise on management.

Question 5   What are you doing and what can you do to help yourself?

Patient's perception: I agreed to hospital admission reluctantly to try to get strength back.

Nurse's perception: Unhappy about being in hospital and losing further independence but should be able to regain some aspects of self-care as is well motivated.

Question 6   What do you expect care-givers, family, friends and others to do for you?

Patient's perception: Neighbours already help with the garden, and the home help cleans, but it is unfair to expect them to do meals and anyway I don't like the food they cook. Meals-on-Wheels food is always cold and awful, not like my own cooking.

Nurse's perception: Dislikes receiving help from others. Unsuitable food often provided, leading to inadequate dietary intake.

SUMMARY

Intrapersonal

Physical   Weight loss, insufficient food intake, reduced function from rheumatoid arthritis.

Psychosocial   Hopes for full independence but is aware this may not be possible.

Developmental   Is now aware that adjustments in lifestyle are required because of physical disability.

Interpersonal

Physical   Dislike of others' cooking has contributed to poor nutritional intake.

Psychosocial   Feels neighbours already contribute enough.

Developmental   Network of support small as no immediate family in district.

Extrapersonal

Physical   Dislikes Meals-on-Wheels. Food unsuitable.

Psychosocial   No alternative services available locally.

Developmental   Dependency may increase because of disease and ageing processes. Needs to plan for the future.

Neuman includes problem identification as part of assessment and, in Mr Smith's case both he and the nurse were able to agree on the difficulties listed below. Since none is immediately life-threatening, the priority was also agreed between the patient and nurse.

1. Loss of independence in preparing own meals.
2. Insufficient calorie intake to maintain weight.
3. Possibility of becoming more dependent in the future.

Neuman points out, however, that when this format is used, reassessment is a continuous process as the client's condition and perceptions alter and intervention is effective in reaching stated goals.

CARE PLANNING   The planning stage using this approach includes:

- a decision as to whether primary, secondary or tertiary action is required
- a statement of goals and the rationale for them
- a prescription

Whenever possible, plans should be made for both immediate and future action, although not all information would be available at the time of an initial assessment.

The goals of care may be directed towards preventing maladaptation, restoring adaptation or maintaining adaptation by either reducing the stresses or strengthening the lines of defence. While it would be hoped that a client can return to his or her previous level of wellness or even improve, this is not always the case and in Mr Smith's situation it would be unrealistic. So for him a new level which he finds acceptable may have to be sought. Box 11.1 shows the goals.

Actions for all three types of goals are included in the care plan but in different categories. Thus all are considered: primary action, aimed at anticipating difficulties before they arise in order to reduce or remove

---

Box 11.1   The problem and goal statements

Problem (i.e. response to Stressor)	Goal (i.e. agreed adaptive behaviour)	
1. Loss of independence in preparing meals due to affects of rheumatoid arthritis	Able to make hot drinks and prepare light meals without aid	Strengthen lines of defence
2. Insufficient calorie intake to maintain weight	Maintain weight at present level	Remove stressor
3. Possibility of becoming more dependent in the future	Identify possible future sources of support	Strengthen lines of defence

them; secondary action, aimed at restoring health; and tertiary action, aimed at maintaining health. Box 11.2 shows Mr Smith's plan.

Neuman emphasises that as care progresses, the situation may alter. During evaluation the actual outcomes of care are reviewed and compared with the stated ones. It may be necessary to revise any of the four steps of the process. In other words, further assessment may be required; the goals may need to be reconsidered; the action may need to be adjusted; or the time span allowed for change readjusted.

A PATIENT CARE STUDY

The following assessment and care plan are for a 40-year-old woman, Mrs Dorothy Baxter, who has just been admitted to hospital to undergo a planned abdominal hysterectomy.

As suggested in the model, biographical data are collected in a fairly standard fashion followed by a semistructured interview and a summary of the information. Emphasis is placed on the shared understanding between the nurse and the patient of the circumstances. The assessment focuses on identifying actual or potential stressors and their effects at an

---

Box 11.2   The nursing action

Primary action	Secondary action	Tertiary action
1.	1. Refer to occupational therapist for assessment, provision of aids and teaching use of aids	1. Arrange home assessment with occupational therapist
	2. Provide opportunities to practise once every day in ward kitchen	2. Draw up a menu plan with Mr Smith for light meals
2.	Discuss food values with Mr Smith and help with menu choice Provide intake of at least 1500 calories per day If hospital menu unsuitable ask dietitian to visit	Teach Mr Smith to plan his own diet within limits of ability in order to maintain his weight
3. Identify local support system available to Mr Smith Discuss possible attendance at local disabled dining clubs		

Ward: *Neuman*	Admission Date: **27·2·95**	Consultant: *Mr Tindle*
Mrs Dorothy Baxter **57 The Beeches** **High Town**		GP: *Dr Hardwick* Tel. No's: **66531**
		House Officer: *Dr Jamieson*
Age: **40**	Marital Status: *Married*	Social Worker *None*
DOB: **30·11·44**	Occupation: *Housewife*	Relatives Staying: *No*
Religion: *C of E*	Baptised:	Relevant Past Medical History:
Likes to be Referred to as: *Dotty*		*No serious illness.* *Dilatation and curettage* *on 15·12·84.* *Heavy bleeding for 18 months.*
NEXT OF KIN: *Husband* Tel. No's: **67841** Name: *Mr G Baxter* Address: *As above*		
Meaningful Others: *Mrs Agnes Bones (sister)* *43 The Elms, High Town* *Tel. 61847*		
Dependents/Siblings: **3** *children* *Peter (18) - at university* *James (16) + Sally (13) - at home*		Allergies/Infectious Diseases: *Shellfish*
TYPE OF ADMISSION:		
Emergency/Waiting List: *waiting list*		
Medical Diagnosis: *Menorrhagia due to fibroids.*		
Reason for Admission: *For abdominal hysterectomy.*		Drugs Taken at Home: *Iron tablet - 1 daily.* *Paracetamol for headaches.*
Surgery/Treatment:		

Figure 11.4   The initial assessment.

intrapersonal, interpersonal and extrapersonal level as well as the current strength of the lines of defence. Figure 11.4 and Box 11.3 show the information recorded following Mrs Baxter's initial assessment.

From the information gathered, Mrs Baxter and the nurse can reconcile any differences of view that they have. For instance, Mrs Baxter may have slightly unrealistic hopes about her rate of recovery and will need

Box 11.3 The in-depth assesment

STRESSORS
a. What do you consider to be your major problem, difficulty or area of concern?
Patient's perception:
The pain with my periods and very heavy bleeding. It got so bad that I couldn't cope with looking after my family. I'd bleed for 3 weeks every month.
Care giver's perception:
Menorrhagia. Anaemia. Looks tired and anxious

b. How has this affected your usual pattern of living or lifestyle?
Patient's perception:
Find it difficult to run the house. Don't go out because of the risk of 'flooding'. Irritable with the children. Tired all the time. Affects my relationship with my husband.
Care giver's perception:
Lethargy and tiredness. Restricted social and personal activities.

c. Have you ever experienced a similar problem previously? If so, what was that problem and how did you handle it? Was it successful?
Patient's perception:
Had a D & C 3 months ago so at least I know about hospitals and am not bothered about operation. My mother came to cope with the children so arrangements worked well but I do miss them and worry that they will be all right.
Care giver's perception:
Good insight into hospital care. Home arrangements well organised. Concerned about missing the family.

d. What do you anticipate for yourself in the future as a consequence of your present situation?
Patient's perception:
Relief from pain and bleeding. Return to my normal self in next to no time. I know I'll have to take it easy and not lift things for a while but I heal very quickly. I don't expect the operation will be very different from the D & C.
Care giver's perception:
Has slightly unrealistic expectations of speed of recovery. Limited understanding of current surgery.

e. What are you doing and what can you do to help yourself?
Patient's perception:
Can look after myself independently at the moment. I take iron tablets and Panadol for the pain. Warm baths seem to help too. I like being independent.
Care giver's perception:
Will need help immediately post-operatively with daily living activities. May find it difficult to depend upon the nurses immediately post-operatively.

Box 11.3   The in-depth assesment—cont'd

f. What do you expect care-givers, family, friends or other to do for you?
Patient's Perception:
*Mother will stay as long as necessary at home. My husband really
wants me back to my old self. I'm sure the nurses and doctors will look
after me when I'm here but I won't need anyone else at home.*
Care giver's perception:
*Good family support. Husband more anxious than he has admitted to
his wife. May need some help for a short while after discharge from
hospital.*
SUMMARY
Intrapersonal factors
Physical:
Menorrhagia, lethargy and tiredness from anaemia.
Psychosociocultural:
Is optimistic about outcome of care.
Developmental:
*Feels secure in her role in the family and wishes to be able to return to
full participation.*
Interpersonal factors
Physical:
Is unable to look after family fully.
Symptoms have limited her physical relationship with husband.
Psychosociocultural:
Social activities limited due to heavy bleeding with tiredness.
Developmental:
*Family are sufficiently independent to support through period of oper-
ation and recovery.*
Extrapersonal
Physical:
Needs are cared for a present.
Psychosociocultural:
No financial or occupational difficulties. Has a supportive family.
Developmental:
No concern about loss of reproductive ability.

to discuss how quickly she will be able to return to her usual 'level of
wellness' (question D). Similarly, because of her fondness for independence, particular attention may need to be paid to the way in which the
immediate postoperative period is dealt with as at that time she will lose
some of her independence and require support from the nurses. These
situations have been recognised within the care plan seen in Figure 11.5,
where problems 1 and 5 have been incorporated in order to increase Mrs
Baxter's understanding, thus hoping to strengthen her own lines of
defence.

Problems	Goals	Primary Treatment (prevention)	Secondary Treatment (intervention)	Tertiary Treatment (follow up)
1. Limited Knowledge about details and outcome of impending surgery.	a) Can explain surgery + care while in hospital. b) Is realistic about length of time required for convalescence.		a) Explain surgery using diagrams. b) Give details of pre and post-op care. c) Discuss arrangements for returning home.	a) Arrange discharge date with patient and family. Discuss rate of return to normal. Check home support for 2 weeks after discharge.
2. Slightly anxious about separation from family.	Can keep in contact with family member at least once a day.		Discuss visiting arrangements with family. Allow free access. Explain phoning procedures.	
3. Anxious about heavy bleeding preoperatively.	Bleeding will be contained by pads.		Give supply of pads in locker. Provide disposal bags. Situate bed near toilet.	
4. Lethargy due to anaemia.	Patient can fulfil activities of daily living without feeling over-tired.		Explain cause of lethargy. Explain and supervise pre-op blood transfusion. 1/2 hrly pulse, hrly BP and T while transfusion in progress.	Explain dietary factors related to iron sources.
5. Impending surgery leading to risks of: a) respiratory distress. b) nausea + vomiting.	Respiratory rate between 1-20. No cough or sputum. No nausea or vomiting post-operatively.	Pre-op visit by physio. 10 deep breaths/hour as soon as alert post-op. NBM from 7 a.m. 28.2.85. Give anti-emetic with analgesic post-op.		

Figure 11.5   The care plan.

Problems	Goals	Primary Treatment (prevention)	Secondary Treatment (intervention)	Tertiary Treatment (follow up)
c) Pain	Pain score of 5 or less on Painometer by 2nd day Post-operatively.	Explain pain levels and use of painometer pre-opera-tively.	Check Pain levels 2 hourly on even hour. Give analgesic if score higher than 4, following prescription.	
d) Deep vein thrombosis	Calf soft and pain free.	Fit elastic stockings. Teach ankle exercises. Advise not to cross legs. Discuss advantages of early mobilisation.	Check calves daily at 10 a.m. Supervise exercises as soon as alert post-op. Leave stockings in situ except for hygiene until fully mobile.	
e) Infection	Maintain temperature of 37°C or less.		Record temperature 6 hrly for at least 48 hours or until stable for 4 consecutive readings. Check wound for inflammation and for dis-charge daily at time of bath.	
f) Shock	BP 120/80 mmHg P 84/min		Record BP and pulse hourly for 6 hours post-operatively. Then reduce to 4 hourly if stable.	

Figure 11.5   The care plan (cont.).

The goal of problem 4, lethargy due to anaemia, is concerned with the removal of a stressor.

The care aimed at preventing complications is considered under primary intervention. Thus the preoperative measures taken to reduce the risks of complications occurring are recorded in this section, shown in problem 5.

Intervention to restore health is recorded under secondary treatment. This is problem 2, where anxiety already exists about family separation. The purpose is to plan intervention to reduce the stressor.

In line with Neuman's recommendations, tertiary care is planned early in the procedure. It is aimed at maintaining health in the future. Thus discharge plans (associated with problem 1) and management of diet to reduce the risks of anaemia are incorporated in this section. Other items may become apparent as Mrs Baxter progresses through her hospital stay and can be added at any time.

The health care systems approach offers an alternative approach to nursing which many nurses may enjoy. It is very broad in its approach, using theories from several fields, but it offers a flexible framework that can easily be adjusted to many fields of nursing work. Although at first sight the framework for assessment may seem to be too vague, with skilled use the amount of information obtained can be great, and the approach ensures that the patient's own perception of his or her condition is not overridden by that of the health care worker.

Learning exercises

1. Sit with a patient you know and ask for his or her help with this exercise. Ask the six assessment questions listed above.
2. Ask the patient what they thought of the exercise and whether they have given you any new information.

Study questions

1. Write notes on the extent to which your own perceptions differed from the patient above and how that has informed the care you will give.
2. Write a short discussion on the use of multidisciplinary assessments.

Chapter 12

A Goal Attainment Model for Nursing

LEARNING OBJECTIVES

On completion of this chapter, the reader will be able to:

1. Differentiate between patient goals and nursing goals
2. Understand the power of communication and teamwork that includes the client
3. Evaluate the success of any plan from the patient's perspective
4. Explain the importance of negotiation in goal attainment

A number of models based on the theory of symbolic interaction have been developed for nursing. The model proposed by Imogene King, an eminent American nursing scholar, focuses on interaction, and has been applied by many American nursing teams. It uses concepts that King found to be recurring in nursing literature, research, teaching and practice.

The model was developed originally through a research project. In the research study, all the interactions between nurses and clients were observed in two different settings from admission to discharge. One group consisted of clients admitted to hospital for surgical procedures, and the other of clients admitted to hospital in an acute crisis, for example, following myocardial infarction. The study set out to answer the following questions:

- What is the nursing act?
- What is the nursing process?
- What is the goal of nursing?
- Who are nurses and how are they educated to practice?
- How and where is nursing practised?
- Who needs nursing in society?

The result of the study was to confirm King's assumptions about the nature of nursing, and led to the development of the model. King's progress was careful. Her first book, published in 1971, was entitled *Toward a Theory for Nursing: General Concepts of Human Behavior*. It was only in her second book in 1981, called *A Theory for Nursing: Systems, Concepts, Process*, that she claimed to have developed a theory for nursing (Meleis, 1991). In 1986 King published a book in which she demonstrated her work's applicability to curriculum design. She (King, 1997) gives an overview of her work and proposes that her theory has several purposes.

(a) To identify concepts that are essential knowledge for nursing as a discipline.
(b) To derive theories and test them in research which may result in scientific knowledge for nursing.
(c) To serve as a structure to develop a curriculum for nursing education.
(d) To implement theory based practice to deliver quality care to all individuals in hospitals, community health care agencies, and in families.

Carter and Dufour (1994) summarise and explore the criticisms of King's work. The objections are that the model is confined to Western cultures, reliant on patient competence and lacks specific guidance for use with the nursing process. The authors draw on examples from practice to refute these points and support King's work.

Figure 12.1 A conceptual framework for nursing: dynamic interacting systems (from King, 1971, with permission).

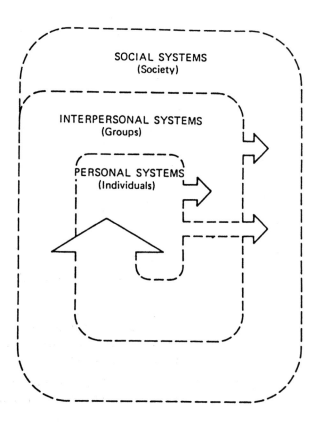

King (1981) arranges her work in three 'open' systems (see Figure 12.1). First the personal systems, which deal with the individual, either nurse or client, and relate to the following concepts: perception, self, body image, growth and development, time and space. Second the interpersonal systems, which deal with people interacting, either one-to-one or in larger groups. The concepts related to the interpersonal systems are: role, interaction, communication, transaction and stress. Third the social systems, which deal with the dynamics of society, its organisation and effect on the environment and people. The concepts related to social systems are: organisation, power, authority, status, decision-making and role. King maintains that all systems have an end product or goal and she proposes that the goal of these systems related to nursing is health.

BELIEFS AND VALUES

The person

People are seen as functioning open systems, who constantly interact with other humans and the environment. Interaction occurs within society, through interpersonal relationships. Such relationships occur according to people's perceptions, which in turn influence their lives and health.

King (1987, p. 108) makes the following assumptions about human beings:

- individuals are social beings
- individuals are sentient beings
- individuals are rational beings
- individuals are reacting beings
- individuals are perceiving beings
- individuals are controlling beings
- individuals are action-oriented beings
- individuals are time-oriented beings

Health

King sees health as related to coping with stress. Her model is holistic in its concerns, encompassing the physical, emotional and social components of people. In her words:

Health is defined as dynamic life experiences of a human being, which implies continuous adjustment to stressors in the internal and external environment through optimum use of one's resources to achieve maximum potential for daily living.

(King, 1981, p. 5)

King believes that health has different meanings for individuals and groups in different cultures, and often for individuals within the same culture. Health can be portrayed as an abstract notion or ideal to which most people aspire. Nurses, who have a major input in helping individuals during life events associated with health, require a broad perspective, which includes an appreciation of the other's world and his/her interpretation of health.

Environment

King (1981) refers to the internal and external environments, both of which create stressors for the individual. As an open system the person is in constant interaction with the environment and adapts to changing circumstances in both spheres.

THE GOALS OF NURSING

The overall aim of goal attainment is to promote health for individuals, families, communities and the world (King, 1996). When the goals of life and health cannot be achieved, such as for the terminally ill, then nurses give care and help individuals to die with dignity. Nursing aims at the achievement of health in individuals by meeting three basic health needs.

1. The need for usable health information at a time when individuals need it and are able to use it.
2. The need for preventive care, to prevent ill health.
3. The need for care when ill.

The specific subgoal to be achieved by nurses in order to meet these health needs is to establish transactions between themselves and clients, their families and other social systems. King sees nursing as predominantly an interpersonal interaction between the nurse and the client. Figure 12.2 shows the process of nursing; a brief explanation of the concepts follows.

Perception

Perception is 'each person's representation of reality. It is an awareness of persons, objects, and events' (King, 1987, p. 109). How people perceive their reality depends on a range of personal circumstances, including: their past, their future hopes, their mood or their ability to see or hear, and so forth. Perceptions are the means by which humans process sensory information and construct understandings of the world.

Judgement

Having perceived the situation, the person makes a judgement about how to act.

Action

Whenever two people meet, some kind of action is involved. It is a sequence of behaviours or activities, which includes mental action in

Figure 12.2 The observable nursing process (after King, 1971).

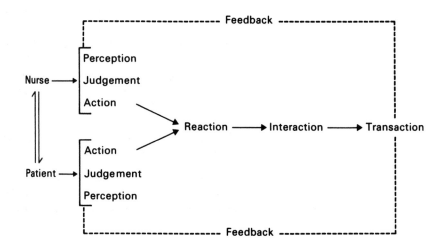

terms of examining the situation from a personal perspective, whether the individual is the nurse or client.

Reaction

This is simply the result of the action. How did the client react to the nurse's suggestion (action). Reaction is the feedback received after taking action.

Interaction

This is an interplay of communication between two or more people. In nursing, it always involves the nurse and client, but may include others.

Transaction

This is reaching some agreement to pursue an action plan to achieve the desired outcome.

King (1987, p. 110) makes the following propositions which give readers a notion of how nurses should behave in order to achieve planned goals.

1. If perceptual accuracy is present in nurse–client interactions, transaction will occur.
2. If nurse and client make transactions, goals will be attained.
3. If goals are attained, effective nursing care will occur.
4. If transactions are made in nurse–client interactions, growth and development will be enhanced.
5. If role expectations and role performance as perceived by nurse and client are congruent, transactions will occur.

King writes that the propositions have been used to formulate research hypotheses so that her ideas can be tested empirically.

KNOWLEDGE AND SKILLS FOR PRACTICE

Nursing is seen as a helping activity, providing a service that meets a social need. The service provides care to individuals and groups who are ill, and it promotes health through education, as shown in Figure 12.3.

The knowledge base for nursing revolves around the three systems and health, including their related concepts. Nurses require specific skills of observation and communication to collect information, to make decisions and to implement a plan of care based on problems amenable to nursing action. Technical skills are seen as an essential part of practice in gathering reliable data about physiological parameters of the health state.

Essentially, King's theory concentrates upon the ability of the nurse and client to communicate and cooperate. Nursing skills and knowledge are channelled towards helping people through the interactive process. An understanding of her process of nursing involves the nurse learning communication skills and understanding how to use them to help the client move towards agreed-upon goals.

King (1981) devotes some space to the notion of decision-making and is generally in favour of a problem-orientated system. She says:

Decision-making in organisations is a dynamic and systematic process by which goal-directed choice of perceived alternatives is made and acted upon by individuals or groups to answer a question and attain a goal.

(King, 1981, p. 132)

Figure 12.3 A diagrammatic representation of King's interaction model (after NDCG, 1973).

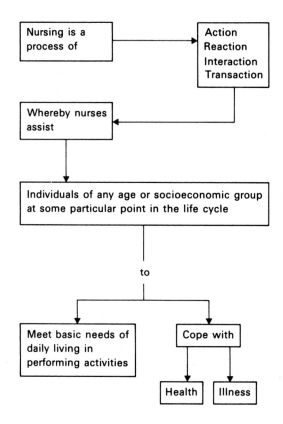

The nursing process consists of action, reaction, interaction and transaction (see Figure 12.2). Basing practice on the knowledge and skills already mentioned, the nurse needs to become skilled in this interactive process before effective professional practice can be achieved.

ASSESSMENT USING AN INTERACTION MODEL

The stages of the nursing process are highly integrated in the model described by King, and relate to the interactive process of perception–action–interaction–reaction–transaction. The steps are circular and occur continuously as nursing takes place (see Figure 12.4). The three systems and their related concepts referred to earlier in the chapter may form the basis for assessment including, of course, health. To help explain the assessment process we return to the example of Mr Smith.

Figure 12.4 The continuous interactive process of nursing.

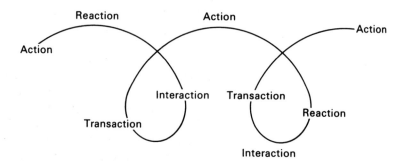

Personal systems (perception, self, growth and development, body image, space and time)

This is an assessment of Mr Smith as an individual. The nurse considers Mr Smith's perception of himself, his world and his current state. Together, the nurse and Mr Smith interact to establish how the current position is viewed by him, and the hopes he has for the future. The perception of Mr Smith towards his own personal predicament reveals his reality. He does not see that he is too thin, but he is bothered by pain in his hands and 'they won't do things anymore' (he is referring to using his hands to cook). He values being independent in his own home and he expects the nurse or doctor to sort his problems out for him.

Interpersonal relationships (human interaction, communication, transactions, role, stress)

Assessment of these systems involves both the relationship between the nurse and client and relationships with others. The quality and extent of relationships concerned in the case of Mr Smith are only superficially considered in the early stages of assessment, but they would develop as the nurse and client interact. Mr Smith seems to expect the nurse to 'sort his problems out'. He lives alone, his neighbours – who are polite to him, and help out in acts such as gardening – are not particularly close to him. He has no family, having lost his wife 20 years ago.

Social systems (organisation, authority, power, status, decision-making)

Through interaction, the nurse and client establish the social system network related to the presenting situation. This includes present and past social systems in Mr Smith's life. It is acceptable to him for neighbours and home helps to keep his home and garden tidy, but it is unacceptable for them to carry out personal services such as providing meals. He feels he has paid his taxes all his life and now deserves a little return from the state.

Health

Health assessment involves getting information from the client and professionals involved to identify stresses. These may include potential or actual stresses, which promote ill health. Rheumatoid arthritis, pain, loss of movement, loss of weight and loss of appetite are all identified as barriers to health in the assessment of Mr Smith.

The nurse considers the differences between his/her perception of Mr Smith's situation and his/her own. They will react and interact in order to find common ground. S/he may need to talk about his idea that he 'hasn't lost that much weight'. They need to come to some consensus so that they can agree upon the problems in this situation and what is the most appropriate plan.

In some practice teams, an open assessment form with these systems and concepts as headings might be appropriate. An example of a more structured approach is shown in Figure 12.5. It focuses on assessment of activities of daily living, modified from those described by Henderson (1966), in relation to King's systems and health. Assessment is by perception and action. Problems are identified through reaction and interaction. Transaction leads to the formulation of a care plan and its implementation.

Evaluating care involves the whole interactive process again, as does any reassessment and replanning. For example, the extract from a care plan in Box 12.1 could only be constructed after the whole of the interactive process has been completed. But the process begins again when the nurse gives the analgesics and milk drink (action and interaction),

Date of admission:	Date of assessment:	Nurse:

MALE ___   AGE   SURNAME . . . . FORENAMES . . . .

FEMALE ___   DATE OF BIRTH . . . . Prefers to be addressed as

. . . .

ADDRESS OF USUAL RESIDENCE

TYPE OF ACCOMMODATION

FAMILY/OTHERS AT THIS RESIDENCE

NEXT OF KIN   NAME   ADDRESS

RELATIONSHIP   TEL. NO.

SIGNIFICANT OTHERS

SUPPORT SERVICES

SIGNIFICANT LIFE CRISIS

REASON FOR ADMISSION

MEDICAL INFORMATION (e.g. diagnosis, past history, allergies)

WEIGHT _____

URINE

TEMP.   PULSE
BP   RESP.

DISCHARGE ARRANGEMENTS: (to be completed on admission)

MAIN SOURCE FOR ASSESSMENT:

PROJECTED DATE OF DISCHARGE:

SIGNIFICANT OTHERS INTERVIEWED: YES/NO

IF YES? DETAILS OF INTERVIEW

ARRANGEMENTS DISCUSSED WITH
RELATIVES: ____   OTHERS ___

HOME HELP _____

D/N
H/V

Figure 12.5   The assessment form.

ADL	PERSONAL SYSTEMS	INTERPERSONAL SYSTEMS	SOCIAL SYSTEMS	HEALTH
BREATHING				
EATING AND DRINKING				
ELIMINATING				
MOVEMENT AND POSTURE				
SLEEP AND REST				
DRESS AND UNDRESS				
BODY TEMPERATURE				

Figure 12.5   The assessment form *(cont.)*.

ADL	PERSONAL SYSTEMS	INTERPERSONAL SYSTEMS	SOCIAL SYSTEMS	HEALTH
SKIN AND PERSONAL HYGIENE				
AVOID DANGER IN ENVIRONMENT				
COMMUNICATION				
RELIGIOUS MATTERS				
WORK				
PLAY				
LEARNING				

Figure 12.5 The assessment form (cont.).

Box 12.1   A care plan item

Problem	Goal	Action
Unable to sleep more than 2 hours at night because of pain in nose	Will sleep for at least 6 hours for 3 nights in succession	1. Give hot milky Ovaltine with analgesics prescribed when patient asks for it 2. Patient can watch television until feels sleepy

observes the client and later seeks his opinion to establish the effectiveness of the strategy (reaction), then decides to continue with the plan or to revise it (transaction).

CARE PLANNING

The care plan is both a statement of the transaction agreed upon by the nurse and client and a guide to the nature of the interactive process to be engaged in while nursing takes place. It is a prescription for action; a means by which to judge reaction; an account of planned interaction. Once transactions are agreed upon, specific goals are set in order to give direction and to be used as yardsticks in determining reaction or, in other words, to evaluate. The specific goals must relate realistically to the goals implicit in the model and should establish transactions between the nurse and client to:

- attain health
- maintain health
- restore health
- give dignified care

Thus the overall goal of this model is holistic health. The goal statements should, as well as being assessable for evaluation purposes, be formulated by the nurse and client and represent a transaction (see Box 12.2).

In this example, nursing has aimed at restoring and maintaining those aspects of Mr Smith's life that he is concerned about and which affect his health. The nursing plan that represents the transaction between nurse and client is shown in Box 12.3.

Evaluation of the care given can be carried out by interaction with Mr Smith to see whether the stated goals have been achieved or not, and whether, in fact, there has been any movement in either of these directions.

The nursing action is written in terms of how the client and nurse will work together to meet the goals (see Box 12.3).

A PATIENT CARE STUDY

Mr Ted Donnelly has been admitted to the medical ward of a General Hospital with acute bronchopneumonia. The initial action of his primary nurse was to record biographical data, and to interact with Mr Donnelly

Box 12.2   The problem and goal statement

Problem (i.e. reaction and interaction)	Goal (i.e. transaction)
1. Losing weight	Will gain weight or remain same weight
2. Unhappy about home help and Meals-on-Wheels providing food	An alternative way of serving a cooked meal will be agreed upon
3. Would like and feels will eventually be able to cook meal everyday	Will be able to cook a meal independently
4. Wants to remain in role of independent adult but not sure if this is possible	Will be able to specifically say what he can be independent in, and what he is likely to be dependent in

to obtain information about the 14 activities of daily living in the context of the three systems and health.

The recordings that were made are noted in Figure 12.6. From this information, the nurse was able to review needs related to:

- giving of information about health
- prevention of ill health
- need for care

She was then able to identify problems in the performance of the activities of daily living related to the client's personal systems, interpersonal systems, social systems and health. In this case, the effects of the past and of the client's attitudes and values had implications for the care to be given. The care is outlined in the care plan (see Figure 12.7).

Box 12.3   The nursing action

Nursing Action
(i.e. action, reaction, interaction and transaction)

1. Discuss and plan daily intake of at least 1500 calories over next 24 hours – each day at 10 a.m.
2. Alternative way of providing a meal each day will be discussed when dietary plan is formulated
3. Refer to occupational therapist for assessment, provision of aids of teaching
4. Review current state of dependence each day

Date of admission: 8·9·96	Date of assessment: 8.9.96	Nurse: Brenda Miles

MALE __X__   AGE 51   SURNAME Donnelly .. FORENAMES Edward William

FEMALE ___   DATE OF BIRTH ......7.8.46......... Prefers to be addressed as

Ted

ADDRESS OF USUAL RESIDENCE	Highway House, High Street, Biggan village
TYPE OF ACCOMMODATION	Detached house - 4 bedrooms, bathroom and toilet on both levels. Central heating.
FAMILY/OTHERS AT THIS RESIDENCE	Wife
NEXT OF KIN	NAME ADDRESS Fiona Donnelly As above RELATIONSHIP TEL. NO. 38198
SIGNIFICANT OTHERS	Daughter - married with two children, lives in S. Africa.
SUPPORT SERVICES	Housekeeper
SIGNIFICANT LIFE CRISIS	When he had to give up work - two years ago.
REASON FOR ADMISSION	Acute bronchopneumonia

MEDICAL INFORMATION (e.g. diagnosis, past history, allergies)
 	
      Cor pulmonale since 1983
               (3 years)
	WEIGHT 12st 4lbs
	
	URINE NAD, SG 1006
	
	TEMP. 39.8°C PULSE 98/min
	BP 160/90 RESP. 36/min
	    mm Hg

	DISCHARGE ARRANGEMENTS: (to be completed on admission) To be discharged home when medical problem resolved. PROJECTED DATE OF DISCHARGE: ? 15·9·96
MAIN SOURCE FOR ASSESSMENT: Ted	
SIGNIFICANT OTHERS INTERVIEWED: YES/NO IF YES? DETAILS OF INTERVIEW	ARRANGEMENTS DISCUSSED WITH RELATIVES:____ OTHERS__ HOME HELP_____ D/N H/V

Figure 12.6 The assessment.

ADL	SOCIAL SYSTEMS	PERCEPTION	INTERPERSONAL RELATIONS	HEALTH STATE AND USUAL PHYSICAL CAPABILITIES
BREATHING	Ashamed of coughing up sputum - feels dirty.	"My cough is worse. I'd give anything for a new pair of lungs."	Conscious that noisy breathing and cough "make it difficult for people - my wife must find me repulsive.".	Very "short of breath" - unable to take more than 20 steps. Coughing up large amounts of sputum.
EATING AND DRINKING	Wife prepares food. Main meal at noon. Likes plain food.	"I eat well." Likes all foods. Drinks tea - whisky at night.		Slightly overweight. Well hydrated.
ELIMINATING	Hates using bedpan or commode.	Is aware of other people noticing odour from elimination.	Embarrassed by need to discuss elimination with others.	Opens bowels daily. Urinalysis - NAD. Does not wake up at night to pass urine.
MOVEMENT AND POSTURE	Restricted in attending valued activities- e.g. golf club.	"Can't do as much as I could because of the breathing."		Can walk slowly from bed to day room and up-stairs. But breathless in doing so.
SLEEP AND REST		"Sleep all the time."		Bed at 10 p.m., up at 6 a.m. Snoozes in morning and afternoon.
DRESS AND UNDRESS		"I don't bother much about appearances as long as I am warm."	"My wife gets annoyed if I don't get dressed during the day."	Independent in dressing.
BODY TEMPERATURE	No difficulty in keeping house warm.			

Figure 12.6   The assessment (cont.).

ADL	SOCIAL SYSTEMS	PERCEPTION	INTERPERSONAL RELATIONS	HEALTH STATE AND USUAL PHYSICAL CAPABILITIES
SKIN AND PERSONAL HYGIENE	No outside assistance at home.	Feels dirty because unable to bathe without help.		
AVOID DANGER IN ENVIRONMENT				Socially isolated.
COMMUNICATION	Limited contact with friends because of poor mobility.	"I miss my nights in the pub."	"I get bad tempered with Fiona because I don't see anyone else."	
RELIGIOUS MATTERS	No formal religious practice.			
WORK	Retired Town Hall clerk. Retired early due to ill health.	"I feel useless and unable to do anything anymore."	Lost touch with friends. Relationship with wife strained through lack of outside stimulation.	Watches TV. Reads Daily Telegraph. No longer able to contribute to household activities.
PLAY	Used to play golf and go to pub 3x week. Gave up golf 3 years ago.			
LEARNING			"I'm too old to change my ways now."	Resistent to changing life style.

Figure 12.6   The assessment (cont.).

DATE	NO.	PROBLEM	GOAL	NURSING ACTION	REVIEW DATE
		Basic need profile-			
8.9.96		Change in usual	Maintain usual		
		daily living	living pattern		
		circumstances			
	1.	Productive cough	Will be able to	a. Provide a single	
			cough up sputum	room when available.	
			easily and	b. Sputum mug in	
			privately.	easy reach.	
				c. Change sputum	
				mug at 10 a.m.,	
				2 p.m., 6 p.m., 10 p.m.	
				d. Refer to	
				physiotherapist	
	2.	Unable to walk far	Will go to toilet	a. Put bed close	
		without becoming	unaided without	to toilets.	
		breathless.	becoming distressed.	b. Provide urinal.	
		Embarassed about			
		possibility of not			
		reaching toilet.			
	3.	Feels "dirty" about	Will express such	a. Signify aware-	
		cough.	anxieties openly	ness of his feelings	
			to nurses.	whenever possible.	
				b. Offer listening	
				time when	
				possible.	

NAME	NO.	PRIMARY NURSE
Mr Ted Donnelly	64	Brenda Miles

Figure 12.7   The care plan.

DATE	NO.	PROBLEM	GOAL	NURSING ACTION	REVIEW DATE
	4.	Unable to bathe unaided.	Skin will be clean.	a. General bath with help of 2 nurses - Mon. and Thurs. mornings. b. Offer wash bowel at waking and before resting.	
	5.	Feels socially isolated because of immobility and feelings of being dirty.	Will express a desire to increase social activity.	a. Offer inform-ation about self-help group for patients with chronic obstructive airways disease. b. Introduce him to patients in similar situation. c. Discuss possi-bility of social activities for the future.	

NAME	NO.	PRIMARY NURSE
Mr Ted Donnelly	64	Brenda Miles

Figure 12.7   The care plan (cont.).

The focus of the care plan is on the achievement of health through helping the client to further develop interpersonal relationships with his social systems network, and to take into account his personal perceptions of his predicament.

The productive cough (problem 1) and the associated feeling of being dirty (problem 3) were considered in the context of Mr Donnelly's usual social systems – his family, his social peers and his friends – and his interpersonal relations with his wife, as well as in its reality as a physical symptom related to health.

Problems 2 and 4 had both health and interactive components, while problem 5, a feeling of isolation, was largely psychosocial.

Thus, the focus of the assessment and the care plan was on the client as an interactive being, viewed within the context of his interaction with others.

Throughout this brief account of Mr Donnelly's care, the interactive process is emphasised. Nursing itself is seen as an interactive activity and the client is seen as an interactive being. An interaction model emphasises this process and King sees it as the overriding concern of nursing.

Learning exercises

1. The next time that you are on duty consider the difference between the things that you are trying to achieve and the goals of the patients you are looking after.
2. Attend a case conference and take note of the roles of the various parties. In particular, where is the client's voice?

Study questions

1. Write a short discussion document that describes the art of negotiation in relation to nurse and client processes.
2. List the advantages of shared goals.

Chapter 13

A Developmental Model for Nursing

LEARNING OBJECTIVES

On completion of this chapter, the reader will be able to:

1. Discuss the professional implications of Peplau's model in relation to the nurse–client relationship
2. Understand the centrality of the nurse–patient relationship to therapy
3. Assess and plan care guided by Peplau's concepts

Hildegard Peplau was one of the earliest American theorists to recognise and respond to the need for changes in nursing practice, and her particular area of interest was psychiatry. Her work dates back to the early 1950s, when she published her thoughts in the book *Interpersonal Relations in Nursing* (1952). It is a measure of the appeal her focus upon interpersonal relationships has that the book was re-issued in 1988. Her work uses developmental, interactionist and human needs theories. Meleis (1991) notes that Peplau was interested in how nurses worked rather than what constituted nursing.

In line with her own beliefs, the views Peplau presented have continued to develop and grow as new knowledge has become available. Growth has occurred both through looking at small aspects of the model in greater depth and by giving fuller explanations to the unity of the whole model. Although her views were written primarily for psychiatric nurses, much of what she has to say can be of use to those working in other fields.

Peplau's work has been described as being influential in creating what is known as second order change, that is in influencing the system of nursing itself. She conducted innumerable workshops for practitioners around the country and was well known throughout the nursing profession in

America. In line with the arguments presented earlier for model-based practice, 'her ideas have provided an architectural design for the practice of a discipline' (Sills, 1978).

The need for a theoretical basis for practice is further emphasised by Peplau's views about professional accountability. She argues that accountability is not a new concept, but one that has always been present in one guise or another. Her reason for highlighting it is to 'prod the professional towards proper behaviour in health care work' (Peplau, 1980). In the past, professional accountability was masked by the nurse's dedication to duty and an expectation that individuals were committed to the service they offered with total devotion and obedience. As time passed this view became outmoded and nurses were rather encouraged to regard decision-making, along with the associated accountability, as a challenging part of practice.

Peplau encouraged the profession to ask questions such as: 'What is it that nurses actually do?' 'What is the specific service they offer?' 'What are the health problems they can treat?' Initially these questions arose from, and were addressed by, the controlling bodies of an occupational group. While this still holds true to some extent, each nurse may be asked to account for her actions to her controlling organisation. Peplau saw some limitations in this system alone. She described it as one which created 'guilty knowledge' – knowledge of practice or malpractice which is not disclosed to the public. Since her early work there has been a growth in professional accountability. It is now quite common for the practitioner to be asked to account for actions and decisions to a wider audience that includes clients and colleagues.

Peplau also stresses the need for accountability to oneself, a personal integrity in being honest about one's actions and being able to justify them. Thus there is a requirement for nurses constantly to update the knowledge base from which they practice, to keep pace with new information, and to be prepared to revise theories. Indeed, Peplau (1987) wrote a short history of nursing science in which she appreciated the work of the later theorists and exhorted nurses to continue to theorise with 'rigour and vigour'.

Peplau argues that the care that a client needs may well be different from the care that a client wants. She suggests that if nurses only respond to what a client wants, they are at risk of providing nothing more than custodial care, customer services or assistance to other health care workers. The skill required to work with someone to review their needs is an interpersonal process requiring considerable expertise and knowledge. Therefore, clarity in the services offered by nurses and constant updating of knowledge and revision of theory are essential if the profession is to offer a nursing service.

BELIEFS AND VALUES

The person

The emphasis of Peplau's approach is on both the patient and the nurse as human beings concentrating on the growth of the client. She identifies the phases through which the partnership progresses in an interpersonal

Figure 13.1   The effect of stress on an individual.

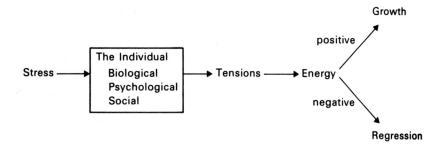

process, and the roles offered by the nurse. The movement through these phases follows a developmental pattern and leads to the growth of those concerned. She sees all individuals as unique people with both biological and psychological components who are capable of achieving new learning and making positive changes. As people are subjected to stress, so tension is created. In turn tension creates energy, and this energy can either be used positively or negatively, leading to growth or to regression respectively. The response to the stress is dependent on its degree and the individual's ability to respond. This in turn is based on the stage of development and past experience of the individual concerned and will be different in every case (see Figure 13.1).

Peplau also recognises that all people have needs which must be met. Thus a physical need may be for food or shelter and a psychological need may be for recognition or sharing. When needs are not met, growth of the individual is inhibited. The presence of needs creates tension and, if needs continue to be unmet, frustration can occur. Individuals strive towards development and growth through learning positive behaviours. If positive behaviours are not achieved, then regression can occur. Since we all live in an unstable environment, we are constantly faced with new situations, new problems to solve and new experiences. Thus human beings continually have the opportunity to carry on developing throughout their lifespan.

Health

As Peplau concentrates on developing the ideas of nursing and interpersonal processes, she gives only cursory consideration to health and the environment. She sees health as a process whereby the person is capable of continuing to grow and develop expertise in areas that contribute to personal and community living. Health is related to the positive use of energy produced by stress.

Environment

The environment is described in terms of extraneous, ever-changing forces surrounding the person and in constant interaction with them. Human development relies upon factors in the environment such as secure economic status and healthy parental environment. She describes the hospital as 'the nurse–patient interpersonal environment'.

THE GOALS OF NURSING

Peplau views nursing as a therapeutic interpersonal process involving a professional closeness or one-way interest in what is happening to another person. She sees the purpose of this relationship as twofold.

First and of immediate concern is the survival of the organism. However, once this goal has been achieved, a second purpose of the service offered by nurses is to help individuals to understand their health problems and to learn from their experiences with them. Stresses cannot, and indeed should not, be avoided, but nurses can help patients to use the stress situations as learning experiences through which they can acquire new patterns of behaviour and thus change.

Peplau (1969) points out that when individuals undergo stress:

> ... *self-concern is almost the exclusive force. The task of the nurse is not to sympathise with this self-concern but rather to aid the patient to bring to bear – to develop through use – his [sic] competence for seeing and understanding his [sic] predicament.*

By assisting people in recognising their own reactions and coping mechanisms, nurses can help them to develop a fuller understanding of themselves and through this to evolve a foresight which will help them to prevent, when possible, future recurrences of illnesses. Thus nursing goes beyond mothering and technical aspects of care into the realms of health teaching and preventive services. The goal is concerned with helping individuals in a creative, productive and constructive way to develop their personality. In achieving this end, Peplau stresses that it is not only the patient or client who will develop but also the nurse through her/his increased understanding of the effects of universal stressors on different unique individuals.

In more recent years, Peplau has expressed a further view about nursing. She sees it not only as an interpersonal process concerned with individual clients, but also as a strong social force (Peplau, 1980). With this change, there is a requirement that nurses become actively involved in planning health care programmes and in setting policies at both local and national levels. Because of nurses' wide and varied contact with people, they are in a position not only to care for the sick but also to make public their views on issues concerned with health care. Thus another goal of nursing can be identified, that of influencing social policy.

KNOWLEDGE AND SKILLS FOR PRACTICE

To Peplau, the essence of nursing is in the relationship between the nurse and the client. She suggests that nursing care occurs within such an interpersonal relationship. In order to help patients to meet their own needs, nurses need first to become aware of themselves, their personal needs and their personal reactions. By doing this, they can manage their own behaviour rather than that of the patient and use themselves as the stimulus or therapeutic agent to which the patients will respond and which will cause them to modify their behaviour. She points out the danger of nurses behaving in such a way as to meet their own personal needs through seeking patient approval. For instance, 'doing something for' a patient may give satisfaction to the nurse and gain thanks from the patient but may not achieve movement towards a goal of development for the patient.

Peplau (1969) suggests that nurses must develop the skill of attaining professional closeness, an attribute only learned through professional schooling. She differentiates professional closeness from physical closeness, interpersonal intimacy and pseudo-closeness. Physical closeness is concerned with the physical act of mothering and is a relatively easy behaviour to acquire. Interpersonal closeness is the two-way interpersonal exchange, usually between two peers, where thoughts and ideas about new experiences are shared together purposely for the benefit of both. Pseudo-closeness is the sympathetic response given in answer to a given situation. 'Isn't that awful' or 'I'm so sorry' are examples of this sort of behaviour. She sees a danger in this type of response since it may block further understanding. While there may appear to be a closeness, it is only superficial.

Professional closeness contains elements of physical closeness and interpersonal intimacy but goes beyond them both. The focus of attention is exclusively upon the client rather than on both participants and a professional's behaviour is adjusted in order to meet the client's needs. Nurses are required to show interest, concern and competence with regard to the client's situation and may still need to learn to manage their own personal responses. In order to achieve this end, Peplau suggests that it is the task of the school to help students to study and understand their own reactions to stressful or difficult situations, such as disfigurement, unpleasant odours or pain, in order that they can control their own reactions. Without attaining this ability, there is a risk of:

- over-involvement at a personal level
- under-involvement with an emphasis on the clinical or technical components of work
- avoidance of clients with difficult problems by allocating them to students or untrained staff

As an alternative, professional closeness allows the nurse to develop an intimate relationship with a patient. The nurse focuses on the patient's personal needs or frustrations and nursing therapy is aimed towards growth of that particular individual.

The type of stimulus the nurse provides in this situation must be based on knowledge. Peplau suggests that this should be broad based and drawn from both the behavioural and the physical sciences and theories of nursing. Thus universal knowledge can be applied and adapted to unique individuals. She suggests that in every situation there is an opportunity for new learning for nurses as they see the different ways people react to universal situations. Peplau also suggests that if there is a mismatch between the nurse's current knowledge and a client's response, then the nurse should be guided as to what further knowledge is needed in order to develop personally or to consider further theories.

While Peplau lays emphasis on the interpersonal nature of nursing, she does not neglect the technical side and points out that nurses must also acquire skills necessary to perform procedures related to

Figure 13.2   A diagrammatic representation of Peplau's development model.

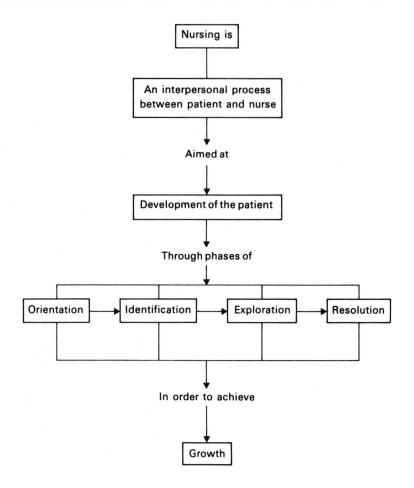

nursing; Figure 13.2 is a diagrammatic representation of Peplau's developmental model.

In line with developmental theory, Peplau suggests that a patient moves through four phases in his movement towards health, which correspond to the four phases of the nursing process. During these phases six roles of nursing emerge.

- *Counsellor* – helps the patient to realise and resolve their problems through personal interaction.
- *Resource* – when the patient requires certain information and the nurse provides it.
- *Teacher* – Peplau (1964) distinguishes between instructional work, where the nurse gives information to the patient and experiential learning, where the patient is encouraged to learn through experience.
- *Technical expert* – relating predominantly to the nurse's ability to use equipment to aid the physically ill.
- *Surrogate* – the patient views the nurse as mother, but gradually learns to see the difference. The patient learns to recognise when to be dependent and independent and eventually the balance between the two.
- *Leader* – the nurse guides the patient towards health.

ASSESSMENT USING A DEVELOPMENTAL MODEL

The orientation phase – assessment

In this phase both the patient and the nurse learn the nature of the difficulty that the patient is experiencing and they develop a mutual trust. The orientation phase is the stage at which data are collected in order that problems can be identified. It may be very rapid or extend over a long period of time, according to the particular nature of the situation.

The identification phase – planning

The second stage is reached when the patient recognises that he or she is forming a relationship with the nurse and the nurse plans the appropriate intervention. Peplau lays emphasis on the fact that since nurses have expert knowledge about nursing, the responsibility lies with them rather than the patients to formulate plans and goals. Her concern about the possible differences between what patients want and what they need is highlighted, and she recognises that the goals of the nurse and the patient may not be the same. Part of the development of the relationship between them will be in the resolution of these variances, the nurse using expert knowledge in helping the patient to have a better understanding and insight into the particular health difficulty concerned.

The exploitation phase – implementation

At this stage of the patient's experience, there is recognition and response to the services that are offered by the nurse. The interpersonal process is fully utilised and both the nurse and the patient move towards mutually recognised goals. The nurse may act as counsellor, resource person, technician or take on any other appropriate role according to the situation.

The resolution phase – evaluation

As the health problem is overcome and the patient no longer requires a nursing service, so the ties that have grown between the nurse and the patient must be broken. The nurse evaluates the situation and learns from the experience in order to be able to apply new knowledge to further situations. The patient returns to an adult state of independence and freedom having, hopefully, grown.

Peplau suggests that there are two basic causes which may lead to a person seeking help from a health care worker when unwell. First, the individual concerned will have a 'felt need' – a problem that has arisen which requires a response. Second, the individual will have expectations of help from the professional person whose advice is sought. During the orientation or assessment phase, these needs and expectations are explored in order to clarify the situation. Peplau suggests that if emphasis at this stage is placed on the disease process and on ways in which it can be overcome, the emphasis of care will also be on the conquering of the disease. Alternatively, if emphasis is placed on the personal growth of the individual, on considering the event which has led to a need for health care as a learning experience of life, then a more genuine consideration of the individual is likely to arise.

Because of the nature of Peplau's views, it would be inappropriate to follow a formal structure during the orientation or assessment phase of development, since the very essence of her approach is based on the relationship that is formed between the client and the nurse. It has been argued that the use of this model is confined to a limited number of clinical settings where the emphasis of care is based on the client's ability to recognise and accept the underlying cause of his or her difficulty. In areas where a greater emphasis is placed on achieving changes in behaviour through other means, the approach may be considered as both time-consuming and inappropriate.

Yet, with the current shift in emphasis towards individuals' rights in managing their own health, there is much to be learned from a model which lays emphasis on helping people to explore why they are facing difficulties. Without such information, the ability to manage in the future may be restricted. While the depth of such exploration can vary considerably, according to the particular situation or indeed the particular wishes of the client concerned, much can be learned by nurses in any setting from a consideration of Peplau's views about personal development and growth. Regardless of the unstructured approach to the assessment in this situation, it is still essential that information gathered during the orientation phase is recorded both for future reference and to assist in professional accountability.

Peplau does not describe or recommend a particular form of record keeping, but the method that we have used to apply the ideas behind her model of nursing is that of process recording using the SOAP format. The format uses the acronym SOAP to describe different stages of the process.

S   This is the subjective experience as described by the client or patient. Direct quotes are often used. If the client is unable to contribute, it is quite acceptable to write 'none'.
O   This is the objective observation that is made by the nurse. Such things as relevant laboratory findings may also be included in this section.
A   This is the formal assessment or judgement made by nurses using both the subjective and objective data. It is the stage at which the information is analysed and at which the problems are identified.
P   This is where a plan of action is decided upon, based on the problem identification and the subjective and objective data that has been gathered.

In some instances this format is extended to include the implementation and evaluation stages of the process. In this situation the following letters are added, making the acronym SOAPIER.

I   The implementation stage of the plan.
E   The evaluation of the plan.
R   The reassessment.

In process recording, each contact between the nurse and the client is recorded using the format described above. Whenever possible the length of the relationship is agreed upon at the beginning of the interaction. For instance, if the client is attending an antenatal clinic, the date for completion would be determined by her expected date of delivery. In an acute surgical ward, the date of discharge may be predicted, whereas in a psychiatric setting the final date may be more fluid and agreed upon at a later date in the relationship.

Because of the different approach that would be used for assessment in this example, the recording of information would take a much less structured approach. In its simplest form, all that is required is a blank sheet of paper. However, it is sometimes helpful to have some sort of guidance to record biographical data and a sheet for use in the process system. Figure 13.3 is an example of a record which may be suitable.

Figure 13.3   An assessment form.

WARD:	Admission Date:
Name:	*Age:*
Address:	*Occupation:*
	Religion:
Tel. No.:	*Likes to be referred to as:*
Next of Kin:	*Meaningful others:*
Name:	
Address:	
Tel. No.:	
Home supports:	
Medical Care:	
Consultant:	*Ward doctor:*
Proposed medical regime:	

Date/Time		Notes	Signature
	S		
	O		
	A		
	P		

Although there is no formal pattern to follow, it may be useful for the nurse to develop a framework which she can use as a mental check list during the orientation phase. An aide-mémoire like this helps to ensure that areas of human needs which may give rise to difficulties are not overlooked. Needs have been written about by many people, for instance Maslow (1954) describes a hierarchy of needs while Henderson (1966) describes 14 activities of daily living which she considers incorporate human needs. The choice may be left with the individual nurse or with the team as to which approach is taken, and may vary according to the type of clinical setting and the emphasis of care. Whichever framework is chosen, it is important that it is shared with all team members in order to facilitate communication.

In the case of Mr Smith, the orientation phase may begin by discussing the circumstances which have led him to seek help. In his case, an activities of living framework may be a useful guide to the discussion. Figure 13.4 is an example of the information gathered about his nutritional needs using the process recording format.

Figure 13.4   A care plan item.

Nursing Notes

Date/Time		Notes	Signature
2/7/95 10 a.m. (admission interview)	S	Is worried about not being able to cook own meals.	
		Says he has lost weight recently.	
		Dislikes food cooked by neighbours or provided by Meals-on-Wheels.	
		Dislikes having to ask other people for help.	
		Has no appetite since he has not been able to cook own food. Cooking for him was 'part of eating'.	
		Worried about how he will cope in future.	
	O	Looks thin and anxious. Can explain his own difficulties well. Dietary intake insufficient to maintain weight.	
	A	Weight 9 st 1 lb (from 9 st 11 lb in May). Unable to hold heavy objects in hands, e.g. saucepans and kettle.	
		Cannot manipulate objects requiring fine movements, e.g. tin opener.	
		Currently has Meals-on-Wheels on Tuesdays and Fridays. Home help cooks on other days and leaves a meal for weekends.	

In this example Mr Smith is able to identify his difficulties quite clearly and the orientation phase or understanding of the difficulty can be established rapidly. In other instances, this phase may take a considerable length of time with repeated interactions and recordings of the process. Even though the difficulties he found have been identified initially for Mr Smith, further assessment may reveal more information, particularly as the trust develops between the client and the nurse.

CARE PLANNING

Progressing to the identification or planning stage, Peplau suggests that, since the nurse has expert knowledge she has the major responsibility for suggesting a plan of action. Continuing to use the process format, both goals and plans may be recorded together. Figure 13.5 shows a plan for Mr Smith.

Unlike some of the other approaches that have been discussed, in this instance the information is recorded on a continual basis, a summary of each contact following the same format. However, as the care progresses, the emphasis of recording will move towards gathering information about evaluation, and reassessment to see whether the need for nursing has been resolved and the relationship can be discontinued.

Figure 13.5   Planning care.

Nursing Notes

Date/Time		Notes	Signature
	P	Goal – Will learn to cook simple meals and hot drinks independently.	
		Refer to occupational therapist for a. advice on suitable aids b. teaching in use of aids	
		Practise use of aids in ward kitchen at least once each day.	
		Goal – Will maintain current weight.	
		Discuss diet and help to draw up a weekly menu which can be prepared independently.	
		Weigh every Friday at 9.00 a.m. in pyjamas.	
		Goal – Will gather information and understanding of services which may be helpful in the future.	
		Discuss possibility of weekly visits to social meeting at disabled centre.	
		Provide information and costing of sheltered housing.	
		Arrange for consultation of social worker.	

Figure 13.6 Biographical data and initial nursing notes.

WARD: Peplau   Admission Date: 3/11/95

Name: Mr Jack Fieldson   *Age:* 68 yrs   DOB: 02.07.27
Address: The Old Barn   *Occupation:* Retired architect
         Mewby on the Hill
                                            Religion: Baptist
Tel. No.: Mewby 83307   *Likes to be
                                            referred to as:* Mr Fieldson

Next of Kin: Daughter   *Meaningful others:*
Name: Mrs Hilary James   Grandchildren – Kathy (6), John (4)
Address: Box Cottage   Mr and Mrs Trevor (neighbours)
         Hawkesbury
         Northumberland
Tel No.: Hawkesbury 43762

Home supports:
  Private home help 3 days weekly
  GP – family friend

Medical Care:

Consultant: Dr Everett   *Ward doctor:* John Reeves

Proposed medical regime:
  For close observation and supervision (suicide risk)
  Drug therapy

Nursing Notes (Excerpt of notes on 1st day of admission)

Date/Time		Notes	Signature
3/11/95 11 a.m.	S	Says he is worried and disturbed by being here and doesn't want to discuss the situation.	
	O	Reluctant to talk. Looking down at the floor. Wringing hands. Physically unkempt.	
	A	Is withdrawn. Ashamed at being in psychiatric hospital. Unable to establish an rapport at this stage.	
	P	Introduce to other patients. Show ward/bed areas. Give time to familiarise himself with environment and see the doctor.	
3 p.m.	E	No change in behaviour.	

Figure 13.6   Biographical
data and initial nursing notes.
(*cont.*).

S   Says he has seen the doctor
    and knows he is depressed but
    nothing can help.
    'This place will make me
    even worse'.

O   Still withdrawn avoiding eye contact.
    No conversation initiated with
    either staff or patients.
    Food on jacket, shirt and around
    mouth.
    Reluctant to join other patients.

A   Apathetic and unhappy.
    In need of constant observation.

P   Re-interview on evening shift.
    Observe closely.

A PATIENT CARE STUDY

Since process recording is obviously a continual operation, only excerpts of the care study are shown below in order to demonstrate the technique. The person concerned is a 68-year-old man, Mr Jack Fieldson, who has recently been widowed. He retired from his work as an architect 2 years ago and lost his wife 6 months ago. Over the last 6 months he has become progressively more withdrawn and depressed and is now no longer able to care for himself. During the orientation phase of nursing, the interactions between Mr Fieldson and the nurse are aimed towards both of them learning more about the nature of Mr Fieldson's difficulties, recognising the cause of the difficulties and developing trust and understanding between them.

The professional schooling of the nurse should enable her to manage her own reactions towards this withdrawn, unresponsive person and to use interactional skills in trying to help him. This should be done without over-involvement but with a professional closeness. A summary of the initial interaction is shown in Figure 13.6, followed by a further summary of the interaction which occurred 5 days later (Figure 13.7).

The first excerpt from Mr Fieldson's progress notes demonstrates the beginning phases of the development of a relationship between client and nurse. Rather than following a formal structure, both the length and initial contact are guided by Mr Fieldson's own responses to the situation and, as can be seen in this beginning stage, the trust which is sought has not yet been established nor has the part that each of the participants will play.

During the second excerpt, the freedom of this approach is again shown. For example, although the frequency of the interactions between Mr Fieldson and his primary nurse are stated, no length of time is prescribed since this would be determined by him. However, in different circumstances, it would be quite feasible to include more details if required. The intensity of the relationship and the strain that is placed on the nurse while being in such close proximity with someone whose mood is low are acknowledged. The work of observing may be shared among other members of the team, while the direct interaction would occur with the primary nurse.

At first sight it may be difficult to see how this approach can be used in settings where the major need has arisen through a physiological disorder.

Figure 13.7 Nursing notes,
5 days after admission.

Date/Time		Notes	Signature
8/11/95 1 p.m.	S	Monosyllabic responses to conversation only.	
	O	Silent tears during lunch. No food eaten. Answers direct questions appropriately but monosyllabically. Does not express any feelings. No movement around ward except when led. No concern for hygiene or appearance.	
	A	Low mood worsening. Suicide risk currently reduced through apathy.	
	P	Review at multidisciplinary team meeting this afternoon.	
	I	Discussed at meeting. Patient not present. Not responding to drug therapy yet. Further action needed. Intensive nursing care. Continuous observation with interaction every 2 hours, or in response to non-verbal approaches, with primary nurse.	

However, the underlying belief in developing a trusting relationship can only be seen as valuable. The approach could be particularly useful in terminal care, in fields where the emphasis of care is towards health education and in work with the disabled. In all these areas it is particularly important that an understanding can develop between both parties and that shared learning about the strengths and needs of the client can occur alongside personal growth for the nurse.

Learning exercises

1. Write a description of a patient with whom you consider you have developed a good relationship in the past.
2. Reflect on this description and identify the element of the relationship that would be considered professional closeness as defined by Peplau.

Study questions

1. From a 'Developmental Model of Nursing' perspective, write a critique of contemporary nursing.

Chapter 14

Humanistic Nursing Theory

LEARNING OBJECTIVES

On completion of this chapter, the reader will be able to:

1. Compare phenomenology and intuitive nursing
2. Identify the phases of engagement with patients that lead to assessment
3. Appreciate the potential of nursing as a therapy

The authors of this theory use the word 'humanistic' with nursing because they see nursing as an interhuman event where the dignity, interests and values of the nurse and the nursed as people are of prime importance. Josephine Paterson and Loretta Zderad are nursing scholars who, before their retirements in 1985, were clinicians in the domains of practice, research and education at the Northport Veterans Administration Hospital in Northport, NY. They described the work in these three domains of nursing as 'clinical nursing' and developed a theory that derived from the experience of clinical nurses.

Paterson and Zderad are considered to be two of the pioneers in nursing theory. In the 1960s and 1970s they set out to explore and describe the nature of nursing as a phenomenon and particularly the nurse/patient relationship. The theory evolved from the descriptions of nursing experienced in all situations regardless of speciality, and the book is peppered with examples from their lives and clinical practice. Their focus on nursing and the nursed (their term for patient) resulted in a detailed examination of nursing and the person, more so than on the other two aspects of nursing's metaparadigms, health and the environment (O'Connor, 1993).

Paterson and Zderad published their book *Humanistic Nursing* in 1976. It represented ideas that had grown from their practice experiences. They took an interpretative route to their theory development, capturing ideas from experience using phenomenological methods. At the time the interpretative perspective which they took was considered 'alternative'.

The dominant trend amongst scholars then was to establish the discipline of nursing through rigorous positivistic methods. It is pertinent that after a period of 10 years, and following the retirement of both of them, the book, which was out of print, was republished in 1988 because there was such a demand for it. The ideas that nursing knowledge is embedded in practice, humanistic ideals are ethics worth pursuing, and nursing is an intensely emotional and interpersonal practice, are now acceptable and even popular. Both Watson (1979) and Parse (1981), later theorists whose work is described in the next two chapters of this book, were influenced by Paterson and Zderad's early work.

PHILOSOPHICAL FOUNDATIONS

Paterson and Zderad are clearly influenced by the existential and phenomenological philosophers and this is evident throughout their work. They explain that existential thought has helped them to understand nursing from an experiential perspective and that phenomenology is the means by which they expose and articulate nursing experience.

A short review of existentialism and phenomenology is appropriate here in order to orientate the reader to the origins of Paterson and Zderad's philosophy and work.

Existentialism

Levinas (1949) offers the following simple definition: 'Existentialism is to experience and think existence'. Barrett (1962) suggests that existentialism is a revolt against rational and mechanistic world views, cultivated by Western philosophers and culminating in the technologically impersonal world of modern times. Paterson and Zderad (1976/1988) had a similar reaction to the traditional scientific approaches to nursing. They described existential experience as: 'Contact with reality with the whole of one's being; [which] involves all that a man [sic] is as opposed to experiencing through one or several faculties'.

Existentialists strive to understand the purpose and meaning of life as experienced by individuals. They believe decisions are made and the shape of the future is formed through people's awareness of their own existence or being. Humans are in an enduring state of development, the hopes and strategies for their future impinge upon individuals as they are now and have been. A person's essence (what the person is) is a product of their existence and therefore existence (the becoming) precedes and shapes the person's ever-developing essence.

Cooper (1990) explains that existing is difficult to conceptualise because it is an art, an impression rather than a quantifiable object. In existing, the human is constantly labouring, contending with choices, is free but responsible, feels anxious, lives in a world that is not predetermined and which seems at times absurd. These things cannot be described in concrete or empirical ways.

While humans are all unique and at times solitary, they also share common features (e.g. they are all unique) and can display solidarity with their fellows. Through dialogue or intersubjectivity, humans work together to overcome hardship and to find meaning in human existence.

Some time ago, MacIntyre (1964) and Barrett (1962) wrote that to an extent the existentialists' works now represent out-moded thought and that their complexity and lack of system make them subject to considerable criticism. Nevertheless, it can be argued that study of their work is worthwhile for the nurse struggling with an emerging paradigm, to discover a discrete knowledge of human experience related to health. It is prudent to consider that the existentialists concentrate on the individual to the detriment of society as a whole, and may overestimate the person's control and contribution towards his/her destiny.

Phenomenology

Phenomenology is both a philosophy and a research methodology. It is a means whereby phenomena are scrutinised as they occur in the world, from the perspective of the subject rather than an external observer. In paying attention to things in this way the subjective experienced world is described, articulated and appreciated. As nurses have unique experiences in their shared world of nursing, Paterson and Zderad have chosen phenomenology as a means of exposing nurses' angular views and using the individual insights to clarify particular phenomena. An existential awareness equips nurses to select phenomena for research. Paterson and Zderad (1976/1988) give the examples of phenomena such as presence, comfort and 'all at once', which have been examined in this way and show how resulting understanding may be used to increase nursing's knowledge base.

BELIEFS AND VALUES

The person

Paterson and Zderad refer to the nurse's humanity as well as the patient's when they discuss the person. The person is a holistic being capable of and responsible for making choices throughout life. For the person, life is a process of becoming (growing, developing oneself). Life is not predetermined for one but is a result of individual choices and actions. The person's particular present experience ('here and now') is influenced by a medley of past events, the present and the future (Paterson and Zderad, 1976/1988). How a person chooses to respond to a situation determines how they are in the world.

Each person is unique, seeing and experiencing the world from a personal angle according to their 'here and now'. However, making and sharing meanings with others is a human need: each human encounter is important and significant in the process of human becoming or, in Paterson and Zderad's terms, 'more becoming'. The person seriously reflects on and contemplates his/her experiences, learning thereby to be conscious of responses and the meanings personally attached to different experiences.

Health

Paterson and Zderad acknowledge that health defined as an absence of disease is inadequate. However, they do not offer an alternative. Regarding health they say that at times nursing is 'health restoring, health sustaining, or health promoting' and that nurses provide health education and supervision for clients. However, health is not necessarily the prime goal of nursing. While nursing is related to health as an absence of disease, they prefer to discuss the notion of well-being and more being as targets of nursing care. Some people cannot aspire to health according to its narrow definition, e.g. the chronically ill, and yet nurses will find their help is required by these people in order to reach their greatest potential for living.

Environment

Great store is set upon the person's situation in the world and relationship with the environment, for whilst Paterson and Zderad concentrate on the nurse/patient relationship, they readily note that nursing dialogue takes place in the complicated world which impacts upon the person's reality. Things in the environment have different meanings for different people. Things that are familiar to the nurse may be strange and uncomfortable for a new client.

Time and space are important concepts. Besides chronological, measured time, they explain time as experienced by both the nurse and the nursed. Nurses may perceive time as speeding by, clients may not. Time spent with a client may seem to be a significant contribution on the part of the nurse. However, it may represent an insignificant amount of time to a client. Personal space is described as the person's 'place'. Space, like time, can be measured, but space as experienced is far more influential in the development of a person's sense of being. Illness may alter the person's perception of space; for example, either the ability to walk far or perhaps to see. Personal space gives one the sense of belonging. Nurses need to be aware not only of their own perception of space but also that of the client.

THE GOALS OF NURSING

Nursing is described as a:

> ... *nurturing response of one person to another in need, it aims at the development of human potential, as well-being and more-being. As something that happens between people, it reflects all the human potential and limitations of the persons involved. As an intersubjective transaction, it holds the possibility for both persons to affect and be affected, the possibility for both to become more.*

(Paterson and Zderad, 1976/1988)

Nursing is a 'lived dialogue', by which Paterson and Zderad mean that the nurse experiences a call for help and responds to the client in a humane and deliberate way; two humans in purposeful two-way communication. The nurse relates with the nursed in a combined interpersonal, or as they term it intersubjective, and business-like or transactional way. As a lived dialogue there is the possibility for both the nurse and the nursed to become more through the shared experience while the shared experience, of course, may have quite different meanings for each according to their angular perspective (where they come from).

Nursing involves the nurse in both being and doing. The 'doing' things in nursing are fairly familiar, but Paterson and Zderad discuss the notion of presence or being and they point out that sometimes presence occurs at the same time as doing. Presence is a way of being with the other; a willingness to be receptive to the other's needs and a communion which conveys that one is quite prepared to be with, to listen to, to concentrate upon, to care for and to love the other. There is a professional element to nursing presence, however, as the nurse is aware of the goals to be achieved through nursing care.

KNOWLEDGE FOR NURSING

I consider my greatest gifts as a human being nurse [are] my ability to relate to other man [sic], to wonder, search, and imagine about my experience, and to create out of what I come to know. My ever developing internalised community of world thinkers dynamically interrelated with my conscious awareness of my experienced nursing realm allow my appreciation of my human gifts and the ever enrichment of myself as a 'knowing place'.

(Paterson and Zderad, 1976/1988)

Paterson and Zderad describe the person as nurse as a knowing place. The person as nurse is a source of knowledge that is unique to nursing and discovered through his/her accounts of experiences. While this is undoubtedly true, the knowledge to be gained from experience is often constrained by the limits of language to portray it. Phenomenology, or the method described by Paterson and Zderad particularly for nursing, phenomenologic nursology, is a means of describing clinical nursing experience and expressing the meanings and knowledge which develop. Paterson and Zderad (1976/1988) describe five phases of their method.

Phase I: Preparation of the nurse knower for coming to know

This is a stage of positive attitudes towards investigation. A curiosity and a willingness to be surprised by new information. It is a time when the nursing researcher puts behind him/her, as much as is possible, preconceived ideas in order to find out more from another perspective.

Phase II: Nurse knowing of the other intuitively

The nurse researcher steps into the other's arena and accepts it as it is presented. The nurse researcher has a closeness with the other and an authentic regard for his/her account. There is no attempt to analyse the other's story, just a willingness to glimpse the particular view from the other's vantage point.

Phase III: Nurse knowing the other scientifically

The information is examined from a distance, it is analysed and interpreted. It is compared with other experiences and similarities and differences are exposed, for the purpose of clarifying the phenomena.

Phase IV: Nurse complementarily synthesising known others

The nurse researcher brings together the information gathered and marks relationships, building up a synthesis of ideas which represents the participants' described raw realities.

Phase V: Succession within the nurse from the many to the paradoxical one

In the last phase the nurse researcher's own particular view is extended through an appreciation of others' experiences. This is as a result of the process through the previous four stages.

Besides nursing's unique knowledge that emanates through the method described above, nurses also use knowledge from the allied sciences and humanities. Paterson and Zderad describe nursing as an art–science. The arts are lauded for helping nurses to understand the human condition and also for being an expressive medium. Study of the arts encourages the nurse to be imaginative and creative. The sciences help nurses to know and make decisions regarding concrete problems dealt with in daily practice. Whilst nurses can learn from the arts and sciences, they also contribute to the general knowledge in the human sciences. Paterson and Zderad (1976/1988) link art and science as art–science to create the impression of the two being indivisible in the practice of nursing.

THE NURSING PROCESS

Paterson and Zderad do not have a prescription for the process of nursing, however, the process of nursing or the experiences of being a nurse informed them when they developed their method for research and their specific nursing theory. Each of the phases in their method relates to their experience in practice.

- *Phase I*: The nurse is open to the experience and is prepared to give concentrated attention to the client. S/he wants to help the other and prepares to understand his/her view of the 'here and now'.
- *Phase II*: Knowing the other is developed through presence. The client and nurse communicate in an authentic way, allowing the nurse to glimpse the other's 'here and now'.
- *Phase III*: The nurse steps back from the situation and reflects upon the experience. S/he analyses the situation and synthesises the components incorporating other ideas from, for example, the literature, to generate ideas or themes.
- *Phase IV*: The nurse compares the present experience with past ones, considering their similarities and differences and thereby enlarges his/her repertoire of understanding.
- *Phase V*: The nurse is able to accept the paradoxes of the chaos of real life and express the new-found knowledge in a way that other nurses can understand and find useful.

The phases can be roughly identified in the following description of a nurse's experience with Mr Smith, the client described in the other chapters, who has been losing weight.

14.11: I telephoned Mr Smith to introduce myself and ask if I might visit him. The referral letter had said that he was 'difficult' and didn't like outside interference. I told him I understood that he was troubled with arthritis and had been losing weight. I said that I would like to spend some time with him to hear from him first hand whether there was a problem and decide whether I might be able to help. He said he would be pleased to see me the following morning at 11 a.m.

15.11: I arrived on time, Mr Smith immediately answered the door and invited me in. I accepted his offer of a cup of tea, which he served on a tray with biscuits. The house is cosy and warm with lots of photographs on the tables and shelves; there wasn't a speck of dust. I complimented him on the cosy feel of the place – he beamed with delight in response and showed me the photograph of his wedding. I told him that the doctor and his neighbours were concerned about his health and asked him to tell me what he thought. I listened intently to his story and noted his expression and gestures. Right from the first referral I had wondered if he couldn't prepare food or whether perhaps he didn't feel like it. From the looks of the neat house and the way he had made the tea, laying a tray, lifting and filling a kettle, undoing the jar with biscuits, I couldn't really see a problem with dexterity or knowing how to look after himself. He talked about his life with his wife, how they kept themselves to themselves and liked life that way. He has no children and admitted that his days were long and lonely now. I had another appointment which I needed to keep so I thanked Mr Smith for his help. He asked when I would come back so I made an appointment for 2 days' time. I asked him what he thought I could do to help if I came back. He said he would think through his problems and give me a list; he said that with a chuckle but I knew he was half serious.

I believe that he doesn't want too much assistance from the neighbours because he doesn't want to give them access to the house and deep down he knows that he is capable of cooking for himself. His main problem seems to be that he has no appetite and therefore has little motivation to make an effort in the kitchen. I need to find out why he has no appetite. I remember a similar case where I moved too quickly to mobilise all the services and found that the person still wouldn't eat when the food was placed in front of her. We eventually found that she had a carcinoma of the stomach. I will try not to jump to conclusions too quickly. I do know that he is lonely and whether or not that is affecting his appetite, it is affecting his quality of life. We need to talk more about this and think of a way most suitable for him to appease it.

In their book Paterson and Zderad demonstrate how they clarify certain phenomena using the phenomenological nursology and illustrate the emergent propositions with experiences from clinical nursing that gave rise to them. This method can be used by clinical nurses to learn more, contribute to nursing's unique knowledge and make their practice more meaningful.

ILLUSTRATIVE EXAMPLES

Instead of a conventional case study we will give some examples of experiences which illustrate a few of the ideas generated by Paterson and Zderad. When they considered the concept of comfort they identified 12 behaviours that contributed to the client's comfort. Some are described below.

I verbalized my acceptance of patients' expressions of feelings with explanations of why I experienced these feelings of acceptance when I could do this authentically and appropriately.

(Paterson and Zderad, 1976/1988)

Example 1

Sarah, Mary's daughter, had come to visit. Mary had been sick for a long time and stayed in the ICU. Her family were extremely worried about her and most attention had focused upon Peter, the husband who doted on Mary and said he would not live without her. She was described by her family as a strong woman and the person who kept them all together.

Sarah sat with her Mother while I pottered around the room, filling in charts, checking the equipment, etc. Gradually I noticed an altercation: Mary couldn't talk as she was on a ventilator but she gesticulated, in an annoyed way, for Sarah to go. Sarah was giving explanations about being busy, etc. but left, tears readily flowing. When I talked to her just outside the room she said it was typical of her Mother expecting her to do all the work. Apparently Mary had told Sarah off for not doing her washing and bringing it up to her, she had told her to go away. This was a bit hard considering that Sarah worked, had come a fair way on public transport and was extremely worried about her Mother. I comforted her and said to come tomorrow when Mary might be in a better frame of mind. She chuckled and said she would come when she had done the washing; there was a pile at home anyway.

When I went back into the room I looked at Mary wondering if she would be upset. She looked at me, eyes blazing, daring me to criticise or try to placate her. I smiled and said 'well, at least you can still lick your children into shape'. She lifted her thumb in agreement and went to sleep. Much later when she was better she said how important it was that Sarah took her place as much as possible. She was furious as the absence of clean washing for her meant that all the other washing wasn't being done either, a symbol that the place was falling to bits without her. I told her how sorry I had felt for Sarah at the time but how I had an inkling she knew what she was about. She laughed and held my hand.

When verbalizations of acceptance were not appropriate, I acted out this acceptance by my behaviour of staying with or doing for when appropriate.

(Paterson and Zderad, 1976/1988)

Example II Sally was unconscious following a cerebral vascular accident. She was breathing spontaneously via a tracheostomy tube. Three of us had just lifted her out into her special chair and arranged her limbs for support and comfort. I talked to her as we were helping her and there was as usual no response at all. When we finished I stayed with her. She was young, younger than me, a successful professional with a loving family. I felt frustrated because I didn't know if she knew I was there or how much I wanted to help. I knelt beside her; comfortable; I held her elbows our forearms touching; my side against her legs and knees. I just knelt and concentrated as hard as I could at communicating with her. I hoped she might respond, I hoped she might know I was there and I hoped she might feel cared for. After a long time I got up, behind me her brother stood quietly not wishing to disturb us. I smiled at him and he solemnly said 'Thank you'. I left him with his sister. I knew what he had thanked me for and its significance.

I expressed purposely, to burst asunder negative self concepts, my authentic human tender feelings for patients when appropriate and acceptable.

(Paterson and Zderad, 1976/1988)

Example III Clary was a new patient. He had been admitted to the ward the night before. The night staff reported that he called for help at least every 5 minutes and whenever he saw someone passing. He was disabled and very large and he always asked to be repositioned which was extremely difficult for the two night nurses to do. Even though they were frustrated the night nurses had always attended him and tried to help.

I discussed my workload with the rest of the team on the morning shift and decided that Clary would be my only patient that morning. I went to him and introduced myself. I explained that I would always work with him when I was on duty and that morning I would spend all my time with him because he was obviously uncomfortable and needed a lot of attention. Clary stayed with us for 5 days and during that time we built up quite a rapport. He learnt that we would attend to him without being called. We used the hoist to help him move so that it was quite easy for two nurses to reposition him. He told me jokes and made me laugh. I told him I enjoyed his company and whenever I could find time went back to sit with him. He began to talk to the other patients in the beds beside him. When he left we all said we would miss him and he smiled.

Learning exercises

1. Make a list of values that you hold about nursing.
2. Compare these with humanistic nursing.

Study questions

1. Write notes on the opportunities that occur each day to get to know patients.
2. Reconsider the work that you do and identify ways that you can make the environment conducive to healing.

Chapter 15

Human Becoming

LEARNING OBJECTIVES

On completion of this chapter, the reader will be able to:

1. Explain the construction of Human Becoming theory

2. Relate the centrality of the patient's perspective to nursing decisions

This chapter looks at the work of one of the more recent nursing theorists, Rosemarie Parse. She still writes extensively but the book that introduces her theory of Man–Living–Health was published in 1981. Subsequently, she renamed this theory Human Becoming and has changed some phrases. In her work she differs from both the positivistic position taken by the natural scientists and the more moderate stance of some of the early nursing theorists who describe the person as a bio-psycho-socio-spiritual organism. Parse (1987) suggests that these early views tend to see the person as an object whose behaviour can be observed, measured and predicted. Alternatively, Parse's frame of reference is one of simultaneity: a view where the person can only be understood as an irreducible, dynamic and complicated whole. She writes that the origins of her work came as 'I began to wonder and wander and ask why not?' (Parse, 1990). This typically lyrical comment gives the reader an impression of simultaneous cogitation, presence, curiosity and movement in the world, which conjures up the unison that she refers to. To many the language she uses will be difficult initially, as many of the terms are unfamiliar and some of the ideas she presents are radically different from those to which most people are used. Nevertheless, she offers an interesting and stimulating perspective on the world of nursing and in particular 'human being's living health' (Parse 1997), and her ideas are worth pursuing.

Parse (1981, 1987, 1992, 1997) acknowledges and appreciates the complexity and unpredictability of the world, seeking to understand the person within the world as a total being who is more than the sum of the parts. Everything she studies is considered from the dynamic perspective of now, history and the future in the context of the universe.

The linked words in the title of her theory 'Man–Living–Health' give the impression of union: the inseparability of people from their being and their construction of health.

This simultaneity view is in harmony with contemporary nursing thought where nurses appreciate and are curious about the subjective and artistic nature of nursing in the context in which it is offered. Parse's work has been used by researchers using qualitative methods. In particular, Parse has worked to develop a method specifically for nursing research (Parse *et al.*, 1985; Parse, 1987, 1990, 1997), which comes directly from her theory of human becoming. This research methodology is informed by phenomenological philosophers.

The fundamentals of Parse's theory include: the person relating to the environment; the person constructing health in his/her world with others; and the person achieving the understanding of the freedom to be and become in an increasingly complicated world. Her assumptions emerge from the principles and concepts developed by Rogers (1970), another eminent and respected nursing scholar, and the thoughts of existential philosophers. She believes that nursing is rooted in the human sciences and sees this situation as preferable to one where nursing knowledge development is dominated by natural sciences and the medical model. She postulates that an anomaly exists between medical and nursing theory. Medicine is primarily concerned with objective knowledge, a concentration which is not conducive to discovering the 'lived in world' experienced by people (Parse, 1981, 1987, 1990, 1997), which is a view that is central to the discipline of nursing.

THEORY CONSTRUCTION

Before relating the underlying assumptions of Parse's work it is necessary to demonstrate how she builds her theory from concepts, principles and tenets. She constructs her work in a logical sequence, introducing first concepts and principles from Rogers' (1970) theory of 'Unitary Man' and then tenets and principles from some of the existentialist philosophers. These foundations are synthesised to form the basic assumptions of her work. Despite this pragmatic breakdown of the work (concepts, principles, tenets), to render it comprehensible, Parse (1987) emphasises the simultaneity of the theory and the reader gets an overall notion of the emphasis on things happening at once and in a complicated way.

The principles and concepts that Parse uses from Rogers' (1970) work are as follows: *helicy, complementarity* (integrality) and *resonancy*, which are the principles; and *energy field, openness, pattern and organisation* (pattern) and *four-dimensionality*, which are the concepts.

In 1997, Parse gave an overview of the theory's evolution. She explains that the nine assumptions underpinned by themes of meaning, rhythmicity and transcendence lead to the three principles of the theory. The nine original assumptions from her early work have been synthesised to become three assumptions about human becoming. Ideas that form the basis of the theory are defined below and enable the reader to understand the assumptions and principles that link and relate to form the model (Figure 15.1).

Rogers		Existential Phenomenology	
Principles	Concepts	Concepts	Tenets
Helicy Complimentarity Resonancy	Energy Field Openness Pattern and Organisation	Coconstitution Coexistence Situated Freedom	Intentionality Human Subjectivity

Assumptions

Human	Becoming
1. The human is coexisting while coconstituting rhythmical patterns with the universe.	5. Becoming is an open process experienced by the human.
2. The human is an open being, freely choosing meaning in situation, bearing responsibility for decisions.	6. Becoming is a rhythmically coconstituting process of human-universe interrelationship.
3. The human is a living unity continuously coconstituting patterns of relating.	7. Becoming is the human's pattern of relating value priorities.
4. The human is transcending multidimensionally with the possibles.	8. Becoming is an intersubjective process of transcending with the possibles.
	9. Becoming is human unfolding.

Principles

1. Structuring meaning multidimensionally is cocreating reality through the languaging of valuing and imaging.	2. Cocreating rhythmical patterns of relating is living the paradoxical unity of revealing-concealing and enabling-limiting while connecting-separating.	3. Cotranscending with the possible is powering unique ways of originating in the process of transforming.

Figure 15.1   Evolution of the theory of human becoming (from Bunting, 1992, p. 7, with permission of Sage Publications, Inc.).

Principles

- *Helicy*. Parse (1981) describes helicy in this way: 'the nature and direction of human and environmental change is continuously innovative, probabilistic, and characterised by increasing diversity …'.
- *Integrality*. This denotes a constant interaction between humans and the environment.
- *Resonancy*. There is a sympathetic vibration and rhythm of energies between the person and environment.

Concepts

- *Energy field*. Both the person and the environment are described as fields that are energised and dynamic. The human field and environmental fields are in constant interaction.
- *Openness*. The person is viewed as an open field not constrained by the confines of the body.
- *Pattern and organisation*. Whilst the person in the environment is ever-changing there is, amidst the seeming irregularity, some pattern which distinguishes the individual. Patterns are formed from the person's behaviours, attitudes and characteristics.
- *Four-dimensionality*. '… man [sic] and environment as four-dimensional energy fields. These energy fields are in simultaneous, continuous, and mutual interaction …' (Parse, 1981). The field domains are not constrained by space or time and the boundaries are constantly moving. The person can stretch out beyond reality to the transcendental world.

Intentionality and human subjectivity are the tenets and coconstitution, coexistence and situated freedom are the concepts Parse used from existential philosophy.

Tenets

- *Intentionality*. This denotes the person's knowledge in the world, by being present and aware. The knowledge enables the person to choose and purposefully to reach possibilities beyond himself or herself.
- *Human subjectivity*. The person's particular relationship with the world through which learning and development occurs in life. The person's growth is affected by the past, the future and the present.

Concepts

- *Coconstitution*. This denotes the person's contribution to the creation of reality. By being in a situation the person affects the milieu and by being open and relating to the environment the person is, in turn, affected by it.
- *Coexistence*. This denotes that the person is never alone in the process of becoming.
- *Situated freedom*. A person chooses both the situations she or he is in and the attitudes adopted. Mindful of the 'history, present, future' matrix, past choices and future aspirations affect choices made in the present. The person is always responsible for the consequences of choices made.

The following three assumptions about Human becoming have been developed by parse from the original nine philosophical assumptions shown in Figure 15.2.

Figure 15.2   Relationship of principles, concepts and theoretical structures of Man–Living–Health (from Parse, 1981, p. 69, with permission).

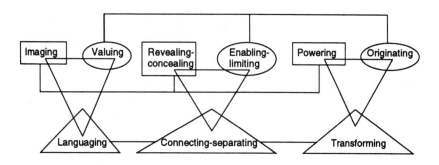

Principle 1: Structuring meaning multidimensionality is cocreating reality through the languaging of valuing and imaging

Principle 2: Cocreating rhythmical patterns of relating is living in the paradoxical unity of revealing-concealing and enabling-limiting while connecting-separating

Principle 3: Cotranscending with the possibles is powering unique ways of originating in the process of transforming

Relationship of the concepts in the *squares*:   Powering is a way of *revealing and concealing imaging*
Relationship of the concepts in the *ovals*:   Originating is a manifestation of *enabling and limiting valuing*
Relationship of the concepts in the *triangles*:   Transforming unfolds in the *languaging of connecting and separating*

Assumptions About Human Becoming (Parse, 1997, p. 32)

- Human becoming is freely choosing personal meaning in a situation, in the intersubjective process of relating value priorities.
- Human becoming is cocreating rhythmical patterns of relating in a mutual process with the universe.
- Human becoming is cotranscending multidimensionally with the emerging possibles.

BELIEFS AND VALUES

Parse's values and beliefs about the person and health are declared in her assumptions, which are derived from a synthesis of the principles, tenets and concepts just outlined (Parse, 1981, 1997). In this manner, Parse weaves her theory from the basic ideas and makes them into a whole that is an indivisible conglomeration that cannot be appreciated in part only.

The person

Parse describes the person as an indivisible, responsible being, forever changing and growing as a result of interaction with the universe. Interaction with others and the universe is a rhythmical pattern of closeness and distance, revealing and concealing, enabling and limiting. Life is created by the person through interactions and choices in a world that unfurls in time towards an increasingly complex future.

Health

Health is constructed by the person and reflects and relates to the person's values and beliefs. Health is a process that reflects the person's evolving relationship with the world and the choices made by the person.

Environment

The environment, or universe as Parse (1992) later refers to it, is an energy field with patterns and organisation that makes it distinct and yet ever-changing. The person and the universe, whilst distant, are constantly together, sometimes near and then farther away. The fluctuating proximity between the person and areas of the universe represent a rhythmical pattern of movement, which ebbs and flows.

THE GOALS OF NURSING

Parse (1981, 1987, 1997) concentrates her attention on the notion of 'human being's living health' rather than defining the why or how of nursing. It is through care for and understanding of the person in the world, exemplified by an ability to stay with the person, that the nurse can guide clients and their meaningful others to choose and make decisions in view of the possibilities. Nursing is a service designed to enable the person to be him or herself, rather than one where the nurse does things, or makes things better for the client. The goal of nursing is for clients to achieve more or improve the quality of their lives according to the individual's, and any meaningful other's, perspective of what constitutes quality of life.

Staying with a person connotes a physical presence but also an ability to accept the other person's perceptions, values and beliefs. It may be that the nurse wishes the person to take a different approach or behave differently, but this may only be done through a process that involves them both constructing new meanings and the person freely choosing a new way.

Parse (1981, 1987) finally develops theoretical structures designed to guide both practice and research and to represent, once again, the interweaving of her ideas regarding 'Human Becoming'. Parse (1987) comments that other theoretical structures could be generated from the matrix of ideas and principles. The theoretical structures are termed by her 'non-directional propositions'. In other words, they are not predicative statements but act as a guide to nursing practice and as a source of questions for research.

Theoretical Structure 1: *Powering is a way of revealing and concealing imaging* (Parse, 1981). The process of relating one's goals and the struggle to achieve them portrays the situation the person finds him or herself in. Through this process of both revealing and concealing information, the person may find new ideas regarding future possibles.

Theoretical Structure 2: *Originating is a manifestation of enabling and limiting valuing* (Parse, 1981). Consideration of values allows the person to understand the limits and opportunities rendered possible by differing perspectives. This view may allow people to consider new ways of being together.

Theoretical Structure 3: *Transforming unfolds in the languaging of connecting and separating* (Parse, 1981). New ways of being together are articulated amongst family members.

KNOWLEDGE FOR NURSING

Parse's work represents an abstract body of knowledge for nursing practice, education and research. She has designed a research method that is specifically for the discipline of nursing. Knowledge is generated concerning the experience of people and rigorously interpreted to describe the essence of particular phenomena of interest to nurses. Participants describe a phenomenon and then, by a process of extraction/synthesis, meaning is transferred from the language of the participants to the language of science (Parse, 1997).

Lee *et al.* (1994) comment that Parse concentrates upon curricula for Master's and Doctoral students. However, Parse proposes that any curricula could be written using 'Human Becoming' as a theoretical structure. Every subject should be approached using the principles and theoretical structures proposed in her work. One example she gives (1981) is of nurses studying Family Health in a Master's programme.

THE NURSING PROCESS

Parse (1987) comments that nursing has not had a methodology for practice which reflects the ontological (what it means to nurses) base of nursing. While it has been used by nurses and Parse describes it as a methodology for practice, the systematic approach to problem solving (the nursing process) is generic and does not relate to the fundamental essences of nursing. She proposes a methodology of nursing practice which stems directly from her theoretical structures, but which is less abstract and more useful for the nurse requiring a guide to work with.

Parse (1987) contends that different theories for nursing practice should result in different practice. To illustrate just how different this theory may be in practice compared to others that have been described in this book, let us return to Mr Smith and his nutritional problem. It should be noted that Parse does not recommend the use of a systematic problem-solving approach to nursing. She considers that the nurse using the problem-solving approach assumes a prescriptive role that is antithetical to the 'Human Becoming' perspective. We think that other

---

Box 15.1   Man–Living–Health practice methodology (from Parse, 1987, p. 167, with permission)

Dimensions
- Illuminating meaning is shedding light through uncovering the what was, is, and will be, as it is appearing now; it happens in *explicating* what is
- Synchronizing rhythms happens in *dwelling with* the pitch, yaw, and roll of the interhuman cadence
- Mobilizing transcendence happens in *moving beyond* the meaning moment to what is not-yet

Processes
- Explicating is making clear what is appearing now through languaging
- Dwelling with is giving self over to the flow of the struggle in connecting-separating
- Moving beyond is propelling toward the possibles in transforming

nurse theorists would counter that whenever possible the nurse, using the nursing process, works in partnership with the client reducing the likelihood of prescriptive practice on the part of the nurse. Another argument may be proffered that the nurse should be prescriptive as s/he must surely know more about health and a rightful role is one of adviser and expert on health matters. However, it should be apparent to readers how fundamentally different this last view is from Parse's regarding the role of the nurse.

Cody and Mitchell (1992) describe a method for nursing practice in three stages, which correspond to Parse's themes of 'meaning, rhythmicity and transcendence'. They are:

- describing the meaning of health from the perspective of the person or family receiving care
- describing patterns of becoming from the person's or family's perspective and mutually planning activities congruent with the values of the person or family
- charting changes in patterns of becoming, as described by the person or family

Mr Smith

A community nurse is invited to visit Mr Smith at home following his discharge from hospital. The nurse sits with him, she notes that he seems to have lost weight, and asks him to tell her what has been happening (in the past, now and the future). Mr Smith is encouraged that she is not giving him advice straight away, but wants to hear his story. He gives an account of what has been happening. In the recount he gets quite angry about interference from the doctor and neighbours. Although his hand movements are restricted he has gradually learnt to compensate and reckons that he can manage most things in the kitchen. Whilst he is lonely without his wife he does not want others to substitute for her company. The nurse asks him what 'lonely' means to him; he is unprepared for this question and cannot answer it. She leaves, making an appointment to return.

At the next meeting he describes lonely as 'how I was before I was married'. His wife was a person who can never be replaced, in a perverse way he wants to miss her, '… by being miserable when she used to go out I could sometimes make her stay with me ….' He thinks that perhaps 'letting things go' is not the best way to deal with her loss, 'she's not here to get cross – I wish she were'. It will simply lead to other losses such as his independence. The nurse and Mr Smith talk about what is going to happen if he continues to eat as he does at present. They consider options and finally Mr Smith chooses to accept some help from Meals-on-Wheels. He does not want a referral to the occupational therapist but they both agree it may be an option in the future. The nurse agrees to keep in contact with Mr Smith once a week. If he loses more weight, or he would like her help, they will review the situation.

CASE NOTES

25.11.95 [Nurse writing] I visited Mr Smith at his invitation. He has lost 5 kg in weight over the past 3 months. He is finding cooking increasingly difficult. The manipulation of kitchen utensils is a problem due to arthritis in his hands, which he has had for over 20 years. He admits that he lacks motivation and appetite. Both of these problems have increased since his wife died 1 year ago. He has talked readily to me and has agreed that I may return when he has had more time to think about his predicament.

signed ....
signed ....

29.11.95 [Mr Smith writing] I have decided to accept Meals-on-Wheels three times a week. It will introduce a little variety into my menu. On the other days I am capable of preparing nutritious snacks for myself. Nurse will return and we will keep an eye on my weight. There are other options if my weight drops any more.

signed ....
signed ....

Whilst Parse's respect for each person's ability and right to make decisions is laudable, the extremes to which she is prepared to take these principles will be novel to most nurses working in traditional settings. Allowing people to make decisions that are, in the nurse's opinion, detrimental to their health is not an easy thing for a nurse to do and could pose moral dilemmas for nurses, even causing them to break organisational rules. For example, they may face a situation of the physiologically unstable patient who decides to discharge him or herself from hospital before seeing a doctor or signing any forms.

There are reasonable objections to Parse's use of language (Holmes, 1990), which she has moderately changed in a later publication (Parse, 1992). We believe that on the whole her language is now in tune with the radical and artistic nature of her work. Cody and Mitchell (1992) report that nurses who use Parse's work in practice do not find the language or abstract notions difficult to come to terms with, so some perseverance is recommended.

CASE STUDY

Carol and Jim have lived together in a 'de facto relationship' for 3 years. Carol works as a shop assistant and her four children live locally but none is living at home. They do not visit but she sees them in town now and again. Jim is a lorry driver. He spends most of the week away from home. He is divorced and his ex-wife and two children live in another city but he does see them regularly. The couple live in Jim's rented apartment.

Carol's profile

From her perspective

- Hard up
- Hard working
- All Jim's got
- Lonely
- A worrier
- Plain

From Jim's perspective

- Keeps house but is a bit untidy
- Good-natured
- Easy to talk to
- Lousy cook
- Spends too much on housekeeping

Jim's profile

From his perspective

- A man's man
- A good friend to my mates
- Work hard – like to relax
- Fond of Carol
- Miss my kids and the life I used to have

From Carol's perspective

- My partner
- Away a lot
- Complains about the house
- Fun to go out with
- Loving – sometimes

Decision-making pattern in the family

Haphazard, Carol makes decisions when Jim is away. If he disapproves he overturns them when he comes back. They don't discuss problems much.

Contextual situation

Carol was admitted to hospital for 2 days. She volunteered to be a bone marrow donor a year ago and has now been called in. She was rather surprised when the call came because frankly she had almost forgotten about volunteering. Now she is terrified. She does not like hospitals. However she is determined to help someone else if she can.

When she walked onto the ward she looked nervous and the nurse noticed that her breath smelt of whisky. Jim looked a little red eyed and had clearly been drinking too. Jim and Carol were shown to the side room which would be hers and they were left there to unpack. Jim was assured that he was welcome to stay as long as he wanted and that food could be provided. The nurse commented that Carol seemed nervous and that she would do whatever she could to help her.

Discussion of nursing practice with Carol and Jim

Carol was easy to talk to, she freely admitted how nervous she was and her determination to carry 'the thing through'. The nurse brought the conversation around to alcohol and asked if they had a drink or two to calm their nerves. They both nodded agreement. The nurse explained that it was necessary for her to find out how much and how regularly Carol drank alcohol to ensure that there was not a health risk for Carol following the anaesthetic. The nurse was not disapproving of their behaviour and therefore did not make the couple feel uncomfortable. She asked Carol to be sure to tell the anaesthetist about her alcohol intake to ensure her safety. There was no problem with proceeding with transplant and Carol made an easy recovery.

The nurse encouraged Jim and Carol to talk with her. Jim stayed in hospital all the time Carol was there. They were both heavy drinkers, with consumptions of well over the recommended amounts. They tended to drink when Jim came home. 'We go straight down the boozer, and I like to keep up with him. We are usually plastered by the time we come home in a taxi.' The nurse asked them about drinking at other times. Jim said he had one in the evening on the road. He was surprised when Carol admitted to having a bottle of whisky in the house. They talked about how their drinking habits had arisen and how their present lifestyles compounded the situation. They talked about the future, but were a bit wary here. The nurse told them that they both drank more than was good for their health and that if they were not able to do without alcohol then many would consider them alcoholics. She asked them if they would like help.

Both Carol and Jim said the problem was not that bad. Jim said that Carol should reduce her intake and that he would help her. The nurse offered them alternative help but they both rejected it. She said it was a pity but their decision. She helped them make a plan to reduce Carol's intake. When Carol was discharged the nurse reminded her that she could always contact her if she needed help. Three months after discharge the nurse wrote to Carol thanking her for her contribution, especially as she had been so nervous and reminding her that she was there if she needed help.

Learning exercises

1. Consider the extent to which you currently understand the experience of the patients you work with.
2. Sit with one patient and ask them to tell you about their experience of being in hospital or needing nursing support in the community.

Study questions

1. Write a story that introduces one of your patients in a holistic way.
2. Reflect on how comfortable you would be sharing this document with the patient.

Chapter 16

Human Science and Human Caring

LEARNING OBJECTIVES

On completion of this chapter, the reader will be able to:

1. Apply the carative factors to contemporary nursing practice

2. Understand the relationship between self-understanding and transpersonal caring

Jean Watson is a noted nurse practitioner, educationalist and scholar whose reputation for creative and imaginative work extends worldwide. Her background is in mental health nursing. She has taught at and led the University of Colorado School of Nursing. In 1986 she opened and directed the Centre for Human Caring. The Centre is a place where people benefit from humanistic nursing, which is guided by a nursing philosophy in tune with Watson's thesis (Neil, 1990; Neil and Schroeder, 1992).

Watson (1979, 1988) constructs nursing as a moral ideal, a humanistic service with a central notion of caring. She has been influenced by a range of theorists from nursing, psychology and the humanities and proffers the idea of nursing as a discipline that draws and generates knowledge through an appreciation of both the arts and sciences. She is especially indebted to the work of Carl Rogers in terms of interpersonal communication, and also uses the theories of human needs. Her regard for human experience and the importance of the meanings people make of their world has been influenced by the existential and phenomenological philosophers.

Originally, Watson's first book *Nursing: The Philosophy and Science of Caring*, published in 1979, was not described as a theory of nursing. However, in the preface to the second printing in 1985, she records that the work provides a theoretical perspective of nursing and caring. As with the other nursing theorists, Watson continues to develop her work.

Nursing: Human Science and Human Care – A Theory of Nursing was published in 1988. In this second book, Watson further differentiates nursing from medicine and explores the ways of knowing and intellectual exploration suited to nursing. Whilst in her early work she refers to science as a method of controlling and predicting nursing work, she later sees science in much broader terms, emphasising an appreciation of 'intuitive, aesthetic, quasirational modes of thought, feeling and action' (Watson, 1988) through qualitative, interpretative methodologies.

Watson (1990) acknowledges that she uses words and notions that some may find embarrassing. It is unconventional to talk, as she does, of nurses loving and being passionate, yet her central thesis is an altruistic ideal of spirited loving and giving to others in order to preserve humanity within the health service. Nurses who retain the ideas of professional distance and non-involvement, and separate their work from themselves in general, may well be uncomfortable with this work.

In 1997 Watson describes the development of the theory and states unequivocally the extent to which the nurses should live the model: '[t]his model now more explicitly acknowledges that the nurse, or practitioner who is working within this theory and its underlying philosophy, needs to cultivate a daily practice for self. Practices such as centering, meditation, breath work, yoga, prayer, connections with nature and other such forms of daily contemplation are essential to the theory's authenticity and success'.

BELIEFS AND VALUES

Beliefs and values are of particular significance in this theory because, as Watson (1988) explains, nursing is not a series of tasks to be performed but a service driven by specific value systems regarding human caring. The values are 'humanitarian, aesthetic, and spiritual, attempting to honor the human dimensions of nursing's work and the inner life world and subjective experiences of the people we serve' (Watson, 1997). The ideals generated from these values are the ones to which nurses aspire and which cause them to choose specific behaviours.

The person

Human beings are viewed as entire entities existing in the world, surrounded by and part of it. Their unique and subjective experience of the physical, natural world and of their own emotions, memories and desires creates their perception of their life in the world. In 1997 Watson wrote '... the evolving work continues to make explicit that humans cannot be treated as objects, that humans cannot be separated from self, other, nature and the larger universe'. A person's perspective, or phenomenological field as Watson (1979, 1988) describes the person's view of the world, and his/her particular experience in it can never be fully understood by another, although empathic understanding by someone may come close. People learn and continue to grow through making meaning of their experiences. Watson describes the development of the human using the analogy of a river, constantly moving and changing yet retaining its form. The person changes with each new awareness. Awareness is affected by the past and in turn affects future perceptions. A person's thoughts can transcend the present and coexist with the past and future, forming a personal conception of reality.

Watson's view of human beings is conventional to a point but she bravely extends her work to include the transcendental self, the soul and spirit of the person. This realm is not commonly addressed by nurses, but one that she insists is important to acknowledge for the nurse's personal growth and for the care of others.

> *The person is not simply an organism or material physical being; the person is also a part of nature, a spiritual being, neither purely physical, nor purely spiritual. A person's existence is embodied in experience, in nature, and in the physical world, but a person can also transcend the physical world and nature by controlling it, subduing it, changing it, or living in harmony with it.*

(Watson, 1988)

Health

Health is related to the authentic self which is experienced when there is harmony between the spheres of the human, that is the mind, body and spirit, and the world. Authentic 'self' is achieved when the subjective inner 'I' relates honestly with the outwardly seen 'me'. This congruity is associated with health.

Watson (1979) claims that health is a difficult concept to define because of its subjective nature; both health and illness are relative concepts according to the experiencing person's perspective. She agrees with ideas such as health as a sense of well-being, an ability to function and relate to others in the world. However she comments that if this is the case then health-care delivery systems are not producing health as an end product of their endeavour. Watson (1979) names three elements associated with health.

1. A high level of overall physical, mental and social functioning.
2. A general adaptive–maintenance level of daily functioning.
3. The absence of illness (or the presence of efforts that lead to its absence).

By far the majority of health care workers are concerned with illness care rather than health care. Indeed she suggests that the realm of medical care is erroneously associated with health care because of its illness orientation.

Illness is described as a disharmony between the inner person and the experiencing person. This disharmony may be brought on by disease, but not always. Inner problems, such as guilt, distress, worry or sadness, can lead to illness which in turn may cause disease or allow a predisposition, for example a genetic weakness, to become manifest.

Environment

The internal and external environments are identified, the internal being related to biophysical, spiritual and mental factors, the external being concerned with such factors as stress and change, and conditions that affect the person, for example, comfort and cleanliness. Human beings are a part of nature and should respect and care for the entire ecosystem.

THE GOALS OF NURSING

Nursing is essentially a transpersonal communication of human caring: the bonding of two individuals in a relationship where the growth and well-being of the other (client) is paramount. The warmth and genuineness of the relationship is established by the nurse's interest in the whole person, in the other's interpretation of his/her world and by having concern for the client's dignity and humanness. In this created and positive climate the client is able to share thoughts and feelings about his/her concerns, and the pair can work together to maintain or re-establish health or help the client to a peaceful death. It is likely that the nurse grows and prospers through the relationship too. However this is not a primary goal of the professional work of the nurse, nor should it be expected.

While it may appear that Watson concentrates on the relationship between one nurse and a client, it is apparent that a caring moment can result from a brief encounter between a nurse and client just as easily as it can as a result of a protracted and involved therapeutic relationship. The poem at the end of the chapter (p. 221) demonstrates this point well.

Watson (1988) thinks that nurses should aim to help people maintain and attain health and a feeling of personhood; in her words, 'harmony within the mind, body, and soul which generates self-knowledge, self-reverence, self-healing, and self-care processes'. This type of care is especially needed in order to recapture our humanity in an increasingly materialistic and mechanistic world.

KNOWLEDGE FOR NURSING

Watson (1979) acknowledges the tremendous differences in various practice settings. However, she still believes that there is a 'core' of knowledge and practice that is relevant to all nurses. Specialised knowledge is required for midwifery, surgical nursing or community nursing; this area-specific knowledge is termed 'trim' by Watson and, although practically essential, is not the essence of nursing, as she believes caring is. There are 10 carative factors that Watson describes. 'Carative' is a word chosen to differentiate nursing care from medical cure. Cure may result or be a part of caring, but this is not necessarily so. The 10 factors form the 'core' of nursing; they are the things that apply to nursing in any setting.

1. **The formation of a humanistic–altruistic system of values**. A philosophy learned through life to accept human values such as love of the other, kindness and concern for others and satisfaction through giving.
2. **The instillation of faith–hope**. Through an effective nurse–client partnership both people develop positive thoughts towards desired outcomes.
3. **The cultivation of sensitivity to one's self and to others**. A self-awareness gives the nurse the ability to communicate his/her own feelings and to help the client do the same.
4. **The development of a helping–trust relationship**. A relationship whereby the client feels the nurse's desire to help and is confident that the nurse is able to help. The relationship is built upon the preceding three carative factors. Watson outlines the following essential components for a helping–trust relationship to develop, which rely on the work of Carl Rogers (1957, 1962).

   - *Congruence*: that is an honesty between what the nurse thinks and *does*.

- *Empathy*: the ability to convey to the client that you have an understanding of their world.
- *Non-possessive warmth*: the client will find no conditions attached to the nurse's warm regard for him/her.
- Effective communication.

5. **The promotion and acceptance of the expression of positive and negative feelings**. In a helpful relationship there is truth, although risk is involved in expressing feelings so honestly. The ability to receive negative expressions of feelings from another is part of the human growth process.

6. **The systematic use of the scientific problem-solving method for decision-making**. Nursing decisions should be sound. The use of the nursing process is a logical means of using available knowledge to the client's best advantage.

7. **The promotion of interpersonal teaching–learning**. The nurse helps clients to know for themselves what promotes their optimum well-being. This carative factor promotes the client's independence.

8. **The provision for a supportive, protective and (or) corrective mental, physical, sociocultural and spiritual environment**. The nurse is aware of the environment and ensures that it is as conducive as possible to the client's well-being. This includes factors such as safety and aesthetic surroundings.

9. **Assistance with the gratification of human needs**. The nurse helps clients to obtain their requirements for health. Watson (1979) adapts Maslow's (1954) hierarchy of human needs for nursing, as illustrated in Figure 16.1. Satisfaction of the lower order needs makes way for the client to achieve the higher order needs.

10. **The allowance for existential–phenomenological forces**. The nurse needs to appreciate that clients need to understand the meaning of their predicaments. Phenomenological perspectives concentrate the person on the meaning of being in the world.

Watson explains that it was in the 1988 book *New Dimensions of Human Caring Theory* that the relationship of the carative factors to '... oneness of being with respect to person, phenomenal field, transpersonal caring relationship, caring occasion and a caring moment' were realised.

In order to care Watson suggests that the nurse needs to know many things and to have talents; talents that include amongst others intelligence, creativity, imagination, astuteness and sensitivity. She claims that nursing is both a science and an art, and together with E. M. Bevis, Watson has discussed and outlined a 'caring curriculum' for nursing (Bevis and Watson, 1989), which carefully involves both perspectives.

To demonstrate expertise with the carative factors, a nurse needs a variety of knowledge; knowledge sometimes derived from other disciplines but made specifically nursing through the practice of nursing. Something Watson terms a nursing qua nursing paradigm rather than a nursing qua medicine paradigm (Watson, 1997). Some areas associated with the carative factors, such as the biophysical needs, are conventional areas of learning for nurses, while others such as the existential–phenomenological experience of people would be new to nursing curricula. The use of traditional scientific facts is most evident in the lower order biophysical needs (see Figure 16.1), for example physiology. On the other hand, when dealing with the higher order needs, for example in helping a person come to terms with his or her death, the nurse will need more complex, albeit less certain, knowledge gleaned from the arts, literature and philosophies.

For Watson (1988) the focus of the discipline of nursing is 'persons and human health–illness experiences that are mediated by professional, personal, scientific, aesthetic and ethical human care transactions' and new nursing knowledge should illuminate these areas. Watson (1988) emphasises the need for nurses to use the qualitative methodologies in pursuit of the discipline. Methodologies that view and celebrate the complexity of human nature and the world, which do not necessarily solve problems but help us to understand the human predicament and expand the discipline's knowledge base, are considered to be most appropriate.

CARE PLANNING

It is difficult to demonstrate care planning for Watson does not write specifically about the organisation or documentation of nursing care. However, she does devote a chapter in her earlier work (Watson, 1979) to the 'systematic use of the scientific problem-solving method for decision-making'. She mentions the nursing process along with the research process as an organised and logical means of solving problems and demonstrating rationale for care to colleagues and clients. We would suggest that the 'lower order needs' (see Figure 16.1) are most conducive

Figure 16.1   Adaptation of Maslow's hierarchy of human needs for nursing (from Watson, 1979, p. 110, with permission).

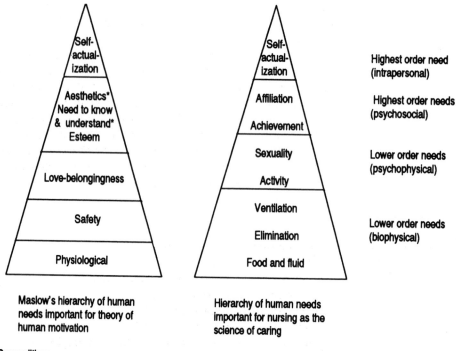

Maslow's hierarchy of human needs important for theory of human motivation

Hierarchy of human needs important for nursing as the science of caring

* Preconditions

Box 16.1   A nursing plan

Subjective information from the client
Objective information, from observation and measurement
Assessment
Plan (care factor)
Intervention
Evaluation

to a systematic approach to problem solving, and problems such as Mr Smith's weight loss can be documented in a nursing process format in a similar way to any of the preceding chapters.

Time spent with Mr Smith when he first arrives allows him and his primary nurse to talk and exchange information. The nurse listens to his explanation of his weight loss; what it means to him. It may mean that he can fit into clothes that he hasn't worn for years or it may be symbolic of the lack of control he feels about his life in general. The nurse also collects objective information like his weight, skin turgor, the fit of his clothes, how much he eats at meals.

The record of nursing in Box 16.2 gives other nurses in the team enough information to get a gist of the care Mr Smith has been receiving and how to carry this on in the primary nurse's absence. In the majority of nursing situations nursing care is given by a number of nurses over a 24-hour period. In these cases it is important that the primary nurses document nursing care in order to account for their decisions and to ensure a continuous service.

For the 'higher order needs' and the other 'carative factors', it is difficult to convey the personal depth of the therapeutic relationship and the meanings expressed by the client in this type of logical format. Indeed it is not always appropriate to document and share personal details which, while they are important to the primary nurse and client, do not need to be related to the rest of the nursing team. The nurse and client need to make a reasonable judgement regarding the amount of information that needs to be communicated to the team in order that they can continue to care for the client when the primary nurse is absent.

PATIENT CASE STUDY

Sunshine acres living centre

The first thing you see up ahead is Mr.
Polanski, wedged in the
arched doorway, like he means absolutely
to stay there, he who shouldn't
be here in the first place, put in here
by mistake, courtesy of that grandson
who thinks he's a hotshot, and too busy raking in

Box 16.2   The assessment

Assessment Talks of the significance preparing his own food has for him. He likes to look after himself. If he shows that he is capable of cooking for himself there is less risk of being put in a home. Really would rather not have 'outsiders' coming into his kitchen 'it isn't always clean and tidy, if you know what I mean': he also thinks that they may grow tired of helping him.
Eats everything that is given to him at meal times. Has some difficulty cutting meat but never asks for help and refuses it when offered: he prefers to 'struggle along'. It takes him about 20 minutes to finish his first course by which time it is cold: he dislikes eating cold food.
Weighs 55 kg and has lost 5 kg since his last Out Patient Appointment.

Plan Set aside at least 10 minutes a day to sit and talk with Mr Smith about matters relating to his nutrition. Go with him, at least once, to see what he learns and how he copes in the Occupational Therapy kitchen. Offer to warm food in the microwave half way through the meal.

Intervention Talked about progress for over half an hour on the first day. Mr Smith is enthusiastic about the help the occupational therapist has given him and is full of ideas for menus at home. Talked also about his fears of becoming dependent and needing to be in a nursing home.

Evaluation [5 days later] Mr Smith appreciates 'his time' to talk. He records what he has eaten and calculates the calorific value to show Judy [primary nurse]. He also describes how he feels about his progress and what he has achieved with the occupational therapist. He is not particularly pleased that for the time being he will need to rely on help from neighbours. However he has said that he would appreciate the odd home-made pie brought around. He has begun to speak about his relationships with friends and the past hurts that have caused him to be wary of relying on friends.

the dough to take time for an old
man. If he had anyplace to go, you know he'd be out
instantly, if he had any
money. So he intends

to stay in that doorway, not missing
a thing, and waiting
for trouble. Which of course
will come. And could be
you – you're handy, you look
likely, you have

the authority. And you're
new here, another young

whippersnapper, doesn't know
ankle from elbow, but has been given
the keys. Well he's
ready, Polanski. So you go right
to him. Mr. Polanski, good
morning you say it in Polish,
which you learned a little of
when you were little, and your grandmother taught you
a little song about lambs, frisking
in a pen, and you
danced a silly little dance with your grandmother
while the two of you
sang. So you sing it

for him, here in the dim, institutional
light of the hallway, light which even you find
insupportable, because at that moment
it reminds you of the light in the hallway
in the resthome where, when your grandmother
died, you weren't
there. So that you're also singing
to console yourself. And at the moment you pay her
this silly little tribute, Mr. Polanski
steps out of the doorway. He
who had set himself
to resist you, he who had made himself
a first, Mr. Polanski,
   contentious
   often combative
   and always inconsolable

hears that you know
the song. And he steps out
from the fortress of the
doorway, begins

to shuffle
and sing along.

Marilyn Krysl

Watson (1990) uses this early version of a poem which was revised
and published in the book *Midwife and Other Poems on Caring* (Krysl,
1989) to communicate to others the caring event. The poem illustrates
well how art can convey feelings and emotions.

Learning exercises

1. Consider your undergraduate curriculum and reflect on the extent to which it addresses the Carative Factors.
2. Reflect on the degree to which you assess accurately the impact that your behaviour has on other people.

Study questions

1. Make notes on each of the Carative Factors.

Chapter 17

Analysing and Evaluating Models for Practice

LEARNING OBJECTIVES

On completion of this chapter, the reader will be able to:

1. Describe the process of critique
2. Write a critique on a published nursing model
3. Discuss the purpose of critiquing models

The purpose behind this book has been to introduce you to the ideas behind nursing models and to outline a number of the more widely used ones in order that you can gain some insight into the breadth and range of different approaches that have been taken. At this stage you may wish to take a more critical look at some of the models and start to make your own judgements about their relative values. To this end a number of nursing writers have developed guidelines on evaluating nursing models and theories. We find the processes described by Stevens (1984) comprehensive, appropriate and easy to follow, and recommend that you read her work if you wish to pursue model and theory evaluation in depth. The process described in this chapter is based on Stevens' work in this area.

One part of evaluation relates to your own personal judgement. Thus, evaluation of a model inevitably includes your feelings about that model. Does it actually 'feel right' to you? Does the central essence of the model 'ring true' and does it fit with your experience and your sense of what nursing is all about?

In addition to this exercising of personal, intuitive judgement, the evaluation of a model using a set of criteria is of use. We find the following simple interpretations we have developed out of Stevens' evaluative criteria useful steps in evaluating a model.

INTERNAL STRUCTURE OF A MODEL

This applies to the description of the model itself. Evaluation of the internal structure of a model involves a close scrutiny of what the author has written. Thus, it focuses on how the author explains and develops her or his perception of reality in nursing, rather than what this actually means to practice. The internal structure of a model can be analysed and evaluated through applying five broad criteria.

Clarity

This is self-explanatory, and simply refers to whether or not the model is easy to understand. The use of difficult language is not necessarily a block to clarity, but if the model is full of obscurity and fails to explain or define the terms used, then it may not meet this criterion for you or your team. You may, for example, find the language used in one model both simple and clear, but some central concepts may not be well defined. Alternatively, you may find a model packed with complex words which make reading it difficult, yet these words may be explained and defined in such a way that, in spite of the use of complex language, the model itself represents a fair degree of clarity.

Consistency

Consistency refers to the use of words and concepts in the same way throughout. In evaluating a model for consistency, the evaluator looks for contradictions. For example, the model may purport to focus on health, yet constantly refer to disease and illness or it may emphasise holism, yet reduce a person to various parts.

Adequacy

A model needs to be adequate for the purposes it sets out to achieve. For example, the author may claim that it is a representation of nursing in general. Questions must then be raised about whether it is sufficiently broad to encompass the nursing of the sick, the extended care of the elderly, the promotion of health in the community, care of those with both physical and mental health problems, and the prevention of ill health in industry.

Logical development

A model should be logical – that is, every tentative conclusion, prediction or position statement included in a model should be supported by both the presentation of the premises on which these are based and clear, supported arguments. Thus, bald statements which are not well supported and argued detract from a model's status. For example, suggesting that all people want to be involved in decision-making in relation to their current health problem without qualification would indicate an unsupported argument. When assessing the logical development of the model, the reader focuses on the sequencing of ideas and concepts and the conclusions drawn in the work.

Level of development

This final component of internal criticism assesses how well developed a model is. For example, you may encounter a model that has been hastily constructed without sufficient thought and rigour and which is little more than a series of unsupported statements that read rather like a 'wish list'. The models discussed in this book are all at a fairly advanced stage of development, though some are still less developed than others.

EXTERNAL VALIDITY OF A MODEL

This concerns the relationship between a model and the 'real world' of practice. Assessing the external validity of a model requires the assessor to move beyond the qualities of the model itself to attempts to see how it measures up to contemporary nursing and society. The external validity of a model can be analysed and evaluated through applying six broad criteria.

Reality convergence

This asks the question: 'Does the reality expressed by the author closely resemble that of the reader?' This will be, of course, influenced greatly by the views held by the assessor. For example, if you are a person who lives life from a largely subjective perspective and who values the perceptions of the person over the measured, objective view of the world, you may find a humanistic model closer to reality than an adaptation model. When assessing a model for reality convergence, such personal views cannot be excluded but an awareness of them is important to judge adequately the degree to which a model achieves this criterion. Reality may also be dependent on your current state of knowledge and it may be that, as you learn more about models, your views will shift.

Usefulness

Models must be of use to practice. In other words, they should be clear about: the concepts central to practice (which assists nurses to prioritise their work); the nature of the person, health and the environment (which gives direction to assessment and intervention); and the goals of nursing (which delineate the nursing role and give direction to nursing care and its evaluation).

Significance

This criterion refers to how important a contribution a model makes to current nursing thought and practice and to the future development of nursing. It involves asking: 'What new clarification does this bring to nursing? What new directions are opened up by the model?' For example, does the model open up opportunities for clarification of the public health role of nurses, or that of independent nurse practitioners, both of which are relatively new areas of work requiring a different perspective.

Discrimination

A model should clearly differentiate the occupation, discipline or activity it describes from others. In the case of a nursing model, it should therefore clearly differentiate nursing from other health-care occupations such as occupational therapy or medicine. This criterion involves asking: 'Does the model describe nursing, or could it easily apply to other occupations? Does it differentiate between a nursing approach to discrete tasks and other approaches (e.g. in areas such as food service, bed making, the distribution of medications)?' Bear in mind, however, that the boundaries of different disciplines are rapidly shifting, and it is not helpful to hold on to too rigid a traditional perspective. It is also worth remembering here that we have in the past lost some components of work to other newer disciplines, and it may be that the time is right to consider whether this was a useful and appropriate move.

Scope

This criterion relates closely to that of adequacy in that it addresses how broad the model is. A nursing model needs to be sufficient in scope to adequately describe all facets of nursing. This includes community care, health education and promotion, illness and accident prevention, the maintenance of a 'normal' lifestyle in extended care, operating theatre activity, high dependency care, acute care and so forth. The scope of a model is therefore assessed by asking: 'To what extent does the model accommodate all of the specialty areas of nursing practice?'

Complexity Although clarity is important in a model, this should not be interpreted to mean that models should be overly simplistic. Given the complexity of nursing, it follows that a well-developed model will reflect this and that it will be sufficiently rich to encompass the richness of nursing. In assessing this criterion, the assessor is looking for sufficient complexity to render the model developed and rigorous.

These steps, drawn from Stevens (1984), are, we believe, useful in analysing and evaluating models for nursing practice and offer a good point from which to start. The outlines offered in this book will give you some insight into which model or models you feel comfortable with, but, having made that judgement, it is important that you also return to the original authors as inevitably the representations here are limited by space but will also have been influenced to some extent by our own interpretations. In future reading you may find other frameworks for analysis of models (e.g. Fawcett, 1989; Meleis, 1991), all of which offer a slightly different perspective, reflecting the particular stance of the writers, a point which we have already highlighted in stressing how the values and beliefs we hold have an impact on both our everyday behaviours and our nursing practice. At the end of the day the decision you make as to which model and framework for analysis you choose has to be an individual choice.

Learning exercises

1. Select a chapter describing a specific nursing model from this book (that is, from Chapters 8–16) and write a critique of the model you select.
2. To what extent, in your experience, do nurses systematically critique nursing models – or any other theoretical text - before accepting or rejecting the ideas presented?

Study questions

1. Why is critique important?
2. Describe the central questions that could be addressed when critiquing a nursing model.
3. List the reasons why critiquing theoretical work is often not pursued by nurses.

Chapter 18

Using a Nursing Model

LEARNING OBJECTIVES

On completion of this chapter, the reader will be able to:

1. Discuss ways in which nursing teams can choose a suitable framework for practice
2. Describe ways of implementing change
3. Describe ways in which the introduction of a change can be evaluated

The purpose of the final chapter of this book is to draw together all the issues that have been raised and to offer some ideas about developing an agreed model or choosing an existing model and implementing it in practice.

To summarise the essence of the book, an understanding and application of model-based practice will:

- Clarify the meaning of nursing
- Identify the value system on which nursing is based
- Give direction to practice
- Identify the role that the nurse should fulfil
- Allow individual nurses to be accountable for their own practice
- Justify the nurse's contribution in a multidisciplinary clinical team
- Point out what knowledge is needed for effective practice
- Highlight areas of practice where research is required
- Require that nurses have some freedom in choosing which model they should practise from
- Guide the development of the curriculum for courses in nursing
- Lead to radical changes in the style of nursing care

Having been introduced to the basis of these points in the preceding chapters, if they are accepted by the reader, then the logical question to address now is 'what to do about it'. The few nurses who work alone need to consider the nature of nursing models and to arrive at a decision about a framework on which to base their practice. They can then incorporate this framework into their work. However, the majority of nurses work in teams, either in wards, departments or community health centres. Inevitably the path they need to follow is a little different in that they will have to talk about ideas and models within the team and make a collective choice about which one to use as a basis for their practice.

CHOOSING A MODEL FOR PRACTICE

Before any nursing team can choose a model to practice from, they will need opportunities to explore various options and to discuss personal models held by individuals within that team. So the first step in choosing a model is to learn about what models for nursing practice are and why they are needed. The purpose of this book is to help nurses in this respect, but learning about topics such as this is often easier in groups where ideas can be shared and issues clarified through pooling of understandings. In our experience, organising group meetings for staff with the purpose of studying various approaches to nursing is often far more productive than one might imagine.

Such meetings offer the opportunity for team members to express their personal views and feelings and discuss those of their colleagues. A whole nursing team seldom has the opportunity of meeting together in this way, yet enabling this to occur is essential because both points of argument and agreements can be identified. Often much less agreement exists than is apparent at first sight, and finding a common solution is the beginning of moving towards model-based practice. A useful approach to take in such meetings is to ask the group to consider their own personal views on each of the three components of the model they use for their practice. Namely:

- Their own views about people
- The goals of their practice
- The knowledge they have and the knowledge they need to achieve those goals

Garbett (1994) has described how he has used focus groups, that is small subgroups who explore a particular issue together, as a means of achieving this end, stressing that everyone's contribution is of equal value. Alternatively, Warfield and Manley (1990) have used a process called 'values clarification' as a starting point for this exercise, which you might like to explore further (Manley, 1992).

Nurses who work in a specific ward, a community 'patch' or a particular department will therefore need to plan and make time for a number of nursing team meetings. The team of nurses must come to some agreement on beliefs and values; the goals of nursing; and what they all need to know, feel and be skilled in order to achieve these goals. Some units have used this type of nursing collaboration to develop their own model for practice (Wright, 1986). The prudent nursing team will also arrange multidisciplinary team meetings or some other means of communication to inform and allow discussion with colleagues about the direction nurses are taking.

We know of several units where each member of the nursing team agreed to read the first five chapters of *Models for Nursing Practice* and then to choose one of the 'model' chapters to study. At subsequent meetings individuals or groups of nurses presented an overview of the model they had chosen. This gave the team an opportunity to consider and compare some different models and to choose one or a combination of one or more that suited the team. Once the model had been chosen of course there was a need for each member of the team to read about it personally and more literature (both primary and secondary sources) about the model was sought.

Through taking a collaborative approach, it is usually possible to agree on a set of valued beliefs, on common goals and on an outline of knowledge, skills and attitudes which the team sees as fundamental to nursing practice. Sometimes this will match almost exactly a specific nursing model that has been described by others. For example, one ward that we are familiar with feels the model developed by Orem (1991) clearly represents real nursing to them, and they now use it as a basis for their practice; another has done the same with Ying's model (1981); and another has chosen the activities of living model developed by Roper *et al.* (1990). Of course there are countless other wards which we do not know about who have selected other specific models.

Some teams find that existing models do not adequately describe reality to them and they decide on an amalgamation of ideas taken from two or more models or on developing a model themselves. Another ward we know of uses the activities of living as a framework for assessment, and applies stress adaptation from Roy's perspective (1984) to these activities; a district nursing team has agreed that nursing to them can only be accurately described by combining the concepts of Orem, Roper *et al.* and Roy. A team of nurses on a psychiatric ward found that none of the models meant much to them and decided that it is too early in their thinking to develop a full-blown one for themselves. They have some agreement on the beliefs and values that underlie 'good' practice in the wards, on some overall goals to be achieved and on some basic knowledge, skills and attitudes that they would like all nurses on the ward to share. All of these approaches are quite acceptable. We are also familiar with a number of nursing teams who have not yet approached their work by considering its essence, and it is often apparent in the sort of nursing work carried out. For example, some using the 'nursing process' have developed assessment forms following what we have called the working party approach. This common approach consists of getting together a small group of staff from the organisation and from the peripheral units of the Health District. They then proceed to attempt to produce some recommendations applicable to the whole unit that everyone else is then supposed to agree with. In the case of the nursing process such working parties have been set up to design what are seen as the all-important forms. All of the members sit around a table and suggest, for example, what headings or questions should go on the assessment form.

The end result of this approach is a form with headings and questions based on a variety of different perspectives but without any clear underlying goal-directed purpose. This form is then sent to nurses throughout the organisation who are required to use it as a standard nursing record. Sadly, when this occurs, there are still some who would suggest that the nursing teams are 'doing the nursing process'. However, without agreement on what the nursing component of the process consists of, more often than not the only change achieved in this approach is different paperwork, with no real change in practice.

To some extent this problem has been exacerbated by the introduction of computerised records, which can be more restrictive as the format is often preset. However, even if this is the situation you are faced with it does not preclude local work to clarify the content in relation to each item. Furthermore, there are usually opportunities even within preset records that allow for flexibility. Hence it may be necessary to be creative in the manner in which such systems are used, but they certainly do not negate the importance of local clarification.

Starting off by agreeing on a model for nursing, rather than concentrating on documentation, is far more in line with the philosophy of the nursing process. It is often less time-consuming than an organisation-wide working party, because a model gives clear structure to assessment and can be undertaken by individual teams. More importantly, however, it leads to a meaningful consideration of how care by nurses is given, and to actual and beneficial changes in practice. The working party approach can lead to no more than a new nursing record, with little chance of any difference in what actually happens to patients. So choosing a model must begin from discussion and education, and is fundamental to introducing changes in nursing practice.

The choice in some areas has also been driven by the model employed in the school of nursing, although we would suggest that it is important that students have the opportunity of exploring a range of different approaches. Nursing students do not have the opportunity to become as involved in the process of choice as nurses who are permanently working in set areas. Therefore they usually need to be aware of the nature, basic structure of and the differences between various models. It is important, however, for students to sort out their own views and choose something which falls in with them. The rotation around clinical units gives them an opportunity to see how various teams of nurses work, and how they apply their own model to patient care.

Choosing a nursing model is not like choosing a new carpet or a dish from the menu of an exclusive restaurant. Such things are 'one off' and once the choice is made, that is it. Choosing a model demands a close scrutiny of ourselves, our patients, other nurses and other health workers. It is not a choice from which there is no going back. As new ideas arrive, new concepts are identified, and patients' needs change, so then does the possible choice of model change. When you buy a new coat the decision is finite, but choosing a model is merely the beginning in a whole cobweb-like chain of ever-growing choices.

IMPLEMENTING A NURSING MODEL IN PRACTICE

If a nursing team finds that it can agree that a certain model represents nursing and that it should form the basis for practice, it is then possible to implement its use within the team.

To introduce this new perspective into the work situation is, in effect, to implement change. Much is written about how to introduce change and a number of theories exist. For a deeper analysis of the change process and strategy for change we direct you to the wealth of literature available elsewhere (cf. Wright, 1989; Marsh and MacAlpine, 1995). We simply want to outline the basis for change and relate this to introducing model based practice by suggesting the approach we have used.

Change refers to the process that brings about alteration in behaviour or substitutes one way of behaviour for another. Some changes occur because of things around us, but most changes cannot effectively occur without being planned. Planned change is usually easier to manage than change that is imposed, haphazard or misunderstood. Nursing in itself can be seen to be an agent of change. It hopes to bring about changes in patients' or clients' behaviour, such as changing dependence into independence, fear into security and so forth. We all know the argument that planned nursing care is more effective than unplanned care, hence the current emphasis in nursing on the use of problem solving. The four steps used in problem solving or the nursing process are useful in providing a framework to plan change. So, in introducing the model of your choice into practice, it is useful to consider it under the following headings.

Assessment

First of all one needs to assess the situation: What is the current situation? Who will be involved in using the model? Who will it affect both within and beyond the nursing team? What changes will it require in such things as work organisation, duty rotas and so on? What resources will be needed, such as new assessment, care planning and evaluation documents? Are these resources available? If so, how can they be obtained and if not, what can be done about it? What needs to be done to overcome problems that will inhibit the introduction of the changes? For example, if lack of understanding by some of the nurses or doctors, physiotherapists and domestic staff is apparent, it may be that the opportunity for learning is necessary before the desired change in practice can be made acceptable to them.

Planning

Having identified the problem, a plan of action can be prepared. For example, group discussions and teaching can be arranged to give a greater understanding of the model, and perhaps the use of the assessment framework. If lack of skills and knowledge or disparity in attitudes in the team have been identified as problems, plans for educational experiences may be developed to overcome them. Meetings with the multidisciplinary clinical team may also be planned. The plan may include target dates for introduction of specific changes and for evaluating them. Incorporated into the plan must also be some means by which the effects of the change will be evaluated. In this way success can actually be measured, leading to encouragement and satisfaction for the nurses concerned.

Implementation   In this step the plan is actually put into action, and the change is regularly monitored, by previously agreed methods, to judge its effectiveness. In the area where one of us works, this approach was taken. The nursing team was given the opportunity to express their own views, learn about a variety of nursing models and select the one they felt closest to. They then planned for educational sessions themselves. These were designed to enable them to become skilled in communicating with patients and to discover and revise their own attitudes to patient care. In addition to these sessions, they planned to meet with the doctors, social workers, physiotherapists and occupational therapists to describe the model and to negotiate the right, within the multidisciplinary clinical team, that nursing has to work in this way and to clarify how this would affect the work and relationships between disciplines.

Evaluation   This plan was implemented and, on evaluation, patients, nurses and the multidisciplinary clinical team had a greater understanding of nursing itself. Patients became more independent and the average length of stay in the wards was reduced. The multidisciplinary clinical team valued the contribution of nursing more highly, with many admissions to the ward being regarded by the team as being best served if the patient's nurse became leader of the multidisciplinary team. The nurses indicated that they were more satisfied with their role than before.

Change, however, does not always run smoothly and perhaps this description sounds deceptively simple. FitzGerald (1994) describes professional developments on an acute medical ward over a three-year period. In this instance the change process was not classical and yet the direction of change informed by theories of change as described above was always aimed towards the teams' shared goals, which reflected their stated values and beliefs.

Some people prefer to go for 'incremental change', that is a step-by-step process where change is managed over a protracted period of time. Others prefer what has been called 'the big bang' (Marsh and MacAlpine, 1995), where considerable time is spent on planning and learning and a single date set for a major change in practice. Neither way is right or wrong, and there are advantages and disadvantages in both approaches. In the former case people may be able to cope more easily with small steps but feel that the process is never ending. In the latter approach the enormity of the change and waiting for action may feel too much for some, but the final achievement can be very fulfilling.

IMPLICATIONS FOR NURSING EDUCATION   Inevitably a shift from one model of practice to another will be of major concern to those nurses working in nursing education. Examination of the curricula of the 1950s and 1960s clearly demonstrates that the implicit model for practice was the biomedical model where the orientation was towards disease and cure. Many of us can vividly remember this emphasis from our own training. Yet a shift has now occurred away from a disease-centred orientation or medical model curriculum towards a client-centred orientation or nursing-focused curriculum. In a 1981 study of 270 American schools, De Back (1981) was unable to find any which still based their curricula on the medical model, which she described as 'organised around disease processes'. The most commonly identified or popular framework was a systems model approach that is 'organised around stability and adaptation of the client'. Such a shift has also taken place in most Western countries such as the United Kingdom, New Zealand, Australia, Scandinavia and continental Europe. However, Street (1990) does warn that some modem curricula have been overtaken by the 'ologies', that is biology, sociology, psychology and so forth, at the cost of time spent on the discipline of nursing itself, a point which is worthy of note as we are striving to clarify the contribution we make to health care.

Torres and Yura (1974) discuss how the model of choice for a particular practice discipline is reflected in the curriculum. They portray a model or conceptual framework as containing theories that reflect the philosophy, goals and desired behaviour for practice (see Figure 18.1). They continue to describe how such a framework can be used in curriculum design, identifying six stages to this end.

- Statement of the philosophy of the programme.
- The broad objectives of the programme.
- The statement of the terminal behaviour flowing from the programme.
- The outline of the conceptual framework.

These initial stages will provide a rationale for the selection of learning experience and a system for classifying knowledge and ordering facts. Once this has been achieved the educator will go on to the following.

- Develop the outcome statements required for each stage of the course.
- Designate the learning experience needed to meet these objectives.

The shift from a disease-centred to a client-centred model has obvious implications for nurse educators not only in the content of what they

Figure 18.1   Curriculum design components.

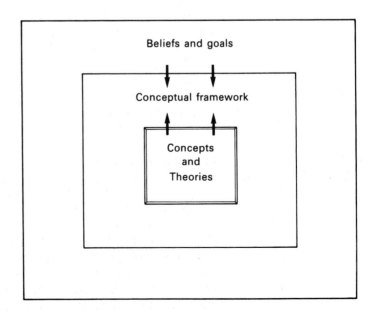

teach, but also in the methods that they employ in their teaching. If there is an emphasis on the patient as an individual, with a right to participate in his or her own decision-making, then there is an implication that the same belief should be reflected in the nurse educator's relationship with the student. The introduction of audit to educational institutions has helped to bring these points to light.

One of the points that has been emphasised throughout this book is that there is no right or wrong model and that individual nurses have the right to choose which one they will base their practice on. Even if they work in a team of nurses, they can contribute their ideas to the group decision. It has also been stressed that it is right for a curriculum to be based on an explicit model: indeed it is impossible to develop a nursing curriculum without some kind of conceptual framework of nursing.

These two points can create a very difficult dilemma for nurse educators, to which there is no simple answer. During their clinical placements, students will be faced with working in a number of different settings, all of which will be using a different model base. If the belief that clinical nurses have the right to choose their own model for practice is accepted, then students will inevitably be exposed to numerous different approaches to care. The challenge for nurse educators is to prepare students to confront a range of approaches.

Several solutions have been offered as a way of meeting this challenge, none of which has proved right or wrong. We can only put forward some of the ideas and leave you to make your own judgement about their merits and deficits.

First, some schools have taken a very eclectic approach, amalgamating ideas from various different models that they believe to be important. In other words they have attempted to develop a single unified model of their own.

A second approach has been to choose a single model on which to base the curriculum. The ideas of other models may be raised, but the direction of the curriculum would be based on one. Undoubtedly, from a curriculum design stance, this is the easiest approach. However, it does raise difficulties in transferring learning to working in settings where a different framework from that used in the curriculum is practised.

A third approach is to divide the curriculum into different components and teach each component using a specific model. For instance, one year may be devoted to learning about the nursing needs of patients who are affected by 'episodic illness', during which a systems approach such as that described by Roy could be used. Another year may deal with the nursing needs of patients requiring continuing care, and a curriculum based on a developmental approach such as that described by Peplau could be used. The framework for the curriculum could be chosen to reflect the one most commonly used in the relevant clinical area.

As new roles such as that of the lecturer practitioner (Lathlean and Vaughan, 1994) take hold, the interrelation between practice and educational settings is being enhanced in such a way that each can learn from, rather than be directed by, the other, hence reducing the impact of some of these difficulties. The interest in such approaches is rapidly growing and will no doubt make an important contribution in the future to the development of both practice and curricula.

Whichever approach is chosen, the important thing is that students are introduced to contemporary nursing theories and given an opportunity to consider their application in practice.

IMPLICATIONS FOR NURSE MANAGERS

Many of the problems that face nurse educators will also affect nurse managers. The management structure that has traditionally been employed in nursing is that of a bureaucracy, based on a hierarchical system with clearly stated rules and regulations or policies which say what nurses can or cannot do according to their level or status. Even though this is changing, as there is a greater degree of devolution of responsibility within practice settings, remnants of this approach still hold fast.

Model-based practice implies it is the individual practitioners or the teams they work in that control the way in which they work. From a management perspective this raises two dilemmas. While managers have the responsibility for ensuring that the organisation fulfils the purpose for which it is designed, that is to supply a nursing service, they have little control over how that service is supplied. Provided that the standards which have been established are fulfilled, the way in which these standards are reached may vary from setting to setting according to which model practice is based on. Inevitably this will alter the function of the manager from one of controlling to one of facilitation – a much more exacting role to fulfil. More flexibility may be needed in setting policies in order to allow for individual variations in different settings. For instance, if the goals of a ward are geared towards independence, it would be inappropriate to make a rule about the use of cot sides for elderly patients. Similarly in a community setting, no rule could be set about the time by which all morning insulins must be given if they are to be planned on an individual basis, although standards such as keeping to appointment times can be made centrally.

So, if a manager's role in controlling the way in which nurses practice is reduced, what is their function? We would see them developing and expanding their role as facilitator, with a much greater emphasis on providing the facilities which allow clinical nurses to practice and develop new ideas. This may involve such things as providing learning opportunities, assessing standards and dependency levels, and ensuring that services and equipment are available, as well as providing the essential moral support for clinical colleagues. Part of that role will be risk assessment, which seeks to ensure safety while encouraging or enhancing innovation. Of course managers also have a vital function in representing nursing at a strategic level. In order to do this they too have an urgent need to be able to be articulate about the manner in which the nursing service contributes to the organisation as a whole, and a working knowledge of models can undoubtedly be of value to them in this arena.

This is not an easy transition, especially as many nurse managers will not have had the opportunity to practise nursing using a nursing model themselves. Yet it can also offer a new and exciting dimension to their work, and the satisfaction of seeing improved patient care.

Figure 18.2 The manager's dilemma, showing facilitation rather than control of practitioners.

IMPLICATIONS FOR NURSING RESEARCH

There has been a rapid increase in the amount of nursing research being carried out over the past 20 years, both by nurses in formal research posts and by clinical nurses themselves. One of the most difficult things to do in research is to define the exact nature of the problem or question, and it is in this area that models of nursing can be so useful.

As we are sure you know by now, models are based on philosophies or beliefs, and goals that reflect theories and concepts. Research is about generating and testing ideas in order to acquire new knowledge. Putting these two thoughts together, the direction of research may be either of the following.

- To refine theories of nursing – what are the related concepts? How do they relate to each other and to nursing itself? Is there an alternative model of nursing?
- To refine theories for nursing. If I do this or that, will it be useful in helping patients to achieve their goals? In using a model, deficits in the knowledge required for practice can be identified.

A third perspective in relation to research is the growing concern that what research has been done is not put into practice. While some may argue that part of this dilemma is caused because the research is not seen as relevant by practitioners (MacGuire, 1990), there is also an argument

that without being clear about the goals of practice it is less easy to identify relevant work.

Working from a model base can help in clarifying any of these aspects
of research, giving it purpose and direction. We know of several clinically based nurses who have developed excellent small-scale research
based on a conceptual framework that is clearly nursing in nature. For
instance, one clinical nurse examined whether teaching relaxation to
people reduces the number of tension-induced symptoms they suffer
(Newing, 1985). Another looked at what problems patients face in fulfilling activities of living following the stress of surgery, regardless of what
the surgery is for. Parse (1990) describes a study exploring the lived
experience of hope based on her theories and there are a growing
number of nursing projects that use her theory to describe phenomena of
interest to nurses. It is clear that an explicit model of nursing can contribute significantly to the work of nurses undertaking research.

Nursing models explicate the theorising, or thinking, of nurses and
thus offer a tentative framework for practice, education, management
and research. It is important, however, to view models for what they are –
merely attempts by nurses to represent what the reality of nursing is to
the writer.

CONCLUSION

In this book we have attempted to introduce you to the ideas inherent in
model-based practice and to offer you some guidance on implementing
and evaluating a model in practice. While the early chapters were largely
theoretical in nature, outlining the common characteristics of nursing
models, we feel that they are an appropriate background to the practical
use of models. Other chapters have tried to show you how some published models can be applied through presenting practical illustrations
based on specific nursing models; how changes in practice can be managed; and how a model can be evaluated.

It is at this stage that we can hand the work over to you. Nobody can
tell you which model to choose or how to implement it. If we presumed
to try to tell you, we would be going against our own beliefs in an individual's right to make choices for him or herself. The model we agree on
tells us that this is the way we should behave!

We cannot pretend that it is easy either to identify the model relevant to
your work or to put it into practice. All we can say is that in our opinion
the path is worth following.

*Science is built up with facts as a house is with stones but a collection of
facts is no more a science than a heap of stones is a house.*

Jules Henri Poincare, *La Science et l'Hypothese*

Learning exercises

1. Identify the model in use in the area in which you are currently placed. Ask nurses in the unit or clinic how this model of practice became the norm.
2. Consider how, in your experience, changing practices or ways of doing things (at work, at school or at home) affects people? How do you cope with change?

Study questions

1. Describe why an openness to change is important.
2. Discuss the change process.
3. List the essential features of an effective approach to implementing change.

References and Bibliography

Allen, D. (1985) Nursing research and social control: alternative models of science that emphasise understanding and emancipation. *The Journal of Nursing Scholarship*, 17(2): 58–64.

Allen, D., Benner, P. and Diekelmann, N.L. (1986) Three paradigms for nursing research: methodological implications. In P.L. Chinn (ed.), *Nursing Research Methodology: Issues and Implementation*. Rockville, MD: Aspen.

Andrews, H. and Roy, C. (1986) *Essentials of the Roy Adaptation Model*. Englewood Cliffs, NJ: Prentice Hall.

Apple, D. (1960) How laymen define illness. *Journal of Health and Human Behaviour*, 1(3): 219–25.

Audit Commission (1992) *Lying in Wait: the Use of Medical Beds in Acute Hospitals*. London: HSMO.

Bardsley, M., Coles, J. and Jenkins, L. (1989) *DRGs and Health Care: the Management of Case Mix*, 2nd edn. London: King's Fund.

Barrett, W. (1962) *Irrational Man*. New York: Anchor Books/Doubleday.

Bauman, B. (1961) Diversities in conceptions of health and physical fitness. *Journal of Health and Human Behaviour*, 2(1): 39–46.

Beitz, J.M. (2001) Overcoming barriers to quality wound care: a systems perspective. *Ostomy Wound Management*, 47(3): 56–64.

Benham, A.J. (1999) Managed care and critical pathway development: the joint replacement experience. *Orthopaedic Nursing*, 18(4): 71–5.

Benner, P. (1984) *From Novice to Expert*. Menlo Park: Addison-Wesley.

Benner, P. and Wrubel, J. (1989) *The Primacy of Caring: Stress and Coping in Health and Illness*. Menlo Park: Addison-Wesley.

Bennett, J.G. (1980) Foreword to symposium on the selfcare concept of nursing. *Nursing Clinics of North America*, 15: 1.

Bevis, E.O. (1978) *Curriculum Building in Nursing*. St Louis: C.V. Mosby.

Bevis, E.O. and Watson, J. (1989) *Toward a Caring Curriculum: a New Pedagogy for Nursing*. New York: National League for Nursing.

Blaxter, M. (1996) Criteria for the evaluation of qualitative research papers. *Medical Sociology News*, 22(1): 68–71.

Botha, M.E. (1989) Theory development in perspective: the role of conceptual frameworks and models in theory development. *Journal of Advanced Nursing*, 14: 49–55.

Boulton, M. and Fitzpatrick, R. (1994) Quality in qualitative research. *Critical Public Health*, 5(3): 19–26.

Boulton, M. and Fitzpatrick, R. (1997) Evaluating qualitative research. *Evidence-Based Health Policy and Management*, 1(44): 83–5.

Brown, C. and Seddon, J. (1996) The social and biomechanical body: can they coexist in nurse education? *Journal of Advanced Nursing*, 23(4): 652–6.

Buckwalter, K. and Kerfoot, K. (1982) Teaching patients selfcare: a critical aspect of psychiatric discharge planning. *Journal of Psychiatric Nursing and Mental Health Services*, 20(5): 15–20.

Bunting, S. (1992) *Rosemarie Parse: Theory of Health as Human Becoming*. London: Sage Publications.

Byrne, M. and Thompson, L. (1978) *Key Concepts for the Study and Practice of Nursing*, 2nd edn. St Louis: C.V. Mosby.

Capra, F. (1982) *The Turning Point: Science, Society and the Rising Culture*. London: Fontana Paperbacks.

Carr, W. and Kemmis, S. (1986) *Becoming Critical. Education, Knowledge and Action Research*. Lewes: Falmer.

Carter, K.F. and Dufour, L.T. (1994) King's theory: a critique of the critiques. *Nursing Science Quarterly*, 7(3): 128–3.

Chant, A. (1989) *The Stem Doctor* (private publication).

Chapple, A. and Rogers, A. (1998) Explicit guidelines for qualitative research: a step in the right direction, a defence of the 'soft' option, or a form of sociological imperialism? *Family Practice*, 15(6): 556–61.

Chessick, R.D. (1980) Some philosophical assumptions of intensive psychotherapy. *American Journal of Psychotherapy*, 34(4): 496–509.

Chin, R. (1980) The utility of systems models and developmental models for practitioners. In J.R. Riehl and C. Roy (eds), *Conceptual Models for Nursing Practice*, 2nd edn. New York: Appleton-Century-Croft.

Chin, P.L. and Jacobs, M.K. (1987) *Theory and Nursing: A Systematic Approach*, 2nd edn. St Louis: C.V. Mosby.

Chinn, P.L. and Kramer, M.K. (1999) *Theory and nursing: Integrated knowledge development*. St. Louis: Mosby.

Chiou, C.P. (2000) A meta-analysis of the interrelationships between the modes in Roy's adaptation model. *Nursing Science Quarterly*, 13(3): 252–8.

Cochrane Collaboration (1993) *Introductory Brochure*. Oxford: Cochrane Collaboration.

Cody, W.K. and Mitchell, G.J. (1992) Parse's theory as a model for practice: the cutting edge. *Advances in Nursing Science*, 15(2): 52–65.

Cody, W.K. and Mitchell, G.J. (2002) Nursing knowledge and human science revisited: practical and political considerations. *Nursing Science Quarterly*, 1.

Commonwealth Department of Health and Family Services (1995) Review of Professional Indemnity Arrangements for Health Care Professionals: *Compensation and Professional Indemnity in Health Care*. Final Report. Canberra: AGPS.

Commonwealth Department of Health and Family Services (1996) Clinical practice guidelines and outcomes. *Better Health Outcomes*, 2(1): 9.

Commonwealth Department of Health, Housing and Community Services (1992) Review of Professional Indemnity Arrangements for Health Care Professionals: *Compensation and Professional Indemnity in Health Care – A Discussion Paper*. Canberra: AGPS.

Commonwealth Department of Human Services and Health (1995) *Taskforce on Quality in Australian Health Care: Interim Report to the Hon Dr Carmen Lawrence MP*. Canberra: unpublished.

Compton, P. (1989) Drug abuse, a self-care deficit. *Journal of Psychosocial Nursing*, 27(3): 22–6.

Cooper, D. (1990) *Existentialism: A Reconstruction*. Oxford: Blackwell.

Copperman, J. and Morrison, P. (1995) *We Thought We Knew: Involving Patients in Nursing Practice*. London: King's Fund.

Craddock, R.B. and Stanhope, N.K. (1980) The Neuman Health Care Systems Model: recommended adaptations. In J.P. Riehl and C. Roy (eds), *Conceptual Models for Nursing Practice*, 2nd edn. New York: Appleton-Century-Croft.

Cullum, N.A. (1994) *The Nursing Management of Leg Ulcers in the Community: a critical review of research*. Report to the Department of Health from the Department of Nursing. Liverpool: University of Liverpool.

Cullum, N., DiCenso, A. and Ciliska, D. (1997) Evidence-based nursing: an introduction ... a journal of evidence-based nursing. *Nursing Standard*, 11(28): 32–3.

Cushing, A. (1993) *A Contextual Perspective to Female Nursing in Victoria, 1850–1914*. Victoria: Deakin University Press.

Davies, C. (ed.) (1980) *Rewriting Nursing History*. London: Croom Helm.

Davis, F. (1975) Professional socialisation as subjective experience: the process of doctrinal conversion among student nurses. In C. Cox and A. Mead (eds), *A Sociology of Medical Practice*. London: Collier Macmillan.

Day, M. (1995) Home Rule. *Nursing Times*, 91(24): 14–15.

De Back, V. (1981) The relationship between senior nursing students' ability for formulating nursing diagnoses and curriculum model. *A.N.S.*, 3(3): 51–66.

De Cecco, J.D. and Crawford, W.R. (1974) *The Psychology of Learning and Instruction*, 2nd edn. Old Tappan, NJ: Prentice Hall.

Department of Health (1990) *Care in the Community: Making it Happen*. London: HMSO.

Department of Health (1991) *The Patient's Charter*. London: DoH.

Department of Health (1993) *A Vision for the Future: the Nursing, Midwifery and Health Visiting Contribution to Health and Health Care*. London: DoH and NHS ME.

Department of Health (1995) *Research and Development: Towards an Evidenced Based Health Service*. London: DoH.

Dickoff, J., James, P. and Weidenbach, E. (1986) Theory in a practice discipline. Part II: Practice oriented research. *Nursing Research*, 17(6): 545–54.

Dingwall, R., Rafferty, A.M. and Webster, C. (1988) *An Introduction to the Social History of Nursing*. London: Routledge.

Dingwall, R., Murphy, E., Watson, P., Greatbatch, D. and Parker, S. (1998) Catching goldfish: quality in qualitative research. *Journal of Health Services Research Policy*, 13(3): 167–72.

Duby, T., Hoffman, D., Cameron, J., Doblhoff-Brown, D., Cherry, G. and Ryan, T. (1993) A randomized trial in the treatment of venous leg ulcers comparing short stretch bandages, four layer bandage system, and a long stretch paste bandage system. *Wounds* 5(6): 276–9.

Duff, L.A., Kitson, A.L., Seers, K. and Humpris, D. (1996) Clinical guidelines: an introduction to their development and implementation. *Journal of Advanced Nursing*, 23: 887–95.

Durdin, J. (1991) *They Became Nurses: A History of Nursing in South Australia 1836–1980*. Sydney: Allen and Unwin.

Eisenberg, J.M. (2000) Continuing education meets the learning organisation: the challenge of a systems approach to patient safety. *Journal of Continuing Education in the Health Professions*, 20(4): 197–207.

Emden, C. and Sandelowski, M. (1999) The good, the bad and the relative. Part two: goodness and the criterion problem in qualitative research. *International Journal of Nursing Practice*, 5: 2–7.

Ersser, S. and Tutton, E. (1991) *Primary Nursing in Perspective*. Harrow: Scutari Press.

Evans, A. and Griffiths, P. (1994) *The Development of a Nursing-led Inpatient Service*. London: King's Fund.

Evidence Based Medicine Group (1992) Evidence-based medicine: a new approach to teaching the practice of medicine. *JAMA*, 268: 2420–5.

Fawcett, J. (1989) *Analysis and Evaluation of Conceptual Models of Nursing*, 2nd edn. Philadelphia: F.A. Davis.

Fay, B. (1975) *Social Theory and Political Practice*. London: George Allen & Unwin.

Fay, B. (1987) *Critical Social Science*. Cambridge: Polity Press.

Field, D. (1972) Disability as social deviance. In E. Freidson and J. Corber (eds), *Medical Men and Their Work*. New York: Aldine Atherton.

FitzGerald, M. (1994) Lecturer practitioners: creating the environment. In J. Lathlean and B. Vaughan (eds), *Unifying Nursing Theory and Practice*. Oxford: Butterworth-Heinemann.

Fitzpatrick, J.J. and Whall, A.L. (eds) (1996) *Conceptual Models of Nursing: Analysis and Application*, 3rd edn. Stamford: Appleton and Lange.

Fraser, M. (1990) *Using Conceptual Nursing in Practice: A Research-Based Approach*, 1st edn. London: Harper and Row.

Fraser, M. (1996) *Using Conceptual Nursing in Practice: A Research-Based Approach*, 2nd edn. London: Harper and Row.

Friedson, E. (1975) *Profession of Medicine*. New York: Dodd, Mead and Co.

Furlong, S. (1995) *Self-Care: Application in Practice*. London: King's Fund.

Game, A. and Pringle, R. (1983) *Gender at Work*. Sydney: Allen and Unwin.

Garbett, R. (1994) Changing philosophy by group interviews. *Nursing Standard*, 8(22): 37–40.

Giroux, H. (1983) *Critical Theory and Educational Practice*. Victoria: Deakin University Press.

Glaser, R. (1962) Psychology and instructional technology. In R. Glaser (ed.), *Training Resources and Education*. Pittsburgh: University of Pittsburgh Press.

Green, J. and Britten, N. (1998) Qualitative research and evidence based medicine. *BMJ*, 316: 1230–2.

Greenhalgh, T. and Taylor, R. (1997) How to read a paper: papers that go beyond numbers (qualitative research). *BMJ*, 315: 740–3.

Griffiths, P. and Evans, A. (1995) *Evaluating a Nursing-led In-Patient Service*. London: King's Fund.

Habermas, J. (1971) *Knowledge and Human Interests* (translated by J. Shapiro). Boston: Beacon.

Hale, C. (1995) Case management and managed care. *Nursing Standard*, 9(19): 33–5.

Ham, C. (1992) *Health Policy in Britain: the Politics and Organisation of the National Health Service*, 3rd edn. London: Macmillan.

Hammond, C., Chase, J. and Hogbin, B. (1995) A unique service. *Nursing Times*, 91(30): 28–9.

Hancock, B. (2000) Are nursing theories holistic? *Nursing Standard*, 14: 37–41.

Harris, J. (1987) QALYfying the value of life. *Journal of Medical Ethics*, 13: 117–23.

Health and Community Services, Victoria (1995) *Towards a New Framework for Quality in Victoria's Hospitals. Issues and Options: A Discussion Paper*. Melbourne: Health and Community Services Promotions Institute.

Heath, H. (1998) Paradigm dialogues and dogma: finding a place for research, nursing models and reflective practice. *Journal of Advanced Nursing*, 28(2): 288.

Heidegger, M. (1962) *Being and Time* (translated by J. MacQuarrie and E. Robinson). New York: Harper and Row.

Henderson, V. (1966) *The Nature of Nursing*. London: Collier Macmillan.

Holmes, C. (1990) Alternative in nursing science foundations for nursing. *International Journal of Nursing Studies*, 27: 187–9.

Honigsbaum, F. (1992) *Who Shall Live? Who Shall Die? Oregan's Health Financing Proposals*. London: King's Fund.

Husserl, E. (1970) *The Crisis of the European Sciences and Transcendental Phenomenology* (translated by D. Carr). Evanston, IL: North Western University Press.

Illich, I. (1975) *Medical Nemesis*. Harmondsworth: Pelican.

Jirovec, M.M., Jenkins, J., Isenberg, M. and Baiardi, J. (1999) Urine control theory derived from Roy's conceptual framework. *Nursing Science Quarterly*, 12(1): 251–5.

Joseph, L.S. (1980) Self care and the nursing process. *Nursing Clinics of North America*, 15: 1.

Kaplan, A. (1964) *The Conduct of Inquiry*. New York: Chandler Press.

Keneley, M. (1988) Handmaidens of medicine: working conditions for nurses in late nineteenth century Victoria. *Journal of Australian Studies*, 22: 57–68.

Kim, H.S. and Kollak, I. (1999) *Nursing Theories: Conceptual and Philosophical Foundations*. Springer: New York.

King, I.M. (1971) *Toward a Theory for Nursing: General Concepts for Human Behaviour*. New York: John Wiley & Sons.

King, I. (1981) *A Theory for Nursing: Systems, Concepts, Process*. New York: John Wiley & Sons.

King, I. (1986) *Curriculum and Instruction in Nursing*. Norwalk: Appleton-Century-Croft.

King, I. (1987) King's theory of goal attainment. In R. Parse (ed.), *Nursing Science: Major Paradigms, Theories and Critiques*. Philadelphia: W.B. Saunders.

King, I.M. (1996) The theory of goal attainment in research and practice. *Nursing Science Quarterly*, 9(2): 61–6.

King, I.M. (1997) King's theory of goal attainment in practice. *Nursing Science Quarterly*, 10(4): 180–5.

Kitson, A., Harvey, G. and McCormack, B. (1998) Enabling the implementation of evidence based practice: a conceptual framework. *Quality in Health Care*, 7: 149–58.

Knaus, W.A., Draper, E.A., Wagner, D.P. and Zimmermen, J.E. (1985) Apache II: a severity of disease classification system. *Critical Care Medicine* 13: 818–29.

Kramer, M. (1990) Holistic nursing: implications for knowledge development and utilisation. In N. Chaska (ed.), *The Nursing Profession: Turning Points*. St Louis: Mosby/Year Book.

Krysl, M. (1989) *Midwife and Other Poems on Caring*. New York: National League for Nursing.

Kubler-Ross, E. (1969) *On Death and Dying*. London: Tavistock.

Lather, P. (1986) Research as praxis. *Harvard Educational Review*, 56: 257–77.

Lather, P. (1991) *Getting Smart: Feminist Res and Pedagogy within the Postmodern*. New York: Routledge.

Lathlean, J. (1989) *Research in Action: Developing the Role of the Ward Sister*. London: King's Fund Centre.

Lathlean, J. and Vaughan, B. (1994) *Unifying Nursing Theory and Practice*. Oxford: Butterworth-Heinemann.

Lauder, W. (2001) The utility of self-care theory as a theoretical basis for self-neglect. *Journal of Advanced Nursing*, 43(4): 545–51.

Lawler, J. (1991) *Behind the Screens*. Melbourne: Churchill Livingstone.

Lee, R., Schumacher, L. and Twigg, P. (1994) Rosemarie Rizzo Parse: Man–Living–Health. In A. Marriner-Tomey (ed.), *Nursing Theorists and Their Work*. St Louis: Mosby.

Lemmer, B., Grellier, R. and Steven, J. (1999) Systematic review of nonrandom and qualitative research literature: exploring and uncovering an evidence base for health visiting and decision making. *Qualitative Health Research*, 9: 315–28.

Levin, L., Katz, A. and Holst, E. (1979) *Self-Care: Lay Initiatives in Health*. New York: Prodist.

Lewis, F.M. and Batey, M.V. (1982) Clarifying autonomy and accountability in nursing service – Part II. *Journal of Nursing Administration*, 12(10): 10–15.

Luker, K. and Kenrick, M. (1993) The evaluation of a clinical information pack and the development of audit criteria for the nursing management of leg ulcers. Liverpool: Department of Nursing, University of Liverpool.

Luker, K. and Kenrick, M. (1995) Towards knowledge-based practice: an evaluation of a method of dissemination. *International Journal of Nursing Studies*, 32: 59–67.

MacGuire, J. (1990) Putting nursing research findings into practice: research utilization as an aspect of the management of change. *Journal of Advanced Nursing*, 15: 614–20.

MacIntyre, A. (1964) *A Critical History of Western Philosophy*. London: Macmillan.

MacLeod, M. (1990) Experience in Everyday Nursing Practice: A Study of 'Experienced' Ward Sisters. University of Edinburgh, unpublished PhD thesis.

Malinski, V.M. (2000) Research-based evaluation of conceptual models of nursing. *Nursing Science Quarterly*, 13(1): 12–17.

Mallow, A. (1943) A theory of human motivation. *Psychological Review*, 50: 370.

Manley, K. (1992) Quality Assurance: the pathway to excellence. In M. Jolley and G. Brykczyriska (eds), *Nursing Care: The Challenge to Change*. London: Edward Arnold.

Manthey, M. (1992) *The Practice of Primary Nursing*, revised edn. London: King's Fund.

Marriner-Tomey, A. and Alligood, M.R. (eds) (2002) *Nursing Theorists and Their Work*, 5th edn. St Louis: Mosby.

Marsh, S. and MacAlpine, M. (1995) *Our Own Capabilities: Clinical Nurse Managers Taking a Strategic Approach to Service Improvement*. London: King's Fund.

Maslow, A.H. (1954) *Motivation and Personality*. New York: Harper and Row.

McFarlane, J. (1978) *The Multidisciplinary Clinical Team*. London: King's Fund.

Meleis, A.I. (1985) *Theoretical Nursing: Development and Progress*. Philadelphia: Lippincott.

Meleis, A.I. (1991) *Theoretical Nursing: Development and Progress*, 2nd edn. Philadelphia: Lippincott.

Menzies, I.E.P. (1960) *A Case Study in the Functioning of Social Systems as a Defense Against Anxiety*. London: The Tavistock Institute of Human Relations.

Moore, J.B. and Pichler, V.H. (2000) Measurement of Orem's basic conditioning factors: a review of published research. *Nursing Science Quarterly*, 13(2): 137–42.

Morgan, G. (1993) The implications of patient focused care. *Nursing Standard*, 7(52): 37–9.

Morris, D.B. (2000) How to speak postmodern medicine, illness, and cultural change. *Hastings Centre Report*, 30(6): 7–16.

Muir Gray, J.A. (1997) *Evidence-Based Healthcare. How to Make Health Policy and Management Decisions*. London: Churchill Livingstone; Ch. 6.

Mullin, V.J. (1981) Implementing the self-care concept in the acute care setting. *Nursing Clinics of North America*, 15: 1.

Murray, R.L.E. and Baier, M. (1996) King's conceptual framework applied to a transitional living program. *Perspectives in Psychiatric Care*, 32(1): 15–19.

NDCG (Nursing Development Conference Group) (1973) *Concept Formulization in Nursing*. Boston: Little, Brown and Co.

Neil, R. (1990) Watson's Theory of Caring in Nursing: the rainbow of and for people living with AIDS. In M. Parker (ed.), *Nursing Theories in Practice*. New York: National League for Nurses.

Neil, R. and Schroeder, C. (1992) Evaluation research within the human caring framework. In D. Gaut (ed.), *The Presence of Caring in Nursing*. New York: National League for Nurses.

Neuman, B. (1980) The Betty Neuman Health Care Systems Model: a total approach to patient problems. In J. Rieffi and C. Roy (eds), *Conceptual Models for Nursing Practice*, 2nd edn. New York: Appleton-Century-Croft.

Neuman, B. (1982) *The Neuman Systems Model: Application to Nursing Education and Practice*. New York: Appleton-Century-Croft.

Neuman, B. (1989) *The Neuman Systems Model*, 2nd edn. New York: Appleton-Century-Croft.

Neuman, B. (1995) *The Neuman Systems Model*, 3rd edn. Connecticut: Appleton and Lange.

Neuman, B. (1996) The Neuman systems model in research and practice. *Nursing Science Quarterly*, 2(2): 67–70.

Neuman, B. and Wyatt, M. (1981) Prospects for change: some evaluative reflections from one articulated baccalaureate program. *Journal of Nursing Education*, 20(1): 40–6.

Neuman, B. and Young, R.J. (1972) A model for teaching total person approach to patient problems. *Nursing Research*, 21(3): 264.

Newing, M. (1985) *Group Processes: a Subjective Exploration*. Oxford: Burford Nursing Development Unit.

NHS Management Executive (1993) *The Evolution of Clinical Audit*. Leeds: NHS ME.

Nightingale, F. (1970) *Notes on Nursing*. Princeton: Vertex.

Norris, C.M. (1979). Self care. *American Journal of Nursing*, 79(3): 486–9.

O'Brien, B. and Pearson, A. (1993) Unwritten knowledge in nursing, consider the spoken as well as the written word. *Scholarly Inquiry for Nursing Practice: An International Journal*, 7(2): 169–82.

O'Connor, N. (1993) *Paterson and Zderad Humanistic Theory*. London: Sage.

Orem, D. (1971) *Nursing – Concepts of Practice*. New York: McGraw-Hill.

Orem, D. (1980) *Nursing – Concepts of Practice*, 2nd edn. New York: McGraw-Hill.

Orem, D. (1985) *Nursing – Concepts of Practice*, 3rd edn. New York: McGraw-Hill.

Orem, D. (1987) Orem's general theory of nursing. In R. Parse (ed.), *Nursing Science: Major Paradigms, Theories and Critiques*. Philadelphia: W.B. Saunders.

Orem, D. (1991) *Nursing – Concepts of Practice*, 4th edn. New York: McGraw-Hill.

Paar, G.H. and Grohmann, S. (2000) Thoughts on a 'general model of psychosomatic rehabilitation' and deductions on treatment intensity and required duration of inpatient treatment. *Rehabilitation*, 39(1): 8–16.

Parse, R. (1981) *Man–Living–Health: A Theory of Nursing*. New York: Delmar.

Parse, R. (1987) *Nursing Science: Major Paradigms, Theories and Critique*. Philadephia: W.B. Saunders.

Parse, R. (1990) Parse's research methodology with an illustration of the lived experience of hope. *Nursing Science Quarterly*, 3: 9–17.

Parse, R. (1992) Human becoming: Parse's theory of nursing. *Nursing Science Quarterly*, 5: 35–42.

Parse, R. (1997) The Human Becoming Theory: the was, is and will be. *Science Quarterly*, 10(1): 32–9.

Parse, R., Coyne, A. and Smith, M. (1985) *Nursing Research: Qualitative Methods*. Bowie, MD: Brady.

Parsons, T. (1951) *The Social System*. London: Routledge & Kegan Paul.

Paterson, J. and Zderad, L. (1976/1988) *Humanistic Nursing*. New York: National League for Nursing.

Pauli, H.G., White, K.L. and McWhinney, I.R. (2000) Medical education, research, and scientific thinking in the 21st century (parts two and three of three). *Education for Health*, 13(2): 165–72; 173–86.

Pearcey, P.A. (1995) Achieving research-based nursing practice. *Journal of Advanced Nursing*, 22: 33–9.

Pearson, A. (1983) *The Clinical Nursing Unit*. London: William Heinemann Medical Books.

Pearson, A. (1988) Theorising nursing: the need for multiple horizons. In Proceedings: Expanding Horizons in Nursing Education. National Nursing Education Conference, Perth, Australia, 1988.

Pearson, A. (1990) *Nursing: From Whence to Where?* Victoria: Deakin University Press.

Pearson, A. (1992) Knowing nursing: emerging paradigms in nursing. In K. Robinson and B. Vaughan (eds), *Knowledge for Nursing Practice*. Oxford: Butterworth-Heinemann.

Pearson, A. (1998) Excellence in care: future dimensions for effective nursing. *NT Research*, 3(1): 25–7.

Pearson, A. (1999) Evidence-based nursing – quality through research. In R. Nay and S. Garratt (eds), *Nursing Older People: Issues and Innovations*. Sydney: Maclennan & Petty, pp. 338–52.

Pearson, A. (2004) Balancing the Evidence. *Health Care Reports*, 2: 45–65.

Pearson, A. and Taylor, B. (1996) Gender and nursing in colonial Victoria 1840–1870. *The International History of Nursing Journal*, 2(1): 25–45.

Pearson, A. and Vaughan, B. (1984). Module I: nursing practice and the nursing process. In *A Systematic Approach to Nursing Care – an Introduction*. Milton Keynes: Open University.

Pearson, A., Punton, S. and Durant, E. (1992) *Nursing Beds: an Evaluation of the Effects of Therapeutic Nursing*. Harrow: Scutari Press.

Pearson, A., Taylor, B. and Coleborne, C. (1997) *The Nature of Nursing Work in Colonial Victoria 1840–1870*. Victoria: Deakin University Press.

Peplau, H.E. (1952/1988) *Interpersonal Relations in Nursing*. New York: G.R. Putman.

Peplau, H.E. (1964) *Basic Principles of Patient Counselling*, 2nd edn. Philadelphia: Smith Kline and French Laboratories.

Peplau, H.E. (1969) Professional closeness. *Nursing Forum*, 8(4): 342–60.

Peplau, H.E. (1980) The psychiatric nurse – accountable? to whom? for what? *Perspectives in Psychiatric Care*, 18(3): 128–34.

Peplau, H.E. (1987) Nursing science: a historical perspective. In R. Parse (ed.), *Nursing Science: Major Paradigms, Theories, and Critiques*. Philadelphia: W.B. Saunders.

Peplau, H.E. (1997) Peplau's theory of interpersonal relations. *Nursing Science Quarterly*, 10(4): 162–7.

Piaget, J. (1932) *The Moral Judgement of the Child*. London: Routledge and Kegan Paul.

Pickersgill, F. (1995) A natural extension. *Nursing Times*, 91(30): 24–7.

Pidgeon, E.C. (1956) Pioneering nursing in Australia. *International Nursing Review*, 3(21): 38–43.

Pietroni, P. (1984) Holistic medicine. New map, old territory. *The British Journal of Holistic Medicine*, 1: 3–13.

Pontin, D. (1999) Primary Nursing: a mode of care or a philosophy of nursing? *Journal of Advanced Nursing*, 29(3): 584.

Popay, J. and Williams, G. (1998) Qualitative research and evidence-based healthcare. *Journal of the Royal Society of Medicine*, 91(Suppl. 35): 32–7.

Popay, J., Rogers, A. and Williams, G. (1998) Rationale and standards for the systematic review of qualitative literature in health services research. *Qualitative Health Research*, 8(3): 341–51.

Rambo, B.J. (1984) *Adaptation Nursing: Assessment and Intervention*. Philadelphia: W.B. Saunders.

Read, S., Jones, N. and Williams, B.B. (1992) Nurse practitioners in A&E Departments: what do they do? *British Medical Journal*, 305: 1466–70.

Reed, P.G. (1996) Transforming practice knowledge into nursing knowledge – a revisionist analysis of Peplau. *Image – the Journal of Nursing Scholarship*, 28(1): 29–33.

Rheil, J. and Roy, C. (1980) *Conceptual Models for Nursing Practice*. New York: Appleton-Century-Croft.

Richardson, G. and Maynard, A. (1995) *Fewer Doctors? More Nurses? A Review of the Knowledge Base of Doctor Nurse Substitution*. York: Centre for Health Economics, University of York.

Robinson, K. and Vaughan, B. (1992) *Knowledge for Nursing Practice*. Oxford: Butterworth-Heinemann.

Roe, B.H., Griffiths, J.M., Kenrick, M., Cullum, N.A. and Hutton, J.L. (1994) Nursing treatment of patients with chronic leg ulcers in the community. *Journal of Clinical Nursing*, 3: 159–68.

Rogers, C. (1957) The necessary and sufficient conditions of therapeutic personality changes. *Journal of Consulting Psychology*, 21: 95.

Rogers, C. (1962) The interpersonal relationship: the core of guidance. *Harvard Educational Review*, 32: 416.

Rogers, M. (1970) *An Introduction to the Theoretical Basis of Nursing*. Philadelphia: F.A. Davis.

Roper, N. (1976) *Clinical Experience in Nurse Education*. Edinburgh: Churchill Livingstone.

Roper, N., Logan, W. and Tierney, A. (1980) *The Elements of Nursing*. Edinburgh: Churchill Livingstone.

Roper, N., Logan, W. and Tierney, A. (1981). *Learning to Use the Process of Nursing*. Edinburgh: Churchill Livingstone.

Roper, N., Logan, W. and Tierney, A. (1985) *The Elements of Nursing*, 2nd edn. Edinburgh: Churchill Livingstone.

Roper, N., Logan, W. and Tierney, A. (1990) *The Elements of Nursing, a Model for Nursing Based on a Model of Living*, 3rd edn. Edinburgh: Churchill Livingstone.

Roper, N., Logan, W. and Tierney, A. (2000) *The Roper Logan Tierney Model of Nursing*. Edinburgh: Churchill Livingstone.

Rose, A.M. (1980) A systematic summary of symbolic interaction theory. In J. Ried and C. Roy (eds), *Conceptual Models for Nursing Practice*, 2nd edn. New York: Appleton-Century-Croft.

Roy, C. (1976) *Introduction to Nursing: an Adaptation Model*. Old Tappan, NJ: Prentice Hall.

Roy, C. (1984) *Introduction to Nursing: an Adaptation Model*, 2nd edn. Englewood Cliffs, NJ: Prentice Hall.

Roy, C. (1997) Future of the Roy Model: challenge to redefine adaptation. *Nursing Science Quarterly*, 10(1): 42–9.

Roy, C. and Fawcett, J. (2002) The nurse theorists: 21st century updates. *Nursing Science Quarterly*, 15(4).

Royal College of Nursing (1990) *The Dynamic Standard Setting System*. Harrow: Scutari Press.

Royal Commission on the National Health Service (1978) *Patient Attitudes to the Hospital Service*. Norwich: HMSO.

Russell, B. (1961) *History of Western Philosophy*. London: Allen and Unwin.

Ryan Belcher, J. and Brittain Fish, L. (1990) Hildegard E. Peplau. In J. George (ed.), *Nursing Theories: the Base for Professional Nursing Practice*. London: Prentice Hall.

Sackett, D.L. and Rosenberg, W.M.C. (1995) On the need for evidence-based medicine. *Health Economics*, 4: 249–54.

Sackett, D.L., Rosenberg, W.M.C., Gray, J.A.M., Haynes, R.B. and Richardson, W.S. (1996) Evidence-based medicine: what it is and what it is not. *British Medical Journal*, 312: 71–2.

Sandelowski, M., Docherty, S. and Emden, C. (1997) Qualitative metasynthesis: issues and techniques. *Research in Nursing and Health*, 20: 365–71.

Schon, D.A. (1987) *Educating the Reflective Practitioner*. San Francisco: Jossey-Bass.

Selye, H. (1978) *The Stress of Life*. New York: McGraw Hill.

Shamash, J. (1995) Measures for comfort and joy. *Nursing Times*, 91(33): 14–15.

Sills, G.M. (1978) Hildegard E. Peplau: leader, practitioner, academic, scholar and theorist. *Perspectives in Psychiatric Care*, 16(3): 22–8.

Sleep, J. (1984) Episiotomy in normal delivery – management of the perineum (parts one and two). *Nursing Times*, 80(47): 28–30; 80(48): 51–4.

Smuts, J.C. (1926) *Holism and Evolution*. New York: Macmillan.

Stacey, M. (1977) Concepts of health and illness: a working paper on the concepts and their relevance for research. In *Social Science Research Council, Health and Health Policy – Priorities for Research*. London: SSRC.

Sterling, S.R. (2001) *Sustainable Education: Re-visioning Learning and Change*. Totnes: Green Books for The Schumacher Society.

Stevens, B. (1984) *Nursing Theory: Analysis, Application, Evaluation*, 2nd edn. Boston: Little, Brown and Co.

Stevenson, L. (1974) *Seven Theories of Human Nature*. Oxford: Oxford University Press.

Stilwell, B. (1987) A nurse practitioner in general practice: working style and pattern of consultation. *Journal of Royal College of General Practitioners*, 37: 154–7.

Street, A. (1990) Nursing practice: high, hard ground, messy swamps and the pathways in between. In *Reflective Processes in Nursing* (Faculty of Nursing Monograph Series). Victoria: Deakin University Press, pp. 1–38.

Taylor, S.G., Geden, E., Isaramalai, S. and Wongvatunyu, S. (2000) Orem's self-care deficit nursing theory: its philosophic foundation and the state of the science. *Nursing Science Quarterly*, 13(2): 104–10.

The Health Supplement (1994) *Process Redesign at the Leicester Royal Infirmary*. The Health Supplement.

The Macquarie Dictionary (1992) McMahons Point, Australia: Macquarie Library.

Thomas, V., Riegel, B., Andrea, J., Murray, P., Gerhart, A. and Gocka, I. (1994) National survey of paediatric fever management practices among emergency department nurses. *Journal of Emergency Nursing*, 20: 505–10.

Tierney, A.J. (1998) Nursing models: extant or extinct? *Journal of Advanced Nursing*, 28(1): 77–85.

Torres, G. and Yura, H. (1974) *Today's Conceptual Framework: Its Relationship to the Curriculum Development Process*. National League for Nursing Publication, 15-1529, pp. 1–12.

Touche Ross and Co. (1994) *Evaluation of Nurse Practitioner Pilot Projects*. London: South Thames RHA/NHS Executive.

Trembath, R. and Hellier, D. (1987) *All Care and Responsibility: A History of Nursing in Victoria 1850–1934*. Melbourne: Florence Nightingale Committee.

Tripp, D. (1987) *Theorising Practice: The Teacher's Professional Journal*. Victoria: Deakin University Press.

UKCC (United Kingdom Central Council for Nursing, Midwifery and Health Visiting) (1992a) *The Scope for Professional Practice*. London: UKCC.

UKCC (United Kingdom Central Council for Nursing, Midwifery and Health Visiting) (1992b) *Code of Conduct for the Nurse, Midwife and Health Visitor*. London: UKCC.

UKCC (United Kingdom Central Council for Nursing, Midwifery and Health Visiting) (1993) *The Council's Proposed Standards for Post Registration Education*. London: UKCC.

Van Slyck, A. (2000) Patient classification systems: not a proxy for nurses 'busyness'. *Nursing Administration Quarterly*, 24(4): 60-5.

Vaughan, B. (1990) Extended roles. *Nursing Standard*, 4(4l): 47.

Vaughan, B. (1992) The nature of nursing knowledge. In *Knowledge for Nursing Practice*. Oxford: Butterworth-Heinemann.

Vaughan, B. and Pillmoor, M. (1989) *Managing Nursing Work*. Harrow: Scutari Press.

Warfield, C. and Manley, K. (1990) Developing a new philosophy in the NDU. *Nursing Standard*, 86(19): 67–9.

Waterworth, S. and Luker, K. (1990) Reluctant collaborators: do patients want to be involved in decisions concerning care? *Journal of Advanced Nursing*, 15: 971–6.

Watson, J. (1979) *Nursing: the Philosophy and Science of Caring*. Colorado: Colorado Associated University Press.

Watson, J. (1988) *Nursing: Human Science and Human Care – A Theory of Nursing*. New York: National League for Nursing.

Watson, J. (1990) Transpersonal caring: a transcendent view of person, health, and healing. In M. Parker (ed.), *Nursing Theories in Practice*. New York: National League for Nursing.

Watson, J. (1999) *Nursing: Human Sciences and Human Care: A theory of nursing*. Sudbury, MA: Jones and Bartlett.

Webb, C. (1997) Evaluating the introduction of primary nursing: the use of a care plan audit. *Journal of Clinical Nursing*, 6(5): 395–401.

Webster, D. (1991) The politics of self care. In R. Neil and R. Watts (eds), *Caring and Nursing: Explorations in Feminist Perspectives*. New York: National League for Nursing.

Welch, J., Parr, S. and Manley, K. (1994) Hopelessness – a nursing diagnosis. *Surgical Nurse*, 7(3): 26–31.

While, A. (1991) *Caring for Children: Towards Partnerships with Families*. London: Edward Arnold.

Whittaker, D.M. (1972) *A Hospital in Wangaratta*. Victoria: Committee of Management, Wangaratta District Base Hospital.

World Health Organisation (1948) *Constitution*. Geneva: WHO.

Wright, S. (1986) *Building and Using a Model of Nursing*. London: Edward Arnold.

Wright, S. (1989) *Changing Nursing Practice*. London: Edward Arnold.

Zderad, L.T. and Belkher, H.C. (1968) *Developing Behavioural Concepts in Nursing*. Atlanta, GA: Southern Regional Education Board.

Index

INDEX 262

KT-367-012

Higher
BIOLOGY

The National Qualifications Examination Paper and the
Scottish Certificate of Education Examination Papers
are reprinted by special permission of
THE SCOTTISH QUALIFICATIONS AUTHORITY

ISBN 0 7169 9342 2
© Robert Gibson & Sons, Glasgow, Ltd., 2000

ROBERT GIBSON · Publisher
17 Fitzroy Place, Glasgow, G3 7SF.

```
┌─────────────────────────────────────────────────────────────────────────┐
│                         IMPORTANT NOTICE                                  │
│                          TO USERS                                         │
│                                                                           │
│   This book sets out the examination papers as they appeared in the       │
│   examinations of 1996–1999 and also the 2000 examination. The style of   │
│   the papers up to 1999 are different from those examined in 2000. The     │
│   content, however, of the old Higher is very similar to the new Higher   │
│   and therefore candidates will find the questions in the old papers       │
│   useful for examination practice.                                        │
└─────────────────────────────────────────────────────────────────────────┘
```

CONTENTS

```
┌─────────────────────────────────────────────────────────────────────────┐
│                       COPYING PROHIBITED                                  │
│                                                                           │
│   Note: This publication is NOT licensed for copying under the            │
│   Copyright Licensing Agency's Scheme, to which Robert Gibson & Sons       │
│   are not party.                                                          │
│                                                                           │
│   All rights reserved. No part of this publication may be reproduced;      │
│   stored in a retrieval system; or transmitted in any form or by any       │
│   means — electronic, mechanical, photocopying, or otherwise — without    │
│   prior permission of the publisher Robert Gibson & Sons, Ltd., 17         │
│   Fitzroy Place, Glasgow, G3 7SF.                                         │
└─────────────────────────────────────────────────────────────────────────┘
```

1996
MONDAY, 13 MAY
9.30 AM – 12.00 NOON

BIOLOGY
HIGHER GRADE
Paper II

INSTRUCTIONS TO CANDIDATES

1. All questions should be attempted: it should be noted however that questions in Section C each contain a choice.

2. The questions may be answered in any order but all answers are to be written in the spaces provided in this answer book, and must be written clearly and legibly in ink.

3. Additional space for answers and rough work will be found at the end of the book. If further space is required, supplementary sheets may be obtained from the Invigilator and should be inserted inside the front cover of this booklet.

4. The number of questions must be clearly inserted with any answers written in the additional space.

5. Rough work, if any should be necessary, should be written in this booklet and then scored through when the fair copy has been written.

6. Before leaving the examination room this book must be given to the Invigilator. If you do not, you may lose all the marks for this paper.

SECTION A

Answer ALL questions in this section.

Marks

1. (*a*) The diagrams below represent some of the structures present in animal and plant cells.

Use letters from the diagrams to match the functions in the table below. (Each letter can be used **once**, **more than once** or **not at all**.)

Function	Letter
Site of m-RNA synthesis	
Site of anaerobic respiration	
Site of protein synthesis	
Transport of protein	
Controls movement of materials into and out of the cell	
Packaging of secretions	

(3)

Marks

(b) The same plant cell was placed in four solutions, each with a different water concentration.

The drawings below show its appearance after several minutes in each solution.

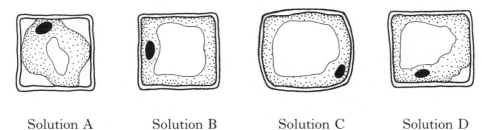

Solution A   Solution B   Solution C   Solution D

Use the letters to complete the table below.

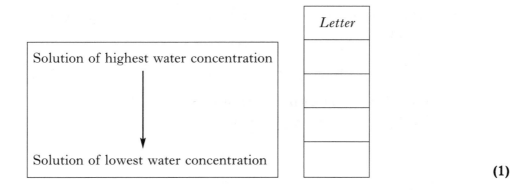

(1)

2. (*a*) The following graph shows the absorption spectrum of a *Marks* photosynthetic pigment and the rate of photosynthesis by a green plant, over the same range of colours of light.

(i) Name a photosynthetic pigment which shows this absorption spectrum.

Pigment _____ **(1)**

(ii) Not all of the light energy which strikes a leaf is absorbed.

State **two** possible fates of the light energy which is not absorbed.

1. _____

2. _____ **(1)**

(iii) Other pigments are involved in photosynthesis.

Explain how the data in the graph support this statement.

_____

_____ **(1)**

(*b*) The following processes occur in either the light-dependent stage or the Calvin cycle.

Place ticks (✓) in the appropriate boxes to indicate the **two** processes which occur in the light-dependent stage.

Processes	Boxes
Formation of GP (PGA)	
Splitting of water molecules	
Generation of ATP	
Release of hydrogen from the reduced hydrogen acceptor (NADPH$_2$)	

(1)

6

(c) A shade plant and a sun plant had the rates of carbon dioxide   *Marks*
exchange by their leaves measured at different light intensities.

The results are shown in the graph below.

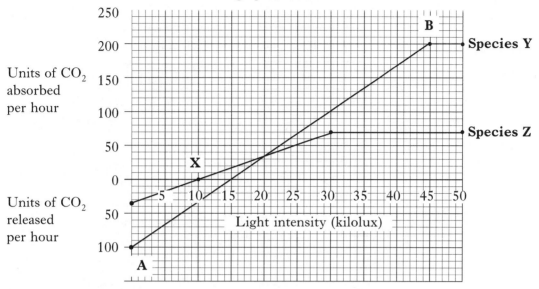

(i) Point **X** on the graph indicates the compensation point for
species Z. By how many kilolux does the value of this light
intensity have to be increased before **species Y** is at
compensation point?

Space for calculation

Answer _____ kilolux   **(1)**

(ii) Which species is a shade plant? Explain your choice of answer.

Species _____

Explanation _____

_____   **(1)**

(iii) From the data, name the environmental factor which limits the
rate of photosynthesis for **species Y** between points **A** and **B**.

Factor _____   **(1)**

(iv) When the rate of photosynthesis is the same for both species of
plant,

1. the value of the light intensity is _____ kilolux

2. the number of units of carbon dioxide absorbed per hour
is _____ units.   **(2)**

7

Marks

3. The diagram below represents an outline of four stages of respiration in muscle cells.

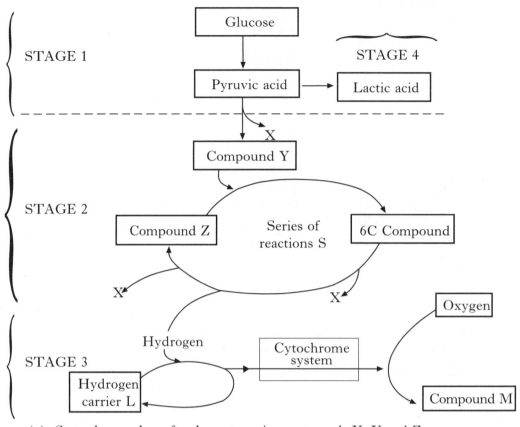

(a) State the number of carbon atoms in compounds X, Y and Z.

    X _____

    Y _____

    Z _____   **(1)**

(b) Name hydrogen carrier L and compound M.

    L _____

    M _____   **(2)**

(c) Identify which **two** stages occur during anaerobic respiration.

    Stage _____ and Stage _____   **(1)**

(d) Name the compound, not shown in the diagram, which is synthesised during the passage of hydrogen through the cytochrome system.

    Name _____   **(1)**

(e) Name the series of reactions S and state their exact location within the mitochondrion.

    Name _____

    Location _____   **(2)**

4. The diagram below represents a stage in protein synthesis.

Marks

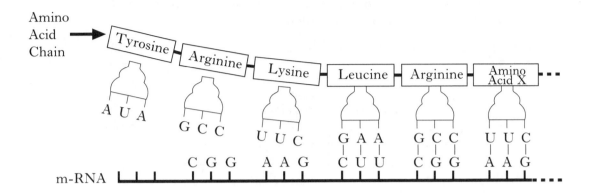

(a) (i) Name the molecules which transport the amino acids to the m-RNA.

_____ **(1)**

   (ii) From the diagram,

   1. identify the codon for the amino acid tyrosine

   Codon _____ **(1)**

   2. identify amino acid X.

   Amino acid X _____ **(1)**

(b) Enzymes are classified as globular protein.

   Give **one** other example of a globular protein.

_____

_____ **(1)**

5. (*a*) The coat colour in mice is controlled by two genes located on different chromosomes. *Marks*

Each gene has two alleles. **A** is dominant to **a**, and **B** is dominant to **b**. The presence of the allele **A** always produces **grey** coat colour.

The other possible genotypes and their phenotypes are shown in the table below.

Genotype	Phenotype
aaBB	Black coat
aaBb	Black coat
aabb	Brown coat

Male mice heterozygous for both genes were crossed with female brown-coated mice.

(i) Complete the table below for this cross.

	Male	Female
Parental phenotype		Brown coat
Parental genotype		
Genotype of gametes		

(1)

(1)

(1)

(ii) What are the possible F$_1$ genotypes?
Space for working

F$_1$ genotypes: ————— ————— ————— ————— **(1)**

(iii) State the expected F$_1$ phenotype ratio.
Space for calculation

Ratio _____ Grey: _____ Black: _____ Brown **(1)**

Marks

(b) In *Drosophila*, the genes for wing length (W), eye colour (E), body colour (B) and presence of bristles (P) are linked.

The table below gives the frequency of recombination obtained in crosses involving different pairs of linked genes.

Gene pair in cross			*Frequency of recombination*
Wing length	×	Eye colour	12 %
Wing length	×	Body colour	18 %
Wing length	×	Presence of bristles	15 %
Eye colour	×	Body colour	6 %
Body colour	×	Presence of bristles	3 %

Use the information to show the position of these genes in relation to each other on the chromosome diagram below.

Use the letters W, E, B and P to identify the position of each gene on the chromosome.

Chromosome   —————⌐———————————————⌐———⌐———⌐———   **(1)**

(c) The diagram below shows a cell from a flowering plant.

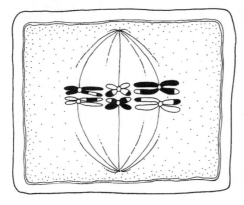

(i) Which **two** features in the diagram show that the cell is dividing by meiosis and not by mitosis?

1. _____

2. _____   **(2)**

(ii) Name a structure in a flower where this cell may be located.

Structure _____   **(1)**

Marks

6. The Galapagos islands and seed-eating finches which live there are described in the following statements.

1. The Galapagos islands are of volcanic origin.

2. The islands are 600 miles from the mainland of South America.

3. Many species of plants and animals which are found nowhere else in the world inhabit the islands.

4. Among the animals there is a wide variety of finch species.

5. Most biologists agree that these species evolved from the one common ancestral species of seed-eating finch.

6. These finch species now occupy many of the niches in the ecosystems of the islands.

7. Similar niches on the mainland are filled by entirely different species of birds.

(*a*)   Use the numbers to identify the **two** statements which suggest that the evolution of these finches is an example of adaptive radiation.

Statement number _____ and _____

(2)

(*b*)   Two of the species of seed-eating finch found on the islands are shown in the diagrams below (drawn to same scale).

Species A   **Species B**

Describe an adaptation of **species A**, shown in the diagram, which allows this species to avoid competing for food with **species B**.

Explain how this adaptation allows **species A** to avoid competition for food with **species B**.

Adaptation _____

_____ **(1)**

Explanation _____

_____ **(1)**

Marks

(c) The diagrams below show the preparation of a cell for somatic fusion.

Plant cell before
treatment

Plant cell after
treatment

(i)   Name the enzyme used in the treatment above.

_____ **(1)**

(ii) What name is given to the cell after treatment?

_____ **(1)**

(iii) What problem in plant breeding has been overcome by the use of somatic fusion?

_____

_____ **(1)**

Marks

7. (*a*) The diagrams show the results of an experiment in which apical buds were removed from plants and the decapitated shoots treated as indicated.

Treatment A   Treatment B   Treatment C

Paste with plant growth substance X

Paste with plant growth substance Y

Paste with no plant growth substance

lateral bud developing

lateral bud developing

(i) Which two treatments, when compared, demonstrate the role of a growth substance in apical dominance? Explain your choice.

Treatments _____ and _____   **(1)**

Explanation _____

_____   **(1)**

(ii) Write the name of the plant growth substance which is responsible for apical dominance.

Name _____   **(1)**

(*b*) The aleurone layers were removed from ungerminated barley grains and immersed in a solution of gibberellic acid.

After 48 hours, the enzyme amylase was found to be present in the solution. This procedure was repeated using a solution of gibberellic acid and actinomycin. Actinomycin blocks mRNA synthesis.

(i) Predict what effect the presence of actinomycin would have on amylase production. Explain your answer.

Effect on amylase production _____

Explanation _____

_____   **(1)**

(ii) Name the part of a barley grain which produces gibberellic acid.

Name _____   **(1)**

8. (*a*) The diagram below shows the metabolic pathways by which *Marks* phenylalanine may be metabolised in the human body.

METABOLIC PATHWAY 1

Phenylalanine ————————————→ **Tyrosine**

|
METABOLIC
PATHWAY 2
↓

Phenylketone

(i) Describe the role of genes in metabolic pathways.

_____

_____ **(1)**

(ii) Metabolic pathway 2 operates only when metabolic pathway 1 is blocked. Explain how such a blockage might occur.

_____

_____

_____ **(2)**

(*b*) The bacterium *Escherichia coli* produces a lactose-digesting enzyme only in the presence of lactose.

The production of this enzyme illustrates the Jacob-Monod hypothesis of gene control in bacteria.

The table below contains statements which refer to events in this control process.

Write **TRUE** or **FALSE** in the table to indicate which events occur in the **absence** of lactose.

List of events in gene control process	*Occurs in the absence of lactose—* ***TRUE*** *or* ***FALSE***
Repressor molecule combines with operator	
Structural gene "switched on"	
Repressor-inducer complex formed	
Regulator gene produces repressor molecule	

(2)

9. (*a*) Enzymes in the liver break down alcohol. *Marks*

The graph below shows the effect of different concentrations of lead on the breakdown of alcohol by these enzymes.

Lead concentration (mM)

Complete the table below by describing the effect of each of the following lead concentrations on the activity of the enzymes.

Lead concentration (mM)	Effect on enzyme activity
0·5	
2·5	
4·5	

(2)

(*b*) State **one** possible effect of each of the following on human fetal development.

1. Excessive alcohol consumption during pregnancy

_____

_____ (1)

2. Use of the drug thalidomide during pregnancy

_____

_____ (1)

10. (*a*) The diagram below shows stages in the control of body temperature in   *Marks*
a mammal.

Stage 1	Changes in body temperature detected in regulating centre in the brain

Stage 2	Corrective mechanisms are activated	
	Changes occur in skin, blood vessels, sweat glands, hair muscles	Changes in adrenaline production alter metabolic rate

Stage 3	Body temperature returns to normal

Stage 4	Corrective mechanisms deactivated

(i) Name the region of the brain in which the temperature regulating centre is located.

Name _____ **(1)**

(ii) How are instructions from the temperature regulating centre relayed to the corrective mechanisms in the skin?

_____

_____ **(1)**

(*b*) The table below lists some of the responses which the body makes to changes in body temperature.

Place ticks (✓) in the appropriate columns to indicate whether each corrective mechanism is in response to an increase or to a decrease in body temperature.

Corrective mechanism	Response to temperature increase	Response to temperature decrease
Reduced activity of sweat glands		
Contraction of hair erector muscles		
Increase in metabolic rate		
Dilation of blood vessels in the skin		

(2)

(*c*) What change in blood glucose concentration results from an increase in adrenaline secretion?

_____ **(1)**

11. (*a*) The diagrams below relate to movement of water in the transpiration stream. Table 1 describes the movement of water at different locations within the plant. *Marks*

Table 1

Location	Movement of water
A	Uptake by root
B	Passage through cortex
C	Ascent in xylem
D	Passage through spongy mesophyll
E	Loss through stomata

Table 2 below contains explanations which relate to the movement of water in some of these locations.

Complete the table.

Table 2

Location(s)	Explanation of water movement
	Columns of water maintained by adhesion and cohesion
	Cells gain water from adjacent hypotonic cells
A	

(3)

Marks

(b) The graph below shows changes in the stomatal aperture of two plant species during 24 hours.

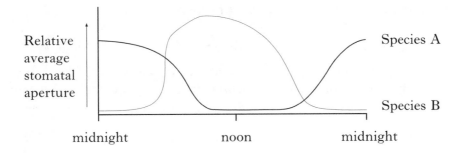

(i) State the change in turgor which takes place in the guard cells of species B between noon and midnight.

_____

_____ **(1)**

(ii) In what type of habitat would the stomatal rhythm shown by species A be an advantage?

_____

_____ **(1)**

(iii) The transpiration stream supplies water to a plant for support and chemical reactions.

State **one** other benefit which the plant obtains from the transpiration stream.

_____

_____ **(1)**

SECTION B

Answer ALL questions in this section.

Marks

12. The diagrams below show stages in the procedure used to extract and identify the photosynthetic pigments present in fresh leaves.

Stage 1 ⟶ **Stage 2** ⟶ **Stage 3** ⟶ **Stage 4**

Extract pigments Separate leaf debris Load pigments on to Develop the
from solution of pigments chromatography paper chromatogram

Position of
pigments

Solvent
level

Solvent
mixture

(a) Describe how the pigments were extracted from the leaf cells in **Stage 1**.

_____

_____

_____ **(1)**

(b) Name a technique used to separate the leaf debris from the solution of pigments at **Stage 2**.

Technique _____ **(1)**

(c) Name the **two** components of the solvent mixture used in **Stage 4**.

Components 1. _____ 2. _____ **(1)**

(d) Explain the importance of the position of the pigments on the chromatography paper as shown in the **Stage 3** diagram.

_____

_____ **(1)**

Marks

(e) During **Stage 4**, the solvent rose to the line indicated by X in the diagram below.

The position of each pigment was measured using a ruler as shown in the diagram.

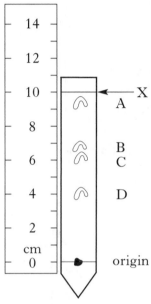

(i) Complete the table below to show the names, the colours and the maximum distances travelled by each pigment.

Letter	Name of pigment	Colour	Maximum Distance travelled (cm)
A		Yellow	9·8 cm
B	Xanthophyll		
C			6·5 cm
D		Green	4·4 cm

(3)

(ii) Occasionally results are obtained in which the pigments are all carried to the top of the chromatography paper.

What error in experimental procedure could account for these results?

_____

_____

(1)

Marks

13. *Dendroica* are birds which nest and feed in fir trees.

Investigators recorded the feeding patterns of three different species of *Dendroica* on tree diagrams as shown below.

Tree diagram

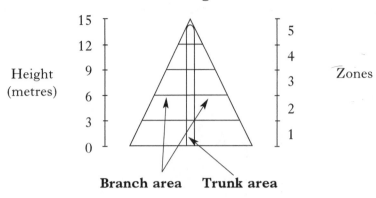

Branch area   Trunk area

Shading in the following tree diagrams shows how often each of the species feeds within different parts of the tree.

Key

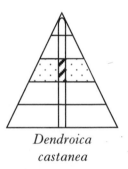

Feeds often

Feeds occasionally

Feeds rarely

Never feeds

Dendroica coronata   *Dendroica tigrina*   *Dendroica castanea*

(a) Which **one** of the species spends most of its feeding time within the trunk area of the tree?

Species _____ **(1)**

(b) Identify the **two** species which feed between a height of 9 and 12 metres.

Species 1. _____ 2. _____ **(1)**

(c) With reference to the feeding zones, describe fully the feeding pattern of *Dendroica tigrina*.

_____

_____

_____ **(2)**

(d) What evidence is there that the three species are able to avoid interspecific competition for food?

_____ **(1)**

22

Marks

The percentage of nests of each species present within each zone is shown in the bar chart below.

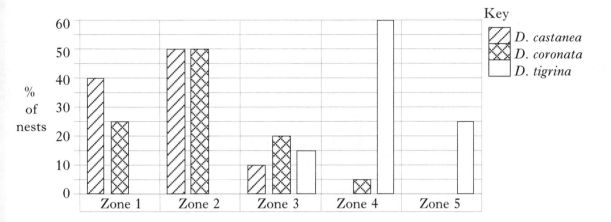

Key
- D. castanea
- D. coronata
- D. tigrina

(e) Between which two species is there the least competition for nest sites?

_____ **(1)**

(f) Which species nests most often in the zone in which it spends most time feeding?

Species _____ **(1)**

(g) In the table below, when each of the statements is matched to each of the three species, only six of the combinations are true.

Identify with the letter **T** in the appropriate boxes in the table the six combinations which are true.

Statement	D. coronata	D. tigrina	D. castanea
Spends most of its feeding time in the outer branches			
Spends time feeding within more than one zone			
May spend some time on the ground when feeding			
Nests in four different zones			

(2)

14. Glucose is stored in muscle tissue in the form of glycogen. Glycogen is the main energy source for respiring muscle tissue.   *Marks*

Endurance time is the time that exercise can be maintained until the muscles become exhausted.

Graph A shows the average endurance time for groups of volunteers with different initial concentrations of glycogen in their muscles.

Graph A

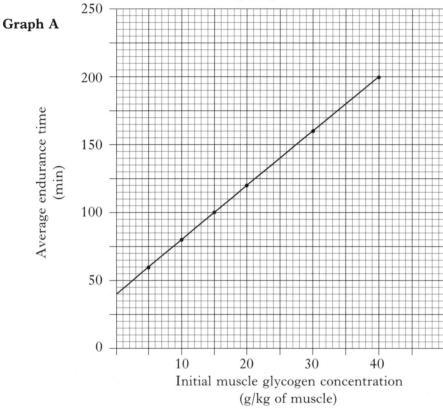

Initial muscle glycogen concentration (g/kg of muscle)

(*a*) From **Graph A**, calculate the difference in the average endurance time between the group of volunteers who started with an initial muscle glycogen concentration of 5g/kg as against the group of volunteers with an initial muscle glycogen concentration of 30g/kg.

Space for calculation

Difference _____ minutes   **(1)**

(*b*) What evidence in **Graph A** shows that glycogen is not the only source of energy available to the muscles?

_____

_____   **(1)**

(*c*) From **Graph A**, predict the initial muscle glycogen concentration of an individual with an endurance time of 240 minutes.

Answer _____ g/kg   **(1)**

Glycogen loading refers to methods used by athletes to increase the concentrations of glycogen stored in their muscles.

Graph B shows the changes in average muscle glycogen concentrations for three groups of volunteers over periods of time.

Each group starts with a common mixed diet and then follows a different procedure. These procedures result in different average glycogen loadings.

Procedure 1
Key
A—B Mixed diet
B—C Carbohydrate only diet

Procedure 2
Key
A—B Mixed diet
B—D Exercise
D—E Carbohydrate only diet

Procedure 3
Key
A—B Mixed diet
B—D Exercise
D—F Fat and protein only diet
F—G Carbohydrate only diet

Graph B

Marks

(*d*) Identify **two** ways in which the average glycogen loading achieved by a carbohydrate only diet can be improved.

1. _____

2. _____   **(2)**

(*e*) Express, as the **simplest whole number ratio**, the average muscle glycogen concentrations achieved at the end of the three procedures.

Space for calculation

Procedure 1 : Procedure 2 : Procedure 3

Ratio   _____ : _____ : _____   **(1)**

(*f*) Calculate the percentage by which the final average muscle glycogen concentration obtained by procedure 3 exceeds that obtained by procedure 2.

Space for calculation

Percentage increase _____   **(1)**

(*g*) From **Graphs A** and **B**, calculate the expected endurance time of a volunteer who had followed procedure 1.

Space for calculation

Endurance time _____ minutes   **(1)**

SECTION C

Both questions in this section should be attempted.
Note that each question contains a choice.

Questions 15 and 16 should be attempted on the blank pages which follow.

Supplementary sheets, if required, may be obtained from the invigilator.

Labelled diagrams may be used where appropriate.

Marks

15. Answer **either** A **or** B.

    A. Give an account of DNA under the following headings:

    (*a*) DNA replication;   6

    (*b*) genetic engineering;   4

    (*c*) gene mutations.   5

    (15)

    OR

    B. Give an account of growth and development in plants under the following headings:

    (*a*) position and activity of meristems;   3

    (*b*) formation of xylem vessels and sieve tubes from undifferentiated cells;   6

    (*c*) importance of magnesium and phosphorus.   6

    (15)

16. Answer **either** A **or** B.

    A. Give an account of how water balance is maintained in fish and in desert mammals.   **(15)**

    OR

    B. Give an account of the principle of negative feedback as illustrated by control of water content and glucose concentration of blood in a mammal.   **(15)**

[*END OF QUESTION PAPER*]

1997
MONDAY, 12 MAY
9.30 AM – 12.00 NOON

BIOLOGY
HIGHER GRADE
Paper II

INSTRUCTIONS TO CANDIDATES

1. All questions should be attempted: it should be noted however that questions in Section C each contain a choice.

2. The questions may be answered in any order but all answers are to be written in the spaces provided in this answer book, and must be written clearly and legibly in ink.

3. Additional space for answers and rough work will be found at the end of the book. If further space is required, supplementary sheets may be obtained from the Invigilator and should be inserted inside the front cover of this booklet.

4. The number of questions must be clearly inserted with any answers written in the additional space.

5. Rough work, if any should be necessary, should be written in this booklet and then scored through when the fair copy has been written.

6. Before leaving the examination room this book must be given to the Invigilator. If you do not, you may lose all the marks for this paper.

SECTION A

Answer ALL questions in this section.

1. The following numbered statements refer to respiration.

    1. In respiration, a high energy compound is synthesised which drives the energy-requiring processes in cells.

    2. In the first stage of respiration, a 6-carbon sugar is broken down to two molecules of a 3-carbon compound.

    3. If oxygen is present, the 3-carbon compound is converted to a 2-carbon compound.

    4. This 2-carbon compound enters a cycle of reactions, during which carbon dioxide and hydrogen are released.

    5. The hydrogen released is transferred to the cytochrome system and it is at this stage that oxygen plays its role in respiration.

    6. In the absence of oxygen, the less efficient process of anaerobic respiration takes place and different metabolic products are formed.

Marks

(a) Name the high energy compound referred to in statement 1.

Name of compound _____   **(1)**

(b) Give **one** example of the energy-requiring processes referred to in statement 1.

Example _____

_____   **(1)**

(c) Which statement describes glycolysis?

Number of statement _____   **(1)**

(d) What is the exact location of the reactions mentioned in statement 4?

_____   **(1)**

(e) Name the compound responsible for hydrogen transfer in statement 5.

Name of compound   _____   **(1)**

(f) Describe the role of oxygen referred to in statement 5.

_____   **(1)**

(g) Explain why the term "less efficient" (statement 6) is used when comparing anaerobic respiration to aerobic respiration.

_____

_____   **(1)**

(h) Name the final metabolic product of anaerobic respiration in human muscle cells.

Name _____   **(1)**

Marks

2. The stages shown below take place when a cell is invaded by a virus.

Stage 1	Stage 2		Stage 4	Stage 5	
DNA of virus enters host cell	Metabolism of host cell is altered	Stage 3	Virus coats are synthesised	New viruses are assembled	Stage 6

(a) Describe the processes which take place during Stages 3 and 6.

Stage 3 _____

_____

_____

Stage 6 _____

_____

_____ **(2)**

(b) Enzymes of the host cell are used during Stage 4.

Name **one** other substance which is supplied by the host cell during this stage.

Name of substance _____ **(1)**

(c) Why are ribosomes required for Stage 4?

_____

_____

_____ **(1)**

Marks

3. In humans, the allele for haemophilia (h) is sex linked and recessive to the normal allele (H).

The family tree below shows inheritance of the condition.

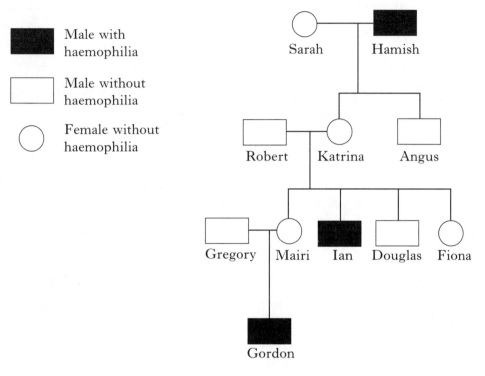

(a) Give the genotype of each of the following individuals.

1. Gordon   _____

2. Gregory   _____

3. Mairi   _____   **(2)**

(b) Individuals heterozygous for the condition are described as "carriers". Name the **two** individuals in the family tree who are **known** to be carriers.

Name 1. _____   2. _____   **(2)**

Marks

4. (*a*) You have to decide whether each of the following statements about nucleic acids is **TRUE** or **FALSE** and **tick the appropriate box**.

If you decide the statement is **FALSE**, you should then write the **correct word** in the right hand box to replace the word **underlined in the statement**.

Statements	True	False	Correct word
During the formation of a new DNA molecule, base pairing is followed by bonding between deoxyribose and <u>bases</u>			
Synthesis of m-RNA takes place in the <u>nucleus</u>			
m-RNA consists of many <u>codons</u>, each consisting of a base, ribose and phosphate			

(3)

(*b*) m-RNA codes for the amino acids which bond to form a protein chain.

The diagram below can be used to identify the amino acids which are coded for by some m-RNA codons.

For example, the m-RNA codons with base sequences CAU and CAC both code for the amino acid histidine*.

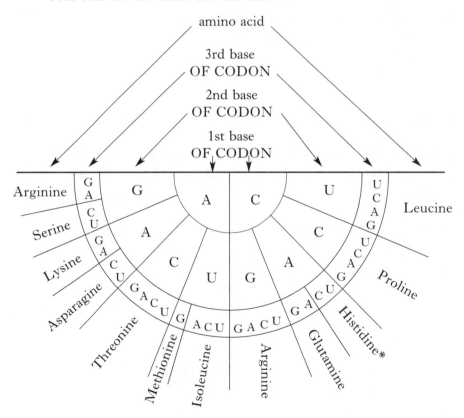

Marks

Use the information in the diagram to answer the following questions.

(i) DNA determines the base sequence on m-RNA.

Which base sequence in DNA would code for the amino acid methionine?

_____ **(1)**

(ii) Which amino acid is carried by the t-RNA molecule which has the anticodon GAC?

_____ **(1)**

(iii) A substitution mutation changes the first base in a codon.

1. Which amino acid will still be inserted correctly into the protein if the first base of one of its codons is changed from A to C?

Amino acid _____ **(1)**

2. Name the **four** amino acids which could still be inserted in the correct sequence despite any substitution in the third base of their codons.

Names 1. _____

2. _____

3. _____

4. _____ **(2)**

Marks

5. (*a*) The diagrams below show **two** possible chromosome mutations which could occur in a chromatid during the process of meiosis.

Normal gene pattern on chromatid | A B C D E F G H I J |

Mutation 1

| A E D C B F G H I J |

Mutation 2

| A B C D C D E F G H I J |

Complete the table below by naming each type of chromosome mutation.

Number	Type of chromosome mutation
1.	
2.	

(2)

(*b*) Name **one** factor, other than chemical agents or temperature changes, which increases mutation rate.

Factor _____

(1)

Marks

6. The diagram below illustrates stages in the control of gene action in bacteria.

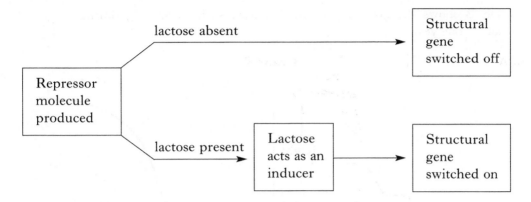

(a) Explain why, if lactose is absent, the structural gene remains switched off.

_____

_____ **(1)**

(b) Explain how lactose acts as an inducer.

_____

_____ **(1)**

Marks

7. The graphs below represent growth patterns in different organisms.

Graph A shows the growth pattern of a locust.

Graph B shows the growth pattern of a tree, such as an oak, during a period of one year.

Graph A   **Graph B**

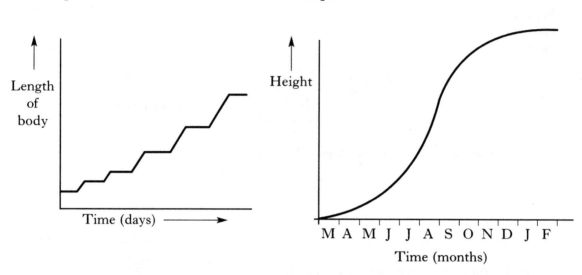

Account for the growth pattern shown by

1. the locust _____

_____

_____ **(1)**

2. the tree. _____

_____

_____ **(2)**

Marks

8. (*a*) The diagrams below show the results of an investigation in which the apical buds of three plants of the same species were treated as indicated.

Treatment A

Apical bud removed. Paste without indole acetic acid (IAA) applied.

Treatment B

Apical bud removed. Paste containing IAA applied.

Treatment C

Apical bud **NOT** removed.

The apical bud produces IAA. **Explain** how the **results** support this statement.

_____

_____

_____ **(2)**

(*b*) Complete the table below, using the appropriate initial letters, to show whether indole acetic acid **alone** (IAA), gibberellic acid **alone** (GA) or **both** (IAA + GA) have a role in each of the processes listed.

Process	Initial Letters
Amylase production by barley grains	
Leaf abscission	
Fruit formation	
Stem elongation	

(2)

Marks

9. (*a*) The diagrams below show four seedlings which have been grown in water culture solutions that differ in the elements they contain.

Experiment A　　**Experiment B**　　**Experiment C**　　**Experiment D**

(i) Identify the elements X and Y.

X _____ 　 Y _____ **(2)**

(ii) Account for the reduced growth in the stem length of the seedling lacking nitrogen.

_____

_____

_____ **(2)**

(iii) If water cultures are not aerated, the uptake of elements is reduced. Account for this fact.

_____

_____

_____ **(2)**

Marks

(b) Many substances affect growth and development in humans.

Insert the appropriate letter from the list of chemical substances into each of the boxes below to match its role in, or effect on, growth and development.

Each letter can be used **once**, **more than once** or **not at all**.

List of Substances   **Boxes**

Name	Letter
Calcium	A
Nicotine	B
Alcohol	C
Vitamin D	D
Lead	E
Thalidomide	F
Magnesium	G
Iron	H

Role in or effect on growth and development	
Inhibits activity of certain enzymes	
Required for the uptake of calcium from the small intestine	
Required for normal growth of teeth and bones	
Required for haemoglobin synthesis	
Retards both physical growth and mental development of the human embryo	

(4)

Marks

10. If a habitat is stripped of its original vegetation, the area is recolonised by plants. The diagram below represents a sequence of plant communities over a period of time in an area where the vegetation had previously been totally destroyed by fire.

| Community A (First colonisers) | → | Community B | → | Community C | → | Climax Community D |

(a) What term is used to describe such a sequence of colonisation?

Term _____   **(1)**

(b) State **two** ways in which the climax community D would be expected to differ from community A.

1. _____

2. _____ **(2)**

(c) Give **one** reason to explain why community C could be established only after the area had been colonised previously by community B.

_____

_____ **(1)**

Marks

11. The flow diagram below shows the sequence of events which results from a decrease in the water concentration of the blood.

Events

(a) Name the exact location of the osmoreceptors.

Location _____ **(1)**

(b) The sentences below refer to the changes which occur after stage 4.

Underline one of **each pair** of alternatives to make the sentences correct.

The kidney tubule becomes $\begin{Bmatrix} \text{less} \\ \text{more} \end{Bmatrix}$ permeable to water. There is

$\begin{Bmatrix} \text{decreased} \\ \text{increased} \end{Bmatrix}$ reabsorption of water into the bloodstream. The effect of

the change in reabsorption of water is to $\begin{Bmatrix} \text{decrease} \\ \text{increase} \end{Bmatrix}$ the rate at which

urine is produced. **(2)**

12. *Ammophila arenaria* (marram grass) grows on sand dunes. Marram grass shows features typical of xerophytes.

Diagram A below shows marram grass growing in a sand dune.

Diagram B below shows a high power view of part of a leaf section of marram grass.

Diagram A

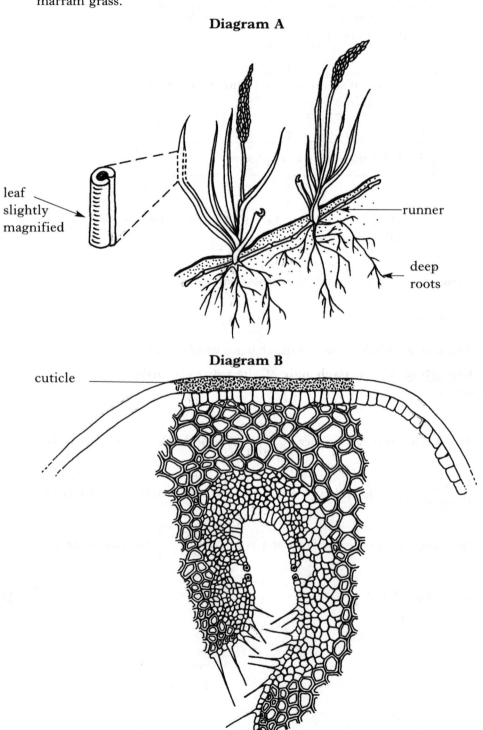

leaf slightly magnified

runner

deep roots

Diagram B

cuticle

Marks

(a) Select **two** features of the leaf shown in the **diagrams** which are typical of a xerophyte. For each feature, explain how water loss is reduced.

Feature 1 _____

Explanation _____

_____

_____ **(1)**

Feature 2 _____

Explanation _____

_____

_____ **(1)**

(b) Explain why marram grass has to have xerophytic adaptations to survive in sand dunes, even though the dunes may be subject to frequent rain.

_____

_____

_____ **(1)**

(c) Explain how a feature labelled in **diagram A** allows marram grass to be an effective first coloniser of sand dunes.

Feature _____

Explanation _____

_____

_____ **(1)**

Marks

13. Bees visit clover flowers to search for nectar and pollen.

Bees were observed feeding from clover flowers within two areas in which the numbers and distribution of flowers were similar.

The distance of the flights made by individual bees when flying from flower to flower was measured.

The results are presented in the pie charts below, and show the percentage of flights made in each distance range within the two areas.

Area 1

Area 2

Key

Flight distance range

■	0– 75 mm
	76–150 mm
	151–225 mm
	over 225 mm

(a) Explain how the search pattern shown for Area 1 suggests that bees are efficient foragers.

_____

_____ **(2)**

(b) In Area 2, there are frequent patches where the flowers have a low nectar and pollen content. As a result, the bees in Area 2 use a different search pattern from those in Area 1.

Explain why the search pattern in Area 2 is of more value to bees when foraging in this area.

Explanation _____

_____

_____ **(2)**

SECTION B

Answer ALL questions in this section.

Marks

14. Dihybrid crosses can be used to show how the independent assortment of chromosomes during meiosis leads to the production of new phenotypes. The following is a summary of a dihybrid cross to the F_2 generation.

Cross 1   Parent A   ×   Parent B

F₁ generation

Cross 2   Members of F_1 crossed

F_2 generation produced

(a) Species which are chosen for use in genetic crosses are usually those which can produce large numbers of offspring.

    (i) Explain why the production of large numbers of offspring is a valuable feature for organisms used in crosses.

    _____

    _____   **(1)**

    (ii) State **two** other features which a species should have if it is to be chosen for use in genetic crosses.

    Feature 1 _____

    _____

    Feature 2 _____

    _____   **(2)**

(b) Precautions are taken during experimental crosses to ensure that only selected individuals are allowed to interbreed.

    With reference to a named organism, describe **one** such precaution.

    Organism _____

    Precaution _____

    _____   **(1)**

45

The following dihybrid cross was carried out with mice.   *Marks*

Parental phenotypes   Black, Straight-haired × Brown, Wavy-haired

F₁ phenotypes   Black, Straight-haired

Members of the **F₁** generation were crossed together

Second cross   Black, Straight-haired × Black, Straight-haired

Results

The table below shows the phenotypes of the **F₂** generation together with their numbers.

Letter	Phenotypes of F_2 offspring	Number of offspring
A	Black, straight-haired	16
B	Black, wavy-haired	6
C	Brown, straight-haired	7
D	Brown, wavy-haired	3

(c)   From the crosses, identify which characteristics are dominant.

_____   **(1)**

(d)   Explain how the results of this cross to the **F₁** generation can show whether the original parents are homozygous or heterozygous.

_____

_____

_____   **(2)**

(e)   Select letters from the table to identify the **two** phenotypes which show that the genes are not linked.

Letters _____ and _____   **(1)**

(f)   The results obtained differ from the theoretically **expected** results.

   (i)   From the **total number** of offspring obtained, calculate the number of offspring which would have been expected to have phenotype C.

   Space for calculation

                                            Number _____   **(1)**

   (ii) Explain why the results obtained differ from the expected results.

   _____

   _____   **(1)**

Marks

15. The Pacific sardine was first exploited by fishermen in 1921.

Graph 1 below shows changes in the annual sardine catch along the Pacific coast of North America. (Catch is measured in tonnes.)

Graph 1

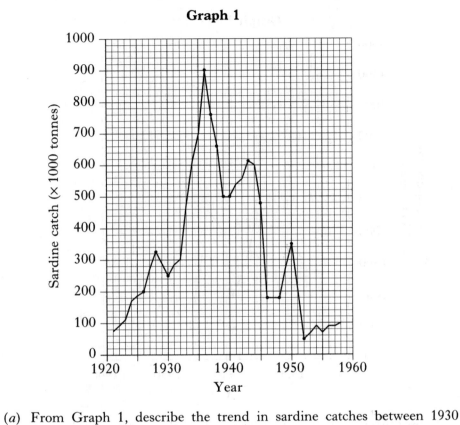

(a) From Graph 1, describe the trend in sardine catches between 1930 and 1946.

_____

_____

_____ **(2)**

(b) Between which years did the largest **decrease** in catch take place?

Tick the correct box.

1934–35 ☐   1935–36 ☐   1936–37 ☐   1938–39 ☐

1944–45 ☐   1945–46 ☐   1950–51 ☐   1951–52 ☐ **(1)**

(c) In how many years was the annual sardine catch greater than 200,000 tonnes?

Space for calculation

Number of years _____ **(1)**

Graph 2 shows changes in the estimated population of sardines in the same area. (Population is measured in tonnes.)

Graph 2

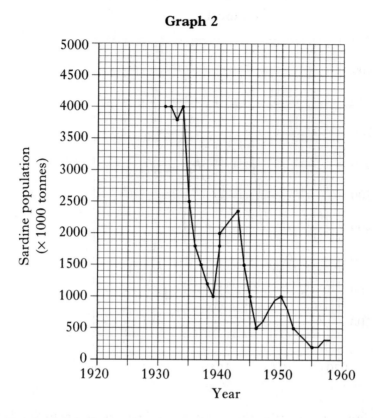

(d) From Graph 2, identify the year in which the sardine population first fell to 10% of its maximum.

Space for working

Year _____ **(1)**

(e) Describe how the data support the statement that after 1936 the sardine population limited the size of the catch.

_____

_____ **(1)**

Marks

(*f*) When the catch was at its lowest in 1952, the percentage of the sardine population lost due to fishing was less than when the catch was at its highest in 1936.

Use the data in Graphs 1 and 2 to show that this statement is correct.

Space for working

Evidence that statement is correct _____

_____

_____ **(2)**

The table below compares the age composition of the sardine populations in 1935 and 1955. (Population is measured in tonnes.)

Age of fish (years)	Percentage of population	
	1935	1955
less than 3	33	61
3	25	29
4	22	8
over 4	20	2

(*g*) Describe how the age composition of the sardine population in 1955 differs from that of 1935.

_____

_____ **(1)**

(*h*) From Graph 2 and the table, calculate the mass of 4 year old fish present in the sardine population in 1935.

Space for working

Mass _____ × 1000 tonnes **(1)**

Marks

16. For survival of a plant species, it is essential that its seeds must not germinate until environmental conditions are favourable. The seeds of European ash do not germinate until almost two years after they have been dispersed.

The data below show the timescale over which three factors are responsible for preventing germination after seeds have been produced in June.

(a) In which two months are impermeability and low temperature reactions the only two factors preventing germination?

Months _____ **(1)**

(b) Ash seeds can be made to germinate earlier than they would normally. Suggest a procedure based on the data which could have this effect.

_____

_____

_____ **(1)**

Marks

An investigation was carried out into factors which affect germination in Norway maple seeds.

The table below shows how many seeds germinated after each treatment.

Letter	Treatment of seeds	Number of seeds planted	Number of seeds germinating
A	Seed coat intact. Stored for three months at room temperature.	248	0
B	Seed coat removed. Stored for three months at room temperature.	228	0
C	Seed coat intact. Stored for three months at 2 °C.	235	188
D	Seed coat removed. Stored for three months at 2 °C.	250	190

(c) From the table, identify the factor which encourages germination in Norway maple seeds in this investigation.

Factor _____   **(1)**

(d) Which treatment gave the greatest germination success?

Space for calculation

Letter _____   **(1)**

The graph shows the results of a further investigation into the percentage germination for Norway maple seeds treated as shown in the table below.

	Letter	Treatment
KEY to Graph	E	Chilled for 4 months Then watered with distilled water
	F	Maintained at room temperature for 4 months Then watered with distilled water
	G	Maintained at room temperature for 4 months Then watered with a 5 mg/l solution of abscisic acid
	H	Maintained at room temperature for 4 months Then watered with a 10 mg/l solution of abscisic acid

Marks

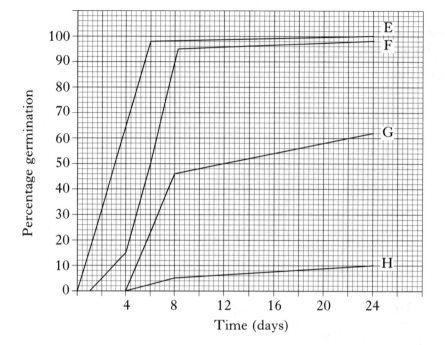

(*e*) From the graph, during which period was the increase in the percentage germination greatest for seeds treated as in F, G or H?

Tick the correct box

0–4 days ☐   4–8 days ☐   8–12 days ☐

12–16 days ☐   16–20 days ☐   20–24 days ☐   **(1)**

(*f*) Calculate the difference between the number of days taken for 50% germination success to be reached in Treatments F and G.

Space for calculation

Number of days _____   **(1)**

(*g*) The abscisic acid concentration in seed coats has an effect on dormancy. What evidence supports this statement?

_____

_____   **(1)**

(*h*) Abscisic acid is present in seed coats. What evidence is there that chilling causes a loss of abscisic acid from seeds coats?

_____

_____   **(1)**

(*i*) Predict the percentage germination in Treatment G after 28 days.

Prediction _____ %   **(1)**

SECTION C

Both questions in this section should be attempted.
Note that each question contains a choice.

Questions 17 and 18 should be attempted on the blank pages which follow.

Supplementary sheets, if required, may be obtained from the invigilator.

Labelled diagrams may be used where appropriate.

Marks

17. Answer **either** A **or** B.

    A. Give an account of membranes under the following headings:

        (a) structure of membranes;   **3**

        (b) entry of materials into the cell;   **7**

        (c) protein transport and secretion.   **5**

          (15)

    OR

    B. The following techniques may be used to produce varieties of organisms. Give an account of these techniques and their benefits:

        (a) genetic engineering of bacteria to manufacture human protein;   **7**

        (b) somatic fusion in plants;   **4**

        (c) selective breeding.   **4**

          (15)

18. Answer **either** A **or** B.

    A. Give an account of natural selection and the evolution of new species.   **(15)**

    OR

    B. Give an account of the light and dark stages of photosynthesis.   **(15)**

[END OF QUESTION PAPER]

1998
MONDAY, 11 MAY
9.30 AM – 12.00 NOON

BIOLOGY
HIGHER GRADE
Paper II

1 (a) All questions should be attempted.

   (b) It should be noted that questions 17 and 18 each contain a choice.

2 The questions may be answered in any order but all answers are to be written in the spaces provided in this answer book, and must be written clearly and legibly in ink.

3 Additional space for answers and rough work will be found at the end of the book. If further space is required, supplementary sheets may be obtained from the invigilator and should be inserted inside the front cover of this booklet.

4 The numbers of questions must be clearly inserted with any answers written in the additional space.

5 Rough work, if any should be necessary, should be written in this booklet and then scored through when the fair copy has been written.

6 Before leaving the examination room, you must give this book to the invigilator. If you do not, you may lose all the marks for this paper.

SECTION A

Answer ALL questions in this section.

Marks

1. The diagrams below show a chloroplast and an outline of the Calvin cycle.

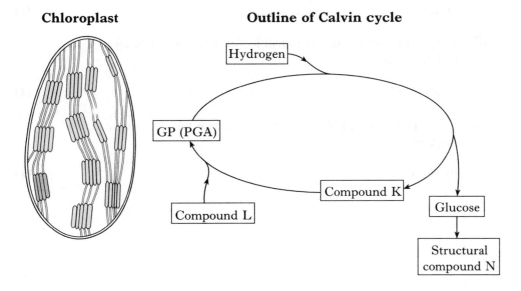

Chloroplast　　　　　　　**Outline of Calvin cycle**

(a) On the diagram of the chloroplast, **put an X** to show where the Calvin cycle takes place. **(1)**

(b) Name compounds K and L in the Calvin cycle.

Compound K _____

Compound L _____ **(1)**

(c) Complete the following sentence by **<u>underlining</u> one** of the words in each group.

Structural compound N is $\left\{\begin{array}{l}\text{starch}\\\text{cellulose}\\\text{glycogen}\end{array}\right\}$ which is deposited in the cell

wall as $\left\{\begin{array}{l}\text{fibres.}\\\text{globules.}\\\text{grains.}\end{array}\right\}$ The cell wall is $\left\{\begin{array}{l}\text{permeable}\\\text{impermeable}\\\text{selectively permeable}\end{array}\right\}$ to water. **(2)**

Marks

(*d*) The hydrogen required for the Calvin cycle comes from the light stage of photosynthesis.

   (i) Name the source of the hydrogen.

      Source _____ **(1)**

  (ii) Name the compound responsible for hydrogen transfer to the Calvin cycle.

      Compound _____ **(1)**

(iii) Name one other product of the light stage which is required for the Calvin cycle.

      Product _____ **(1)**

Marks

2. (*a*) Two types of ribonucleic acid (RNA) are involved in protein synthesis. Complete the blanks in the following table to show the types of RNA, their functions and location(s) in a cell.

Type of RNA	Function	Location(s)
		1. Cytoplasm 2. _____
	Transfers amino acids to ribosomes	Cytoplasm

(2)

(*b*) The m-RNA codons for some amino acids are given in the table below.

Codon	Amino acid
AGA	arginine
CUC	leucine
ACA	threonine

State the order of bases on the deoxyribonucleic acid (DNA) which would result in the assembly of the following amino acid sequence.

leucine—threonine—arginine

_____

(1)

(*c*) Describe the function of the rough endoplasmic reticulum and the Golgi apparatus in a cell.

Rough endoplasmic reticulum _____

_____

(1)

Golgi apparatus _____

_____

(1)

Marks

3. (*a*) An investigation into an antibody is summarised below.

(i) Name the cells in the rabbit which produce antibodies.

_____ **(1)**

(ii) Specific antibodies are formed in response to foreign antigens. How do the results of the investigation support this statement?

_____

_____

_____ **(2)**

(*b*) The list below refers to structures and compounds involved in the defence of organisms.

List	Letter
antibody	A
cyanide	B
lymphocyte	C
lysosome	D
nicotine	E
resin	F
tannin	G

Use the letters from the list to identify:

(i) the cell organelle associated with phagocytosis;

Letter _____ **(1)**

(ii) the **four** chemical substances produced by plants for their defence.

Letters _____ **(1)**

Marks

4. The diagram below represents a pair of homologous chromosomes as they appear in a plant cell during meiosis.

The letters indicate the positions of three genes on the chromosomes.

Points 1 and 2 show the position of chiasmata which may result in crossing-over.

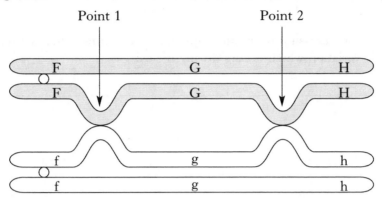

(*a*) State a location in a flowering plant where cells undergo meiosis.

Location _____ **(1)**

(*b*) Meiosis in the cell described above produces gametes with various genotypes. The grid below shows these genotypes.

1	2	3	4
FGH	FGh	FgH	Fgh
5	6	7	8
fgh	fgH	fGh	fGH

Use the **numbers** from the grid to answer the following questions.

(i) Which **two** genotypes are **not** recombinants?

Numbers _____ and _____ **(1)**

(ii) Which **two** genotypes result from crossing-over at Point 1 only?

Numbers _____ and _____ **(1)**

(iii) Which **two** genotypes result from crossing-over at both Points 1 and 2?

Numbers _____ and _____ **(1)**

Marks

(c) Between which two genes on the chromosomes shown opposite would the highest frequency of recombination take place?

Tick the correct box.

Between F and G ☐   Between G and H ☐   Between F and H ☐   **(1)**

(d) Apart from crossing-over and mutation, state **one** other source of genetic variation which occurs during meiosis.

_____   **(1)**

Marks

5. (*a*) Tetracycline is an antibiotic which kills bacteria.

Strains of bacteria which are resistant to tetracycline have evolved.

The information below shows stages in the evolution of tetracycline resistance in bacteria.

Stage 1 | Original population of bacteria

Stage 2 | A mutant bacterium arose in the population. The mutant had an abnormal membrane protein which prevented tetracycline entering the cell

Stage 3 | The population of bacteria was exposed to tetracycline

Stage 4 | Natural selection led to the evolution of a resistant population of bacteria

(i) Explain how gene mutation would lead to the production of the abnormal membrane protein described in *Stage 2*.

_____

_____

_____ **(2)**

(ii) Explain how tetracycline acts as an agent for natural selection and how this leads to the evolution of a resistant population of bacteria.

_____

_____

_____

_____ **(2)**

(*b*) Name an agent which causes gene mutations.

_____ **(1)**

6. The maps below show the positions of land masses in the Southern Hemisphere at three times in the past.

The chart below shows the stages in the evolution of three species of flightless birds in the land masses of the Southern Hemisphere following isolation.

140 million years ago *100 million years ago* *70 million years ago*

Key to maps

A —Africa
B —South America
C —Australia
D —Antarctica
E —India

common ancestral form

evolution of the ostrich (Africa)

evolution of the rhea (S. America)

evolution of the emu (Australia)

140   120   100   80   60   40   20   0

Million years before present

Marks

(a) What type of isolation mechanism is shown by the maps?

_____   **(1)**

(b) From the chart, how many millions of years separated the isolation of the emu from the isolation of the ostrich from the rhea?

Number _____   **(1)**

(c) Use the information in the maps and chart to account for the evolution of these three species from a common ancestral form.

_____

_____

_____

_____   **(2)**

Marks

7. The information below shows some of the procedures used in genetic engineering to insert a gene from a donor organism into a bacterial cell.

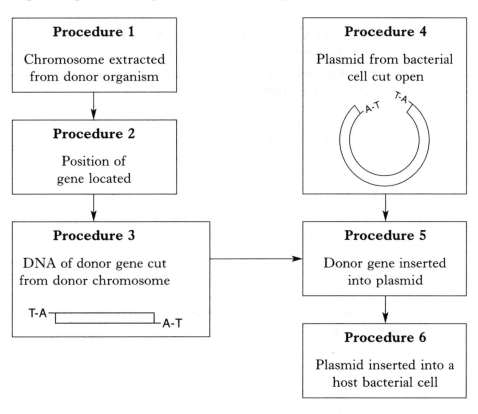

(a) Endonuclease enzymes and ligase enzymes are used in some of the above procedures.

   (i) Identify the **two** procedures which use **endonuclease** enzymes.

   Procedures _____ and _____ **(1)**

   (ii) Identify the procedure which uses **ligase** enzymes.

   Procedure _____ **(1)**

(b) Name a technique which could be used in **Procedure 2** to locate the position of a gene on a chromosome.

   Technique _____ **(1)**

(c) Which feature, shown in the procedures, allows insertion of the isolated donor gene into the open plasmid during **Procedure 5**?

   _____

   _____

   _____ **(1)**

Marks

8. (*a*) Complete the table below to show the effects of macro-element deficiency in plants.

Element omitted	Symptoms of deficiency	Importance of element
	1. Overall growth reduced 2. Early death of older leaves	Membrane transport
Phosphorus	1. Overall growth reduced 2. Leaf bases red	
Magnesium	1. Overall growth reduced 2. _____ _____	

(4)

(*b*) The following graph compares the uptake of nitrate ions by barley roots in the presence and absence of oxygen.

Account for the effect of oxygen on the uptake of nitrate by the roots.

_____

_____

_____

_____

(2)

Marks

9. (*a*) The diagrams below show the results of experiments on the growth of plant shoots.

Experiment 1

Experiment 2

(i) How do the results support the statement that the shoot tip is the site of production of IAA?

_____

_____ **(1)**

(ii) If a shoot is illuminated from one side, IAA is transported to the dark side. Explain how this fact accounts for the phototropic response of a shoot.

_____

_____

_____

_____ **(2)**

(*b*) Give one application of plant growth substances.

_____

_____ **(1)**

Marks

10. (*a*) The flow chart below represents part of the homeostatic control of blood glucose concentration in a human.

Normal blood glucose concentration →
Increase in blood glucose concentration → Detected by receptor cells → Corrective mechanism 1 → Normal blood glucose concentration

Normal blood glucose concentration →
Decrease in blood glucose concentration → Detected by receptor cells → Corrective mechanism 2 → Normal blood glucose concentration

   (i) State the location of the receptor cells.

   _____ **(1)**

   (ii) Complete each box in the table below by inserting the word **increases** or **decreases**.

	Insulin concentration	*Glucagon concentration*
During corrective mechanism 2		

   (1)

   (iii) In corrective mechanism 1, glucose is removed from the blood and is converted into a storage carbohydrate.

   Name the storage carbohydrate and name the organ in which it is stored.

   Name _____

   Organ _____ **(2)**

(*b*) The following statements refer to endotherms and ectotherms.

   Tick the appropriate box to indicate if the statement is **true** for endotherms **and/or** ectotherms.

	Endotherm	*Ectotherm*
Can only regulate body temperature through change in behaviour		
Body temperature held constant independently of external environmental temperature		
Metabolic rate increases with increase in external temperature		

   (2)

Marks

11. When an area of land is cleared of vegetation and left to be colonised, succession takes place.

The table below gives information about two plant species which grow at different stages in this succession. Other changes which take place during this succession are also shown.

	Stage in succession	
	Early succession	*Late succession (climax)*
Plant species	Rosebay willowherb	Beech
Information on plant species	Fast growing with bright pink flowers. The fruit releases many, light, hairy seeds.	A large tree reaching 30 metres in height. Leaves form a dense canopy. The fruit is a nut and is eaten by animals such as rabbits.
Biomass of community	---------- increasing/decreasing/does not change --------➤	
Complexity of food webs	---------- increasing/decreasing/does not change --------➤	

(a) Show the effect of succession on biomass and complexity of food webs by underlining **increasing**, **decreasing** or **does not change** in the table above. **(1)**

(b) (i) Select a feature of rosebay willowherb and explain how this feature helps the plant to be an efficient early coloniser.

Feature _____

Explanation _____

_____

_____ **(1)**

(ii) Select a feature of beech and explain how this feature helps to prevent other plant species from succeeding it.

Feature _____

Explanation _____

_____

_____ **(2)**

Marks

12. Freshwater and salt water bony fish have adaptations which maintain the water concentration of their body fluids at a constant value.

(*a*) Name the process responsible for the movement of water into and/or out of cells.

Process ———————————————— **(1)**

(*b*) **Underline** the correct answer in the statement below.

Salt water fish are $\left\{\begin{array}{l}\text{hypertonic} \\ \text{hypotonic} \\ \text{isotonic}\end{array}\right\}$ to their environment. **(1)**

(*c*) In the list below, **tick** (✓) the **four** boxes which show features of osmoregulation in freshwater fish.

List	Tick (✓)
High glomerular filtration rate	
Few glomeruli present	
Active uptake of salts at gills	
Concentrated urine produced	
Low urine volume produced	
Low glomerular filtration rate	
Dilute urine produced	
Many glomeruli present	
Active secretion of salts at gills	

(2)

Marks

13. The grid below refers to types of behaviour which birds use to obtain food and to defend themselves.

A	B	C
Cooperative hunting	Behaviour which reduces interspecific competition	Dominance hierarchy
D	E	F
Territorial behaviour	Social defence	Behaviour which reduces intraspecific competition

The table below contains some examples of bird behaviour.

Use the letters from the grid to identify the type of behaviour described in each example.

Each letter can be used **once**, **more than once**, or **not at all**.

Example of behaviour	*Letter(s)*
Pelicans, searching for food, form a circle around fish, then dip their beaks into the water simultaneously.	
The Sooty Tern feeds on larger fish than other species of Tern which live in the same area.	
In a population of Great Tits, birds with the widest stripe on their breast feed first when food is scarce.	

(3)

SECTION B

Answer ALL questions in this section.

14. Animals may show escape responses when first exposed to certain stimuli. These responses may alter as a result of habituation.

    In a laboratory experiment, twenty snails of the same species were observed for 20 minutes. During part of the experiment, a stimulus (X) was applied to the animals at 2 minute intervals. Throughout the experiment the number of animals showing an escape response was noted at 2 minute intervals.

    The results are shown below.

Time (minutes)	0	2	4	6	8	10	12	14	16	18	20
Stimulus applied	none	none	none	none	stimulus X	stimulus X	stimulus X	stimulus X	stimulus X	stimulus X	stimulus X
Number showing escape response	0	0	0	0	20	19	20	14	8	0	0

(a) Why was it good experimental procedure to wait for 8 minutes before applying the stimulus for the first time?

_____

_____ **(1)**

(b) Results can be invalid if the stimulus is not applied correctly.

State **one** precaution which should be taken when applying the stimulus.

_____

_____ **(1)**

(c) Explain how the results indicate that habituation has occurred in this experiment.

_____

_____ **(1)**

(d) Habituation is a **short term** change in behaviour.

Describe an experiment which would demonstrate this feature of habituation.

_____

_____ **(2)**

In a further experiment, a different stimulus (Y) was applied instead of *Marks*
stimulus X.

The results are shown below.

Time (minutes)	0	2	4	6	8	10	12	14	16	18	20
Stimulus applied	none	none	none	none	stimulus Y	stimulus Y	stimulus Y	stimulus Y	stimulus Y	stimulus Y	stimulus Y
Number showing escape response	0	0	0	0	20	19	19	20	20	19	20

(e) State how the response of the animals to stimulus Y differs from that to stimulus X. Suggest why this difference may be important for animals in coping with danger.

Difference in response _____

_____ **(1)**

Importance _____

_____ **(1)**

In another experiment, stimulus X was applied, but a third stimulus (Z) was substituted from 18 minutes.

The results are shown below.

Time (minutes)	0	2	4	6	8	10	12	14	16	18	20	22	24
Stimulus applied	none	none	none	none	stimulus X	stimulus X	stimulus X	stimulus X	stimulus X	stimulus Z	stimulus Z	stimulus Z	stimulus Z
Number showing escape response	0	0	0	0	20	19	8	1	0	19	19	7	0

(f) Identify a feature of habituation which is shown by the results of the third experiment, and explain how this feature would be beneficial to animals.

Feature _____

_____ **(1)**

Explanation _____

_____ **(1)**

Marks

15. Between 1970 and 1995, thousands of kilometres of hedgerow were cut down to make larger fields for growing and harvesting crops.

The table below shows the length of hedgerow present in the United Kingdom at four dates.

Year	Length of hedgerow (km)
1970	515 000
1984	412 000
1990	371 000
1995	309 000

(a) Calculate the percentage reduction in the length of hedgerow between 1970 and 1984.

Space for calculation

Answer ＿＿＿＿＿ %　　**(1)**

(b) During which period did half of the total hedgerow destruction take place?

Tick the correct box.

1970–1984 ☐　　　1984–1990 ☐　　　1990–1995 ☐　　**(1)**

The graph below shows how crop yield and several abiotic factors change with distance from a hedge.

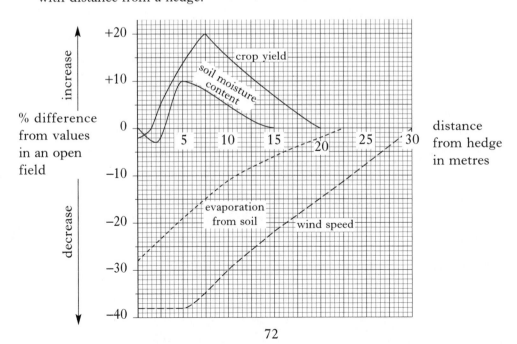

72

Marks

(c) What is the evidence that wind speed is not the only factor which affects evaporation of water from the soil?

_____

_____ **(1)**

(d) The yield of the crop in the open field is $0.8\,kg/m^2$.

Calculate the crop yield at a distance of 7.5 metres from the hedge.

Space for calculation

Crop yield _____ kg/m^2 **(1)**

(e) Up to what distance from the hedge does its presence lead to a decrease in crop yield when compared to the values in an open field?

Distance _____ metres **(1)**

(f) Describe how soil moisture content changes with distance from the hedge.

_____

_____

_____

_____ **(2)**

(g) Between which of the following distances from the hedge does evaporation change most?

Tick the correct box.

0–5 m ☐   5–10 m ☐   10–15m ☐   15–20m ☐ **(1)**

(h) **Tick** the appropriate box to show whether the statement below is **True** or **False**.

	True	**False**
When compared to an open field, an increased soil moisture content is always accompanied by an increased crop yield.	☐	☐

(1)

Marks

16. The population density of red deer in Scotland varies from area to area.

Population density affects survival, growth and fertility of the deer.

The bar chart shows the results of population surveys in areas with low population densities and areas with high population densities.

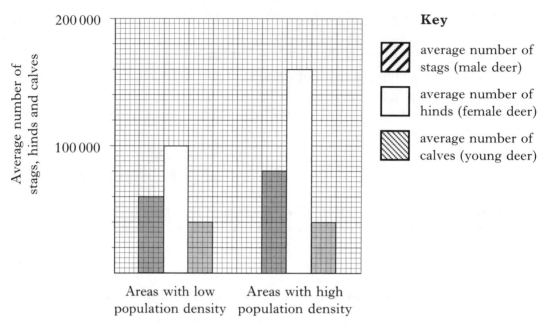

(*a*) The ratio of hinds to stags in areas with low population densities was 5 hinds : 3 stags.

Calculate the simplest whole number ratio of hinds to stags in areas with high population densities.

Space for calculation

Ratio _____ Hinds : _____ Stags **(1)**

Marks

Graph 1 below shows the results of a study in which areas with different population densities were compared.

In each area, measurements were made of the following:

(i) the percentage of calves which died;

(ii) the average mass of antlers per stag.

Graph 1

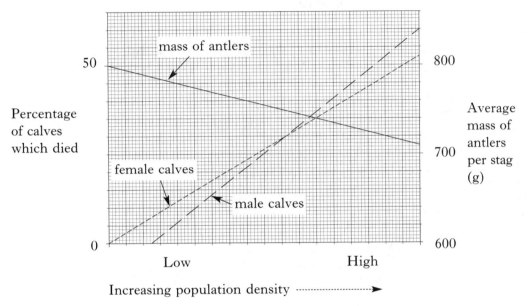

(b) What evidence from Graph 1 suggests that growth of the deer is affected by population density?

_____

_____ **(1)**

(c) The proportion of stags in areas with high population densities is less than in areas with low population densities.

Explain how the data in Graph 1 could account for this difference.

_____

_____

_____ **(1)**

Graph 2 shows a comparison of fertility in deer populations in eight different locations in Scotland.

In each location, measurements were made of the population density and the percentage of one-year-old hinds which were pregnant.

Populations living in woodland and open hill areas were compared.

Graph 2

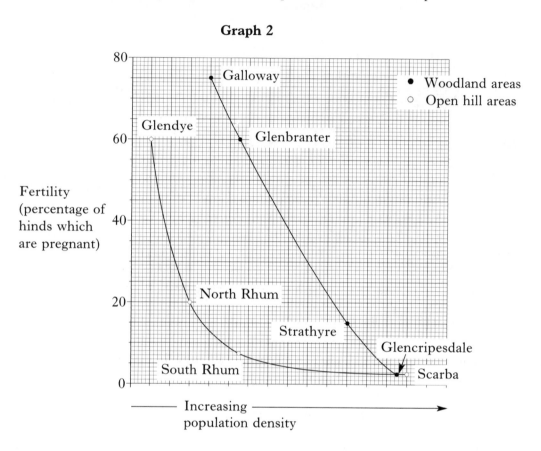

(d) Use the data in Graph 2 to describe the effects of increasing population density on fertility in open hill areas.

_____

_____

_____

_____

(2)

Marks

(*e*) Name the **two** locations shown in Graph 2 which should be compared to support each of the following statements.

1. A woodland population has a higher percentage of pregnant hinds than an open hill population of a similar density.

   Locations ———————— and ———————— **(1)**

2. An open hill population has a lower population density than a woodland population in which the percentage of pregnant hinds is similar.

   Locations ———————— and ———————— **(1)**

(*f*) How could the data in Graph 2 account for the difference between the percentage of calves present in areas with low and high population densities as shown in the bar chart?

———————————————————————————————

———————————————————————————————

——————————————————————————————— **(2)**

SECTION C

Both questions in this section should be attempted.
Note that each question contains a choice.

Questions 17 and 18 should be attempted on the blank pages which follow.

Supplementary sheets, if required, may be obtained from the invigilator.

Labelled diagrams may be used where appropriate.

Marks

17. Answer **either** A **or** B.

    A. Write notes on each of the following:

    (*a*) position and activity of meristems;   5

    (*b*) formation of annual rings;   5

    (*c*) the plant growth substance gibberellic acid.   5

                                                                              (15)

    OR

    B. Write notes on each of the following:

    (*a*) the Jacob-Monod hypothesis;   6

    (*b*) phenylketonuria;   4

    (*c*) the role of the pituitary gland.   5

                                                                              (15)

18. Answer **either** A **or** B.

    A. Give an account of the production of ATP in cell respiration.   **(15)**

    OR

    B. Give an account of the transpiration stream and explain how
           xerophytes are adapted to reduce water loss by transpiration.   **(15)**

[END OF QUESTION PAPER]

1999
WEDNESDAY, 12 MAY
9.00 AM – 11.30 AM

BIOLOGY
HIGHER GRADE
Paper II

1 (a) All questions should be attempted.

   (b) It should be noted that questions 16 and 17 each contain a choice.

2 The questions may be answered in any order but all answers are to be written in the spaces provided in this answer book, and must be written clearly and legibly in ink.

3 Additional space for answers and rough work will be found at the end of the book. If further space is required, supplementary sheets may be obtained from the invigilator and should be inserted inside the front cover of this booklet.

4 The numbers of questions must be clearly inserted with any answers written in the additional space.

5 Rough work, if any should be necessary, should be written in this booklet and then scored through when the fair copy has been written.

6 Before leaving the examination room, you must give this book to the invigilator. If you do not, you may lose all the marks for this paper.

SECTION A

Answer ALL questions in this section.

1. (*a*) The diagram below illustrates movement of molecules of substances A and B across the membrane of a human kidney cell.

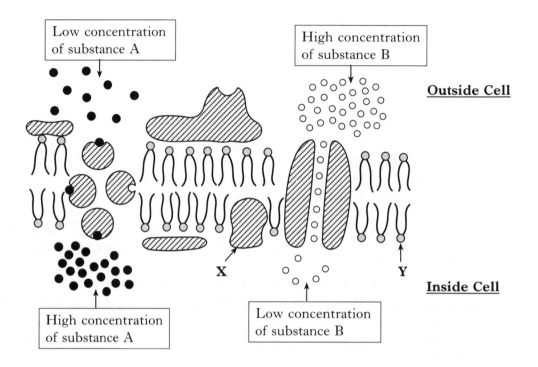

Marks

    (i) Identify membrane components X and Y.

       X _____

       Y _____ **(1)**

    (ii) Name the methods by which substances A and B **enter** the cell.

       Method for A _____

       Method for B _____ **(2)**

  (*b*) Some membrane molecules act as antigens. When a kidney is transplanted into a patient, antibodies are produced in response to these antigens. Name the cells responsible for antibody production.

    _____ **(1)**

Marks

2. The diagram below shows invasion of a bacterial cell by a virus.

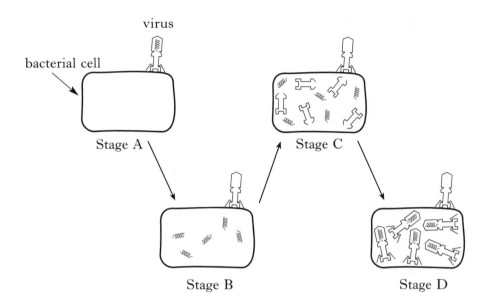

(*a*) Describe what happens between the following stages.

1 Stages A and B _____

_____

_____ **(1)**

2 Stages B and C _____

_____

_____ **(1)**

(*b*) State what takes place after stage D is complete.

_____

_____ **(1)**

Marks

3. (*a*) The diagram below shows an outline of some stages in cell respiration.

Storage carbohydrate

↓

Glucose

↓

Pyruvic acid → Anaerobic respiration

↓

Krebs cycle

(i) Name the storage carbohydrate of **each** of the following cell types.

Liver cells _____

Potato tuber cells _____　　**(2)**

(ii) Name the sequence of reactions by which glucose is converted to pyruvic acid. State the location of this reaction sequence within a cell.

Name _____　　**(1)**

Location _____　　**(1)**

(iii) Describe the role of NAD in cell respiration.

_____

_____　　**(1)**

Marks

(b) The diagram below shows energy transfer within a cell.

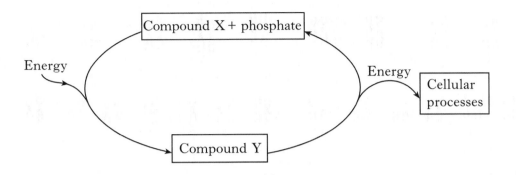

(i) Identify compounds X and Y.

X _____

Y _____   **(1)**

(ii) Give **one** example of a cellular process which requires energy release from compound Y.

_____   **(1)**

(c) Name **two** products of anaerobic respiration in yeast cells.

_____ and _____   **(1)**

4. (*a*) The diagram below shows two human karyotypes.

Individual A | Individual B

Marks

(i) State which individual is male and give a reason for your answer.

Individual _____

Reason _____

_____ **(1)**

(ii) Karyotype A shows a mutation which affects chromosome set 21. Complete the table below to name the organ in which this mutation may occur and the inherited disorder which results.

Organ where mutation occurs	
Name of inherited disorder	

(2)

(iii) A pair of homologous chromosomes are the same size and shape. State **one** other feature which allows a pair of chromosomes to be described as homologous.

_____

_____ **(1)**

Marks

(b) In a certain organism, genes A, B, C and D are located on the same chromosome. The percentage recombination between pairs of these genes is shown in the table below.

Gene pair	Percentage recombination
A and B	20
A and C	5
B and D	5
C and D	30

(i) Use the information above to indicate the position of genes A, B, C and D in relation to each other on the chromosome diagram below.

Space for calculation

Chromosome _____ **(1)**

(ii) How can recombination lead to variation in the genotype of gametes?

_____

_____ **(1)**

Marks

5. The diagram below represents part of a DNA molecule during replication.

(*a*) What is the first event in the process of DNA replication?

_____ **(1)**

(*b*) From the diagram, identify components 1 and 2.

1 _____

2 _____ **(1)**

(*c*) Identify the type of bond labelled as X on the diagram.

_____ **(1)**

(*d*) From the diagram, identify each of the bases 3, 4 and 5.

Base 3 _____

Base 4 _____

Base 5 _____ **(2)**

Marks

6. (*a*) The diagram below shows the DNA base sequence which codes for the amino acids in part of a haemoglobin molecule.

					*
DNA	CAT	GTA	AAT	TGA	CTT

mRNA	____	____	____	____	____

Amino acid
sequence --- valine --- histidine --- leucine --- threonine --- proline ---

   (i) Complete the diagram to show the base sequence on the mRNA synthesised from this DNA.

   (1)

   (ii) If the base A was substituted for the base T at the point indicated by *, how would the amino acid sequence in the haemoglobin differ?

   _____ **(1)**

   (iii) Name **two** other types of gene mutation.

   _____ and _____ **(1)**

   (iv) What name is given to a triplet of bases found on a strand of mRNA which codes for one amino acid?

   _____ **(1)**

(*b*) The diagram below represents part of a metabolic pathway within a cell.

Compound A ----------► Compound B ----------► Compound C

Enzyme 1   Enzyme 2

Gene 1   Gene 2

Which compound could accumulate within the cell if a mutation occurred in Gene 1?

Explain your answer.

Compound _____

Explanation _____

_____ **(2)**

Marks

7. (*a*) Somatic fusion is a technique used in plant breeding.

The flow diagram below shows an outline of this process.

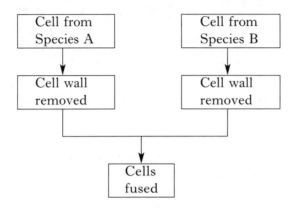

(i) Name the enzyme used to remove cell walls.

_____ **(1)**

(ii) What term is used to describe a cell formed after the cell wall is removed?

_____ **(1)**

(iii) What problem in plant breeding is overcome by somatic fusion?

_____

_____ **(1)**

(*b*) Human insulin can be produced by genetic engineering techniques. Enzymes are used at different stages in this process.

Complete the blanks in the following table to show the enzymes used and their function.

Name of enzyme	Function in process
Endonuclease (restriction enzyme)	
	Joins DNA molecules

(1)

(*c*) Name a technique used to locate genes on a human chromosome.

_____ **(1)**

Marks

8. The diagram below shows a cross section through xylem vessels forming annual rings in the trunk of a tree.

(a) Which letter identifies the vessels formed in the spring?

Give a reason for your answer.

Letter _____

Reason _____

_____ **(1)**

(b) The formation of xylem vessels follows the pattern shown below.

mitosis in meristematic cells ⟶ cell differentiation ⟶ formation of xylem vessels

(i) Name the meristematic tissue responsible for the formation of annual rings.

_____ **(1)**

(ii) Describe **two** structural changes that take place as a cell becomes differentiated to form part of a xylem vessel.

1. _____

_____ **(1)**

2. _____

_____ **(1)**

(c) Other cells in the stem become differentiated to form phloem tissue. How can the formation of different tissues during development be explained in terms of gene activity?

_____

_____ **(1)**

9. The graph below shows the annual variation in the light intensity at the canopy and ground layers in a deciduous woodland.

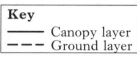

Key
——— Canopy layer
– – – Ground layer

Canopy layer

Ground layer

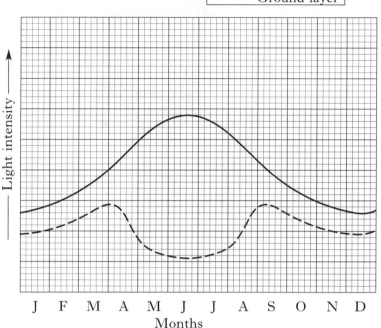

Light intensity

J F M A M J J A S O N D
Months

Marks

(a) Account for the changes in light intensity at the ground layer throughout the year.

_____

_____

_____ **(2)**

(b) (i) Complete the following sentences by **underlining** one of the words in each group.

Ground layer plants are $\left\{ \begin{array}{c} \text{sun} \\ \text{shade} \end{array} \right\}$ plants. Compared to canopy

plants, their net gain of carbohydrate is $\left\{ \begin{array}{c} \text{greater} \\ \text{less} \end{array} \right\}$ at lower light

intensities. **(1)**

(ii) What name is given to the light intensity at which the rate of photosynthesis is equal to the rate of respiration?

_____ **(1)**

Marks

(c) The graph below shows the rate of photosynthesis under different conditions.

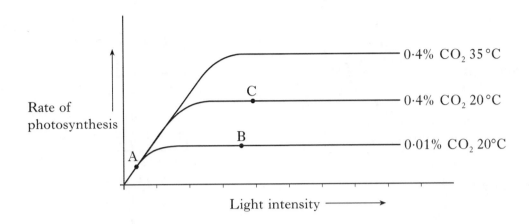

Use the information in the graph to complete the table below.

Tick (✓) **one** box in each row to indicate the factor that is limiting the rate of photosynthesis at points A, B and C.

Graph point	Temperature	Light intensity	CO_2 concentration
A			
B			
C			

(2)

Marks

10. The flow diagram below shows the effects of two hormones on growth and development in the human body.

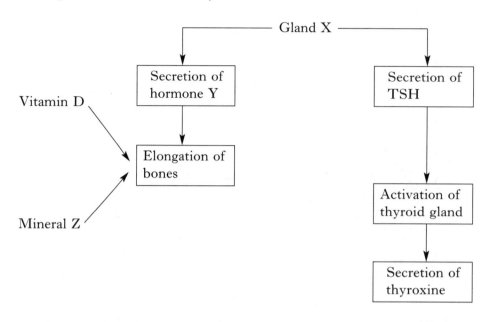

(a) Name gland X, hormone Y and mineral Z.

Gland X _____

Hormone Y _____

Mineral Z _____   **(2)**

(b) State the role of vitamin D in promoting bone growth.

_____

_____   **(1)**

(c) The control of thyroid activity is an example of negative feedback control. Given this information, predict the effect of an increase in thyroxine on gland X.

_____

_____   **(1)**

Marks

11. (*a*) Breeding behaviour in certain mammals is influenced by photoperiod. The graphs below show how the mating activity of sheep and ferrets is affected by changes in photoperiod during the year.

(i) Describe the relationship between photoperiod and the onset of mating activity in sheep.

_____

_____ **(1)**

(ii) It is several months after mating before lambs are born whereas ferrets give birth only weeks after mating.

Suggest how the timing of mating activity is advantageous for survival of the young of both species.

_____

_____

_____ **(2)**

(*b*) Under certain conditions the growing stem of a plant may show etiolation.

(i) Under what environmental conditions would etiolation occur?

_____ **(1)**

(ii) Describe **one** way in which an etiolated plant differs in appearance from a normal plant.

_____ **(1)**

12. The grid below shows some of the factors that are involved in the flow of water through a plant.

A turgor of guard cells	B adhesive forces	C diffusion along a concentration gradient
D cohesive forces	E osmosis	F light intensity

(a) **Use the letters** from the boxes above to answer the following question. Which **two** factors contribute to movement of water molecules as a continuous column within xylem vessels?

Letters _____ and _____   **(1)**

(b) Describe how changes in factor A can affect the rate of transpiration.

_____

_____

_____   **(2)**

(c) Stomata open as conditions change from dark to light.

Why is this important to plants?

_____

_____   **(1)**

(d) State **one** benefit of transpiration to plants.

_____

_____   **(1)**

13. The graphs below show some of the changes that take place in fully-grown leaves during a 10 day period in autumn.

    Graph 1 shows changes in the mass of protein and chlorophyll per cm² of leaf area.

    . **Graph 2** shows changes in the rate of photosynthesis, expressed as the rate of carbon dioxide uptake.

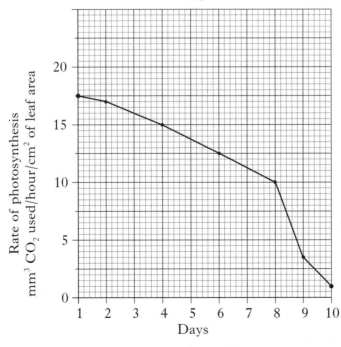

Marks

(a) From **Graphs 1** and **2**, what is the rate of photosynthesis when chlorophyll content is at a maximum?

_____ mm^3 carbon dioxide used/hour/cm^2 of leaf area   **(1)**

(b) From **Graph 2**, calculate the volume of carbon dioxide used in 10 hours by a leaf with a surface area of 20 cm^2 on Day 6.

Space for calculation

_____ mm^3 **(1)**

(c) Express the relationship between the masses of protein and chlorophyll per cm^2 of leaf area on Day 10 as a simple whole number ratio.

Space for calculation

_____ protein : _____ chlorophyll   **(1)**

(d) From **Graph 1**, calculate the percentage decrease in the mass of protein per cm^2 of leaf area from Day 4 to Day 9.

Space for calculation

_____ %   **(1)**

(e) In **Graph 1**, the protein content of leaves is expressed in mg of protein/cm^2 of leaf area.

Why could this method of expressing protein content **not** be used to give a fair comparison between the leaves of different plant species?

_____

_____   **(1)**

(f) Chlorophyll content of leaves may limit the rate of photosynthesis. Use the data to comment on this statement.

_____

_____

_____   **(2)**

Marks

14. In humans, changes in the level of exercise bring about change in pulse rate and stroke volume (the volume of blood pumped from the heart in one heartbeat).

Graph 1 shows how pulse rate and stroke volume change with level of exercise.

Level of exercise is measured as rate of oxygen uptake.

Graph 1

(a) What is the pulse rate and the stroke volume when the rate of oxygen uptake is 1·6 litres/minute?

Pulse rate _____ beats/minute

Stroke volume _____ cm³ **(1)**

Marks

(b) Calculate, in litres, the total volume of blood leaving the heart in one minute when the rate of oxygen uptake is 0·6 litres/minute.

Space for calculation

_____ litres **(1)**

(c) Calculate the increase in the rate of oxygen uptake when the pulse rate is increased from 70 beats/minute to 140 beats/minute.

Space for calculation

_____ litres oxygen/minute **(1)**

(d) What evidence from **Graph 1** would support the statement that there is a limit to the volume of blood that the heart can hold?

_____ **(1)**

Ventilation rate is calculated as the volume of air inhaled during one minute.

Graph 2 shows how ventilation rate changes with level of exercise.

Graph 2

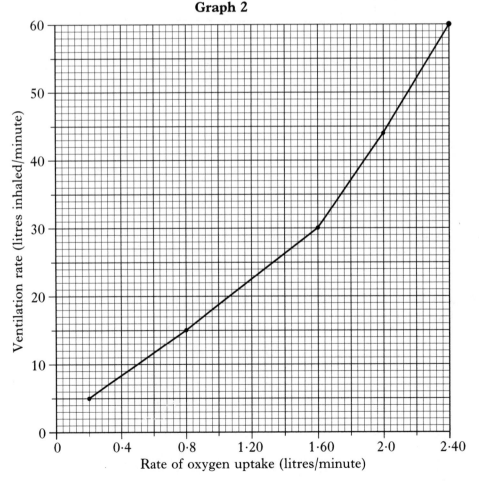

Marks

(e) Given that 20% of air is oxygen, calculate the volume of the oxygen inhaled per minute when the rate of oxygen uptake is 2·4 litres/minute.

Space for calculation

_____ litres   **(1)**

(f) What additional information would be required to calculate the average volume of air taken in during each breath over one minute?

_____

_____   **(1)**

(g) Using information from **Graphs 1** and **2**, complete the table below by writing **T** if you think that the statement is **true** and **F** if you think that the statement is **false**.

Statement	T or F
As rate of oxygen uptake increases, the rate of increase in stroke volume decreases	
The rate at which pulse rate changes is lowest at low rates of oxygen uptake	
When ventilation rate doubles, the rate of oxygen uptake always doubles	

(3)

15. An investigation was carried out into the effect of different concentrations of indole-acetic acid (IAA) on growth in length of shoot tips.

Two 10 mm lengths of shoot tip tissue were immersed in solutions containing different concentrations of IAA.

A control experiment was set up with two 10 mm lengths of shoot tip tissue immersed in distilled water.

The results obtained are shown in the table below.

- Promotion (+) in growth is obtained when the growth is greater than in the control.

- Inhibition (−) in growth is obtained when the growth is less than in the control.

Concentration of IAA solution (molar)	Average length of shoot after 24 hours (mm)	Average difference in length compared to control (mm)
Control	**12·0**	
10^{-9}	12·0	0·0
10^{-8}	13·0	+1·0
10^{-7}	14·0	+2·0
10^{-6}	15·0	+3·0
10^{-5}	16·0	+4·0
10^{-4}	14·5	+2·5
10^{-3}	13·0	+1·0
10^{-2}	12·0	0·0
10^{-1}	11·0	−1·0

Increasing concentration

Concentration of IAA solution (molar)

Marks

(a) Complete the graph for the results obtained for average difference in length of shoot tips compared to control at different concentrations of IAA. **(2)**

(b) Identify the range of IAA concentrations that promote shoot growth.

From: _____ molar   to: _____ molar   **(1)**

(c) State **one** way in which the design of the experiment could be changed to increase the reliability of the results.

_____

_____   **(1)**

(d) Predict the effect of an IAA concentration of 10^{-10} molar on shoot growth.

_____

_____   **(1)**

(e) Explain why −2 mm would be the greatest value for inhibition of growth in shoots.

_____

_____   **(1)**

(f) Suggest why the shoot tips were left in the solutions for 24 hours.

_____

_____   **(1)**

(g) Why must the plant tissue used in the investigation be taken from the tip of the shoot?

_____

_____   **(1)**

Marks

(*h*) The concentration of IAA is varied in the investigation. Other variables, however, must be kept constant.

Name **two** variables that must be kept constant during the investigation.

1. _____

2. _____ **(2)**

(*i*) Describe the importance of the control experiment in this investigation.

_____

_____

_____ **(1)**

(*j*) Describe the effect of IAA on cells in the shoot tip.

_____

_____ **(1)**

SECTION C

Both questions in this section should be attempted.
Note that each question contains a choice.

Questions 16 and 17 should be attempted on the blank pages which follow.

Supplementary sheets, if required, may be obtained from the invigilator.

Labelled diagrams may be used where appropriate.

Marks

16. Answer **either** A **or** B.

    A. Write notes on each of the following:

        (*a*)   the need to maintain body temperature within tolerable limits;   **2**

        (*b*)   control of water concentration in the blood of a mammal;   **6**

        (*c*)   control of blood glucose concentration in a mammal.   **7**

                                                                      (15)

OR

    B. Write notes on each of the following:

        (*a*)   foraging behaviour in animals;   **4**

        (*b*)   social mechanisms in animals for obtaining food and for defence;   **6**

        (*c*)   defence mechanisms in plants.   **5**

                                                                      (15)

17. Answer **either** A **or** B.

    A. Give an account of the process of photosynthesis.   **(15)**

OR

    B. Give an account of the role of isolation mechanisms and natural selection in the evolution of new species.   **(15)**

[END OF QUESTION PAPER]

NATIONAL
QUALIFICATIONS
2000

MONDAY, 29 MAY
9.00 AM – 11.30 AM

BIOLOGY

HIGHER

SECTION A—Questions 1–30 (30 marks)

Instructions for completion of Section A are given.

SECTIONS B AND C (100 marks)

1   (a)   All questions should be attempted.

(b)   It should be noted that in **Section C** questions 1 and 2 each contain a choice.

2   The questions may be answered in any order but all answers are to be written in the spaces provided in this answer book, and must be written clearly and legibly in ink.

3   Additional space for answers and rough work will be found at the end of the book. If further space is required, supplementary sheets may be obtained from the invigilator and should be inserted inside the **front** cover of this book.

4   The numbers of questions must be clearly inserted with any answers written in the additional space.

5   Rough work, if any should be necessary, should be written in this book and then scored through when the fair copy has been written.

6   Before leaving the examination room you must give this book to the invigilator. If you do not, you may lose all the marks for this paper.

SECTION A

Read carefully

1 Check that the answer sheet provided is for Biology Higher (Section A).

2 Fill in the details required on the answer sheet.

3 In this section a question is answered by indicating the choice A, B, C or D by a stroke made in **ink** in the appropriate place in the answer sheet—see the sample question below.

4 For each question there is only **one** correct answer.

5 Rough working, if required, should be done only on this question paper—or on the rough working sheet provided—**not** on the answer sheet.

6 At the end of the examination the answer sheet for Section A **must** be placed inside the front cover of this answer book.

Sample Question

Which of the following molecules contains six carbon atoms?

A Pyruvic acid

B Glucose

C Ribulose bisphosphate

D Acetyl co-enzyme A

The correct answer is **B**—glucose. A **heavy** vertical line should be drawn joining the two dots in the appropriate box in the column headed **B** as shown in the example on the answer sheet.

If, after you have recorded your answer, you decide that you have made an error and wish to make a change, you should cancel the original answer and put a vertical stroke in the box you now consider to be correct. Thus, if you want to change an answer D to an answer B, your answer sheet would look like this:

If you want to change back to an answer which has already been scored out, you should enter a tick (✓) to the **right** of the box of your choice, thus:

SECTION A

All questions in this section should be attempted.

Answers should be given on the separate answer sheet provided.

1. The graph shows the rates of respiration and photosynthesis in a plant, over a 24 hour period.

At which of the following times is there the greatest net production of carbohydrate?

A   0800 hours

B   1200 hours

C   1400 hours

D   1800 hours

2. The graph shows the effect of varying carbon dioxide concentration on the rate of photosynthesis in a plant.

Which line in the table shows factors which could be limiting the rate of photosynthesis at points X and Y?

	Limiting factor at X	Limiting factor at Y
A	temperature	carbon dioxide concentration
B	light intensity	temperature
C	carbon dioxide concentration	temperature
D	carbon dioxide concentration	carbon dioxide concentration

3. Those cells of seaweed which actively absorb iodide ions from sea water would be expected to have large numbers of

A   mitochondria

B   chloroplasts

C   ribosomes

D   vacuoles.

4. Which of the following correctly identifies the sequence in which organelles become involved in the production of a hormone for secretion?

 A Nucleus → Ribosome →
    Golgi Apparatus → Rough E.R.

 B Ribosomes → Rough E.R. →
    Golgi Apparatus → Vesicles

 C Nucleus → Rough E.R. →
    Vesicles → Ribosomes

 D Ribosomes → Vesicles →
    Rough E.R. → Golgi Apparatus

5. Cyanogenesis in *Trifolium repens* is a defence mechanism against

 A grazing

 B bacterial invasion

 C fungal infection

 D water loss.

6. Which of the following is **not** a plant response to invasion by other organisms?

 The production of

 A resin

 B nicotine

 C antibodies

 D tannins.

7. Lysosomes are involved in the defence of the body as they

 A carry out phagocytosis to engulf bacteria

 B produce antibodies to destroy viruses

 C contain lymphocytes

 D allow phagocytes to digest bacteria.

8. An enzyme and its substrate were incubated with various concentrations of either copper or magnesium salts.

 The time taken for the complete breakdown of the substrate was measured.

 The results are given in the table.

Metal concentration $(mol \ l^{-1})$	*Time needed to break down substrate* (Seconds)	
	Copper salts	*Magnesium salts*
0	39	39
1×10^{-8}	42	21
1×10^{-6}	380	49
1×10^{-4}	1480	286

 Which line in the table below describes correctly the effects of high concentrations of these metals on enzyme activity?

	High concentration of copper salts	*High concentration of magnesium salts*
A	promoted	promoted
B	promoted	inhibited
C	inhibited	inhibited
D	inhibited	promoted

Questions 9 and 10 refer to the information below.

In tomato plants, dominant allele **P** determines purple stem and allele **p** determines green stem. In addition, dominant allele **F** determines a cut-edged leaf and allele **f** determines a smooth-edged leaf.

The following table shows two crosses of tomato plants.

PARENT CROSSES	NUMBER OF PROGENY			
	Purple and cut	Purple and smooth	Green and cut	Green and smooth
1 Purple, cut × purple, smooth	219	207	64	71
2 Purple, cut × green, cut	722	231	0	0

9. What are the most probable genotypes for the parents in cross 1?

   A PpFF × PPff

   B PpFF × Ppff

   C PpFf × PPff

   D PpFf × Ppff

10. What are the most probable genotypes for the parents in cross 2?

   A PPFf × ppFF

   B PPFf × ppFf

   C PpFf × ppFF

   D PpFf × ppFf

11. Huntington's chorea is a non-sex-linked dominant condition in which muscle coordination and mental abilities are gradually lost. Usually the symptoms do not appear until the person is approaching middle age.

   A woman's father is heterozygous for this condition. Her mother is normal. What are the chances of her inheriting this condition?

   A 1 in 1

   B 1 in 2

   C 1 in 3

   D 1 in 4

12. Which of the following describes the chromosome complement of a white blood cell?

   A Polyploid

   B Diploid

   C Haploid

   D Nil

13. The following table refers to the mass of DNA in certain human body cells.

Cell type	Mass of DNA/cell $(\times 10^{-12} g)$
liver	6·6
lung	6·6
P	3·3
Q	0·0

From the information in the table, cell types P and Q are, respectively

   A a kidney cell and an ovum

   B a nerve cell and a mature red blood cell

   C a mature red blood cell and an ovum

   D an ovum and a mature red blood cell.

14. The table below shows the number of chromosomes in human gametes from both normal and abnormal meiosis.

An autosome is any chromosome other than a sex chromosome.

Gamete	Number of autosomes	Type of sex chromosome
A	23	X
B	22	X
C	22	Y
D	23	Y

Which ovum, when fertilised with a normal sperm, will result in a child with Down's Syndrome?

15. The diagram below represents the areas of interbreeding of 4 groups of birds. Interbreeding takes place in the shaded areas.

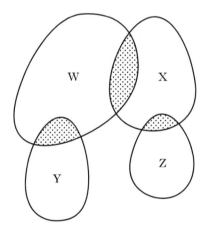

How many species are present?

A   1

B   2

C   3

D   4

16. In an investigation into the population size of peppered moths, 50 moths were captured in a woodland area, marked and released. One day later, another 50 moths were captured and 10 of these were found to be marked.

All the marked moths had survived in the area during the 24 hour period. What is the estimated moth population in the woodland area?

A   60

B   90

C   250

D   500

17. Which of the following adaptations are likely to occur in a desert mammal?

A   Short loops of Henlé and a low concentration of ADH

B   Short loops of Henlé and a high concentration of ADH

C   Long loops of Henlé and a low concentration of ADH

D   Long loops of Henlé and a high concentration of ADH

18. Which of the following is an example of competition within a species?

A   Poppies growing amongst wheat

B   Maize plants growing in a field

C   Bracken growing around seedling pine trees

D   Rabbits and sheep feeding on grass in the same field

19. Which of the following statements about habituation is correct?

A   It is a temporary change in behaviour.

B   It occurs only in young animals.

C   It is an example of social behaviour.

D   It is a permanent change in behaviour.

20. Two plants of different species had their carbon dioxide (CO_2) uptake and output measured in relation to light intensity. The results are shown below.

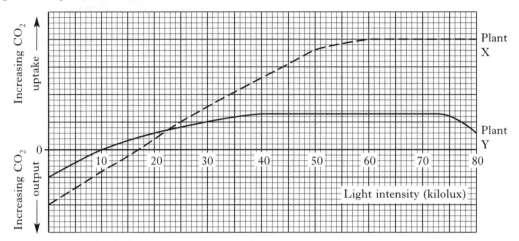

Which of the conclusions in the table below would be a correct interpretation of the graphs?

	Type of plant	*Light intensity at which Compensation Point is reached*
A	Plant X is a shade plant.	17 kilolux
B	Plant X is a sun plant.	60 kilolux
C	Plant Y is a sun plant.	40 kilolux
D	Plant Y is a shade plant.	10 kilolux

Questions 21 and 22 refer to the diagram of a transverse section through a dicotyledon stem shown below.

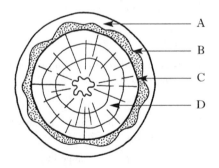

21. In the diagram of a transverse section of a dicotyledon stem shown above, where is a meristematic layer to be found?

22. In which region of the stem would the structure shown in the diagram below be found?

23. Which of the following plant cells is **not** formed as a result of differentiation?

A Cambium cell

B Companion cell

C Phloem sieve tube

D Xylem vessel

24. Part of the *E. coli* chromosome is shown in the diagram below.

The product of the regulator gene normally binds with the operator. If a mutation occurs in the regulator gene such that its product can no longer bind with the operator, which of the following occurs?

A Transcription of genes R and S only when the appropriate substrate is present

B No transcription of genes R and S at any time

C Continuous transcription of genes R and S

D Intermittent transcription of genes R and S

25. An investigation into the influence of different concentrations of IAA on the development of certain plant organs was carried out. The growth-inhibiting or growth-promoting effects are shown below.

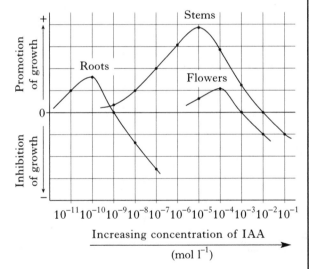

The graph shows that an IAA concentration of

A 10^{-3} mol l^{-1} promotes flowering and stem growth

B 10^{-5} mol l^{-1} causes increase in stem length and flower production

C 10^{-7} mol l^{-1} increases growth in roots and stems

D 10^{-9} mol l^{-1} inhibits stem growth and promotes root growth.

26. The flow diagram below outlines the processes which occur in the human body to speed up the metabolic rate.

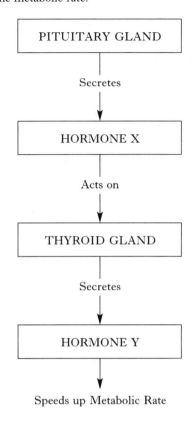

Hormones X and Y are

	X	Y
A	Thyroid Stimulating Hormone (TSH)	Thyroxine
B	Growth Hormone	Thyroid Stimulating Hormone (TSH)
C	Thyroxine	Thyroid Stimulating Hormone (TSH)
D	Thyroid Stimulating Hormone (TSH)	Growth Hormone

27. In a germinating barley grain, gibberellic acid stimulates the production of

A soluble sugar by the endosperm

B amylase by the endosperm

C soluble sugar by the aleurone layer

D amylase by the aleurone layer.

28. The table below gives information concerning three macro-elements X, Y and Z.

Macro-elements	Symptom of deficiency	Role of the macro-element
X	Chlorotic leaves Reduced growth	Required for chlorophyll production
Y	Reduced growth Leaf bases red	Required for ATP and nucleic acids
Z	Chlorotic leaves Reduced growth	Formation of proteins and nucleic acids

Which of the following correctly identifies X, Y and Z?

	X	Y	Z
A	Magnesium	Nitrogen	Phosphorus
B	Nitrogen	Potassium	Magnesium
C	Magnesium	Phosphorus	Nitrogen
D	Nitrogen	Magnesium	Potassium

29. Drinking a large volume of water will lead to

A increased production of ADH and kidney tubules becoming more permeable

B decreased production of ADH and kidney tubules becoming more permeable

C decreased production of ADH and kidney tubules becoming less permeable

D increased production of ADH and kidney tubules becoming less permeable.

30. The graph below shows the variation in prey and predator numbers recorded over a ten week period.

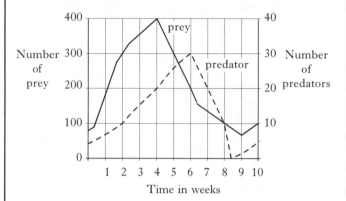

In which week is the prey to predator ratio largest?

A Week 2

B Week 4

C Week 6

D Week 8

Candidates are reminded that the answer sheet MUST be returned INSIDE the front cover of this answer book.

SECTION B

All questions in this section should be attempted.

1. The pathway below represents an outline of stages in respiration in a mammalian cell.

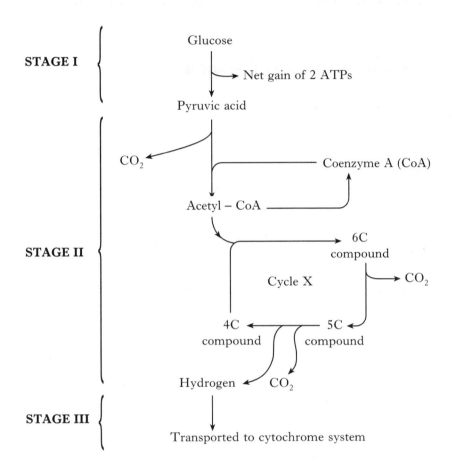

(a) Complete the table below by inserting the number of carbon atoms present in each substance.

Substance	Number of carbon atoms
Glucose	
Pyruvic acid	
Acetyl group	

2

(b) Explain why the gain of 2ATPs in **STAGE I** is described as being a **net** gain.

_____

_____

1

Marks

(c) Name cycle X in **STAGE II**.

Name _____   **1**

(d) Name the carrier that transfers hydrogen to the cytochrome system.

Name _____   **1**

(e) Name the final hydrogen acceptor in **STAGE III**.

Name _____   **1**

2. (*a*) Slices of beetroot, rhubarb and celery tissues were immersed in sugar *Marks* solutions of different concentrations. After 30 minutes the number of plasmolysed cells in a sample of 50 cells was counted under a microscope.

Concentration of sugar solution $(mol\,l^{-1})$	Number of plasmolysed cells in a sample of 50 cells after 30 minutes		
	Beetroot tissue	Rhubarb tissue	Celery tissue
0·30	0	10	5
0·35	4	16	8
0·40	10	25	14
0·45	20	40	30
0·50	35	45	40
0·55	50	50	50

(i) From the table, identify the solute concentration of the cell contents of rhubarb tissue in which 50% of the tissue cells show plasmolysis.

_____ $mol\,l^{-1}$

1

(ii) Explain how the results for celery tissue at a concentration of $0·35\ mol\,l^{-1}$ suggest that the cells do not all have the same cell sap concentration.

_____

_____

1

(iii) Which of the tissues has cells with the highest solute concentration?

Tissue _____

1

(iv) From the results, calculate the percentage increase in the number of plasmolysed cells which would occur in beetroot tissue when moved from a $0·45\ mol\,l^{-1}$ to a $0·50\ mol\,l^{-1}$ sugar solution.

Space for calculation

Answer _____ %   **1**

(*b*) The descriptions in the list below refer to either the cell wall or the cell membrane.

Complete the table, using the letter **W** for descriptions of the cell wall and **M** for descriptions of the cell membrane.

Description	Letter
Destroyed by boiling	
Made up of fibres	
Fully permeable	
A fluid mosaic	
Contains proteins	

2

(*c*) The graph shows the effect of change in the oxygen concentration on the rate of absorption of potassium ions from solution by the roots of barley seedlings.

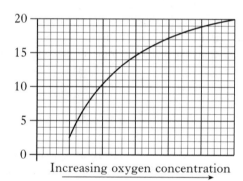

Account for the effect of increased oxygen concentration on the absorption of potassium ions from solution.

_____

_____

_____ **2**

3. (*a*) In an investigation into the sequence of reactions that occur in photosynthesis, unicellular green algae were kept in the dark for 24 hours and then exposed to light for varying periods. After each period of illumination an extract of the algal cells was obtained. The chromatograms developed from these extracts are shown below together with the length of the period of illumination.

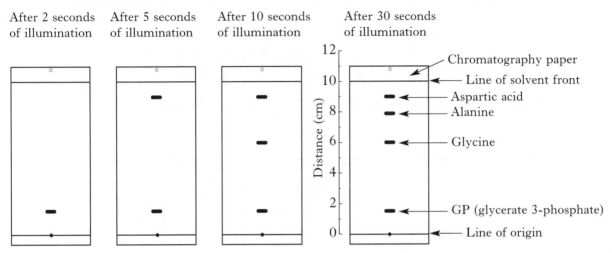

Marks

(i) From the chromatograms, state the sequence in which these chemical compounds were formed.

Sequence _____ → _____ → _____ → _____ **1**

(ii) The Rf value of a compound can be calculated from a chromatogram and then used to identify the compound. The formula for calculating the Rf value is shown below.

$$\text{Rf value} = \frac{\text{Distance travelled by compound from origin}}{\text{Distance travelled by solvent from origin}}$$

From the chromatogram, using the formula, calculate the Rf value of glycine.

Space for calculation

Rf value for glycine = _____ **1**

Marks

(b) The graph below shows the relative concentrations of glycerate 3-phosphate (GP) and ribulose 1, 5-bisphosphate (RuBP) in a chloroplast during changes in light and dark conditions.

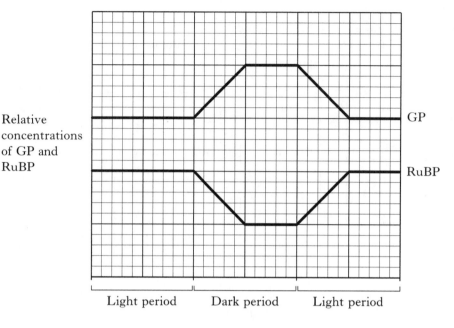

Relative concentrations of GP and RuBP

GP

RuBP

Light period   Dark period   Light period

(i) What evidence from the graph supports the statement that GP can be converted to RuBP in the light?

_____

_____   **1**

(ii) Name the **two** chemical compounds produced in the light dependent stage that are required for the conversion of GP to RuBP.

Compound 1 _____ Compound 2 _____   **1**

(iii) Other than being converted to RuBP, GP is also converted to a 6 carbon sugar. Name this 6 carbon sugar.

Name _____   **1**

(iv) Within which region of the chloroplast does the inter-conversion of GP and RuBP occur?

Region _____   **1**

Marks

4. (*a*) The diagram below represents the four different nucleotides of DNA. The bases of the nucleotides are bonded in pairs.

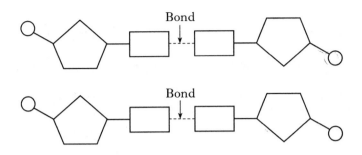

(i) Name the type of bond which links the base of one nucleotide to the base of another.

Name _____   1

(ii) **On the diagram:**

1 insert the appropriate letters or names of the four different nucleotides;   1

2 draw lines to show how adjacent nucleotides are bonded in a DNA molecule.   1

(*b*) Complete the table below to show structural differences between the nucleic acids DNA and RNA.

Structure	Type of nucleic acid	
	DNA	RNA
Number of strands present		
Type of sugar in nucleotide		

1

(c) The diagram below shows part of one strand of a DNA molecule and the results of four different types of gene mutation which can occur within this molecule.

Complete the table below by naming the type of gene mutation which has occurred in each case.

Mutation number	Type of gene mutation
1	
2	
3	
4	

2

(d) Name **one** mutagenic agent.

_____ **1**

(e) Haemophilia in humans results from a gene mutation.

The allele for haemophilia (**h**) is sex-linked and recessive to the normal allele (**H**) for blood clotting.

The family tree below shows inheritance of the condition.

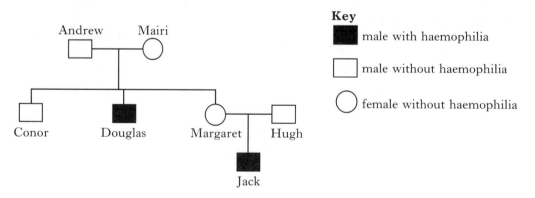

Give the genotype of each of the following individuals.

Conor _____ Douglas _____ Margaret _____ **2**

Marks

5. The diagram below shows the structure of a virus that invades and replicates within plant cells.

nucleic acid ⎯⎯

coat ⎯⎯

(*a*) Name the type of chemical substance that forms the viral coat.

Name _____

1

(*b*) Stages in the invasion of a plant cell by a virus are listed below.

Using the appropriate letters, place the stages in the correct sequence.

Letter	Stages
A	Assembly of new viruses
B	Synthesis of viral coat
C	Entry of viral nucleic acid into cell
D	Replication of viral nucleic acid

Sequence ____ → ____ → ____ → ____

1

(*c*) The sequence below shows transmission of a virus through **two** generations.

1 Virus infects a plant cell.
2 First generation of viruses released.
3 New plant cells infected.
4 Second generation of viruses released.

The figures for transmission success of the virus to new plant cells are shown below.

50 viruses are released from any infected plant cell.
30% of released viruses infect new plant cells.

If a single virus infected a plant cell, calculate the number of viruses expected to be released in the second generation.

Space for calculation

Number _____

1

6. Read these statements about enzymes and answer the questions which follow. *Marks*

  1. Enzymes play a vital role in the life of all organisms. Their activity can be affected by environmental factors such as the presence of lead.

  2. Enzymes are proteins and are coded for by genes.

  3. Occasionally a gene mutation occurs and the effect of this is the production of an abnormal enzyme.

  4. An abnormal enzyme may cause a block in a metabolic pathway.

  5. Certain bacteria produce the enzyme β-galactosidase which breaks down lactose.

  6. Production of this enzyme is normally prevented by the activity of a regulator gene.

(*a*) What is the effect of lead referred to in statement 1?

_____

_____ 1

(*b*) To which class of proteins do enzymes belong (statement 2)?

_____ 1

(*c*) Explain how a gene mutation would lead to production of an abnormal enzyme (statement 3).

_____

_____ 1

(*d*) Explain how the activity of the regulator gene has the effect described in statement 6.

_____

_____ 1

(*e*) Which statements describe the cause of a disorder such as phenylketonuria?

_____ 1

7. The diagram below represents a stage in the process of meiosis.

The letters E or e, F or f and G or g show the positions of the alleles of three genes.

Homologous pairs of chromosomes align and form points of contact as shown by X and Y.

(a) What name is given to points X and Y?

_____ 1

(b) Crossing over may take place at points X and Y.

In the table below tick (✓) the boxes to identify which combinations of alleles would result from crossing over at point X only, and crossing over at both points X and Y.

Combination of alleles	Crossing over at point X only	Crossing over at points X and Y
eFg		
EfG		
eFG		
Efg		
EFg		
efG		

2

(c) Crossing over is a feature of meiosis that leads to variation.

Name **one** other feature of meiosis that leads to variation.

_____

_____ 1

Marks

Marks

(*d*) In a certain organism, the genes P, Q, R and S are located on the same chromosome. The table below shows the frequency of recombination between different pairs of genes.

Gene pairs	Frequency of recombination %
P and Q	8
P and R	14
Q and R	22
Q and S	4
S and P	12

Use the information in the above table to show the positions of genes P, Q, R and S in relation to each other on the chromosome diagram below.

Chromosome --

1

Marks

8. (*a*) A salmon was transferred from fresh water to salt water.

The graph below shows the changes in the drinking rate of the salmon.

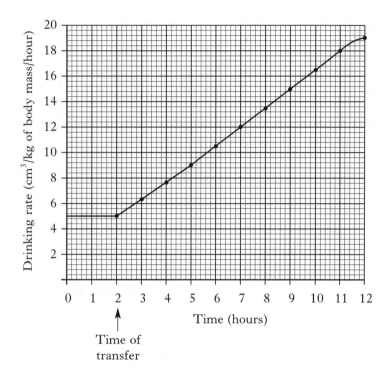

(i) Calculate the volume of water drunk by a salmon weighing 2·5 kg over the two hour period before it was transferred to salt water.

Space for calculation

_____ cm³   **1**

(ii) Calculate the percentage increase in the drinking rate nine hours after transfer.

Space for calculation

_____ %   **1**

(iii) Describe the activity of the chloride secretory cells of the gills while the salmon is in the fresh water environment.

_____

_____   **1**

Marks

(iv) Complete the following sentences by **underlining** one of the words from each pair.

When the salmon is in salt water, water $\left\{ \begin{array}{c} \text{leaves} \\ \text{enters} \end{array} \right\}$ by osmosis.

The reason for this is that its tissues are $\left\{ \begin{array}{c} \text{hypertonic} \\ \text{hypotonic} \end{array} \right\}$ to the salt water. **1**

(v) In the table below tick (✓) the boxes which show the changes in kidney function which occur when the salmon is transferred to salt water.

Kidney function	*Increase*	*Decrease*	*Stays the same*
Rate of filtration			
Rate of production of urine			

1

(b) The diagram below represents a cross section through a leaf that has sunken stomata.

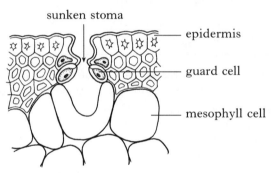

(i) Describe the conditions of the environment in which plants with sunken stomata may be found.

Explain how this adaptation would be advantageous to survival in these conditions.

Conditions _____

Explanation _____

_____ **2**

(ii) Explain the effect of an increase in turgor of the guard cells on the rate of transpiration.

_____

_____ **1**

9. The apparatus shown below was used to measure the rate of transpiration of a leafy twig at different temperatures.

Marks

The changes in mass recorded can be used to calculate the mass of water lost in transpiration over a 10 minute period of time.

(a) Explain why the twig was cut off under water when the apparatus was being set up.

_____

_____   **1**

(b) The apparatus was left at each temperature for 15 minutes before starting to measure the transpiration rate.
Explain why this precaution was good experimental procedure.

_____

_____   **1**

(c) Identify **one** environmental factor that must be kept the same at each temperature in order to make the results obtained valid.
Explain why this factor must be kept constant.

Environmental factor _____

Explanation _____

_____   **1**

Marks

The table below shows the results of the investigation.

Temperature (°C)	Change in mass per 10 minutes (g)
5	1·5
10	3·0
15	4·5
20	5·5
25	6·0

(*d*) Using the results, plot a line graph of change in mass per 10 minutes against temperature in the grid below.

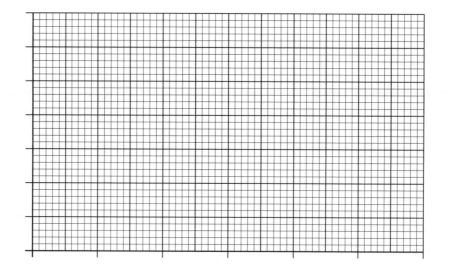

2

(*e*) From the results, predict the change in mass for 10 minutes at 30°C and justify your prediction.

Predicted change in mass _____

Justification _____

_____

2

10. Indole acetic acid (IAA) and gibberellic acid (GA) are plant growth substances which have effects on the growth and development of flowering plants.

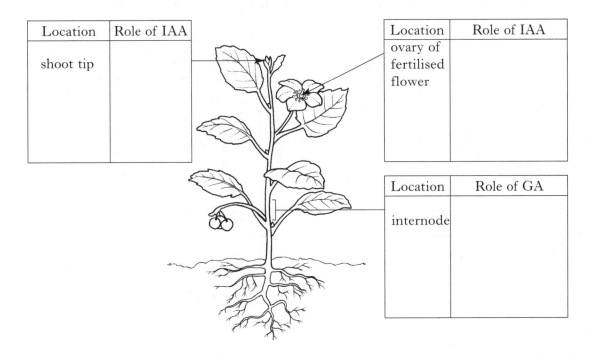

Location	Role of IAA
shoot tip	

Location	Role of IAA
ovary of fertilised flower	

Location	Role of GA
internode	

Marks

(a) Complete the boxes above to describe the roles of IAA and GA in the locations shown in the diagram.

2

(b) Give **one** application of a plant growth substance in horticultural practice.

_____

1

(c) A change in the photoperiod can initiate the flowering process.

(i) What is meant by the term photoperiod?

_____

_____

1

(ii) State **one** way in which a change in photoperiod affects behaviour in birds.

_____

_____

1

11. After an area of farmland was abandoned it was colonised initially by herbs and grasses. In the following 80 years there were changes in the plant community as shown in the graphs below. Changes in the depth of organic material in the soil are also shown.

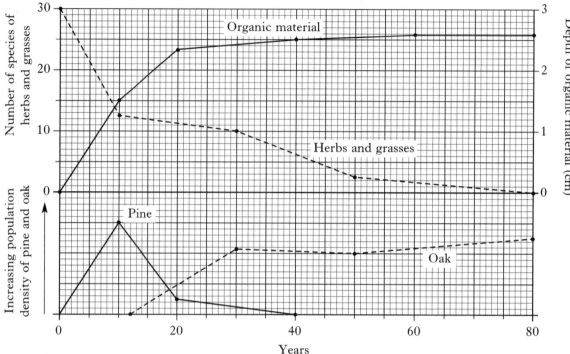

Marks

(a) What evidence in the data indicates that succession has taken place?

_____

_____ **1**

(b) Oak seeds can only germinate successfully if there is enough organic material to protect them from drying out.

On the basis of the data given, what is the minimum depth of organic material required by the oak seeds?

Depth ——————— cm   **1**

(c) Oak woodland forms the final community in this succession.

State the name given to this community and describe a feature of such a community.

Name ————————————————

Feature ——————————————————————

_____ **2**

12. Until the 1970s, whales in the Antarctic Ocean were hunted as a source of food and other raw materials. Amongst those hunted were the Blue whale (20–30 metres long), Fin whale (15–25 metres long), Sei whale (10–15 metres long) and Minke whale (7–10 metres long).

The profit from larger whales is greater than from smaller whales.

Changes in whale population can be monitored by examining records of the number of whales caught each year. The information is shown in the table below.

Year	*Number of whales caught (thousands)*			
	Blue	*Fin*	*Sei*	*Minke*
1930	27	10	0	0
1940	11	18	0	0
1955	3	6	8	0
1965	0	0	18	0
1975	0	0	2	12

(*a*) Whalers targeted less profitable species of whale when the numbers of the more profitable species declined.

What evidence in the data supports this statement?

_____

_____ **1**

(*b*) (i) Wild populations can be monitored because of their importance as a source of food or raw materials.

State **one** other reason why wild populations are monitored.

_____

_____ **1**

(ii) Name **two** density dependent factors which may affect the numbers in a wild population.

Factor 1 _____

Factor 2 _____ **1**

13. The list below shows some changes which occur in animals as a result of changes in body temperature.

Marks

A	fall in body temperature	**E**	increase in metabolic rate
B	increase in sweat production	**F**	erection of hair
C	decrease in metabolic rate	**G**	constriction of blood vessels
D	hair flattening	**H**	decrease in sweat production

The diagram below shows part of the control system for body temperature in a mammal.

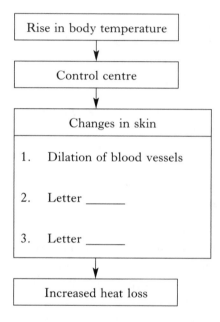

(*a*) Complete the diagram by inserting the appropriate letters from the list to show the changes which occur in the skin as a result of a rise in body temperature.

1

(*b*) Choose a letter from the list to show the effect of an increase in environmental temperature in an ectotherm.

Letter _____

1

(*c*) State how instructions are passed from the control centre to the skin.

_____

1

14. When the concentration of glucose in the blood rises, there is an increase in the concentration of insulin in the blood. As the insulin concentration increases, the rate of glucose uptake by liver cells increases.

These relationships are shown in **Graph 1** and **Graph 2**.

Graph 1

Graph 2

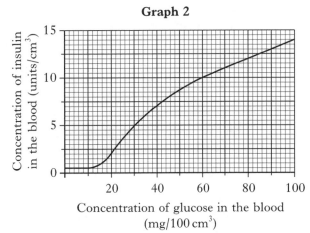

Marks

(a) From **Graph 1**, which change in the concentration of insulin in the blood caused the greatest increase in the rate of glucose uptake by the liver?

Tick (✓) the correct box.

From 0–5 units/cm³ ☐   From 5–10 units/cm³ ☐

From 10–15 units/cm³ ☐   From 15–20 units/cm³ ☐   **1**

(b) The volume of blood in a normal, healthy individual is 5 litres.

From **Graph 2**, calculate the mass of glucose present in the blood at an insulin concentration which remains constant at 10 units/cm³.

Space for calculation

_____ mg   **1**

(c) From **Graph 1**, calculate the percentage change in the rate of glucose uptake by the liver when the concentration of insulin in the blood increases from 10 units/cm³ to 20 units/cm³.

Space for calculation

_____ %   **1**

Marks

(d) From **Graphs 2** and **1**, calculate the rate of glucose uptake by the liver when the concentration of glucose in the blood is $60\,mg/100\,cm^3$.

Space for calculation

_____ µg/g of liver/hour   **1**

(e) What happens to glucose which is taken up by liver cells?

_____   **1**

Graph 3 shows the changes in concentration of glucose in the blood of an individual with a normal pancreas and one with a defective pancreas.

Graph 3

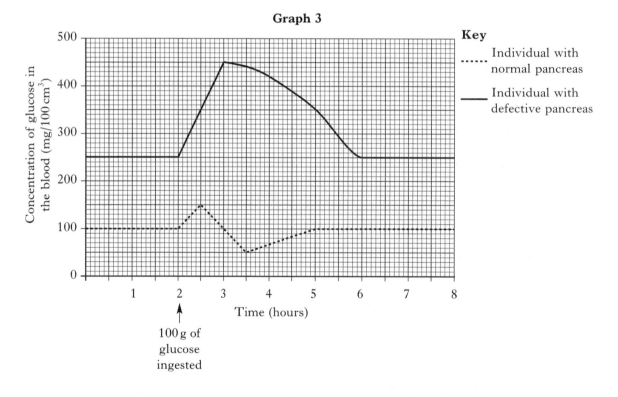

(f) From **Graph 3**, describe the changes in the blood glucose concentration of the individual with a normal pancreas after ingestion of 100 g of glucose.

_____

_____

_____   **1**

2000

Marks

(g) From **Graph 3**, calculate the difference between the times taken for the concentration of glucose in the blood of the two individuals to return to a stable level from their maximum levels.

Space for calculation

Difference in time _____ **1**

(h) From **Graph 3** and **Graph 2**, calculate the concentration of insulin in the blood of the individual with the normal pancreas when their blood glucose level is stable.

Space for calculation

Concentration of insulin in the blood _____ units/cm^3 **1**

SECTION C

Both questions in this section should be attempted.

Note that each question contains a choice.

Questions 1 and 2 should be attempted on the blank pages which follow.

Marks

Supplementary sheets, if required, may be obtained from the invigilator.

Labelled diagrams may be used where appropriate.

1. Answer **either** A **or** B.

    A. Write notes on each of the following:

        (i) insulin production by genetic engineering;   **6**

        (ii) the technique of somatic fusion in plants and one of its benefits.   **4**

  OR   **(10)**

    B. Write notes on each of the following:

        (i) foraging behaviour in animals;   **4**

        (ii) social mechanisms in animals for obtaining food and for defence.   **6**

                                                           (10)

In question 2 ONE mark is available for coherence and ONE mark is available for relevance.

2. Answer **either** A **or** B.

    A. Give an account of *m*RNA synthesis and the role of *m*RNA in protein synthesis.   **(10)**

  OR

    B. Give an account of the role of isolation mechanisms in the evolution of new species.   **(10)**

[END OF QUESTION PAPER]

Printed by Bell & Bain Ltd., Glasgow, Scotland.